Fat *is not* A Four-Letter Word

CHARLES ROY SCHROEDER, Ph.D.

Fat is Not a Four-Letter Word

Library of Congress Cataloging-in-Publication Data

Schroeder, Charles Roy
Fat is not a four-letter word / Charles Roy Schroeder, Ph.D.
p. cm.
Includes bibliographical references and index.
ISBN 1-56561-000-8 : $14.95
1. Fat—Health aspects. 2. Adipose tissues. 3. Reducing.
4. Nutrition.
I. Title.
QP752-F3S36 1992 92-3352
613.2—dc20 CIP

Edited by: Patricia Richter
Design: Dan Norquist
Printed in the United States of America

10 9 8 7 6 5 4 3 2 1

Published by: CHRONIMED Publishing
P.O. Box 47945
Minneapolis, MN 55447-9727

For My Wife Judy

whose lush beauty and loving nature
inspired me
to write this book

ACKNOWLEDGEMENTS

From my credentials alone, one would understandably think me an unlikely candidate for writing this book. I never personally suffered antifat insults and ridicule; nor have I ever had to diet. In fact, although by nature I am a bit thin, a lifetime of exercise has given me a fairly muscular appearance. Further, all of my professional training and employment has been in the areas of health and fitness — areas which constantly preach an antifat message.

Not surprisingly, having grown up in a country that is constantly bombarded with powerful antifat propaganda, I too had strong antifat attitudes for most of my life. And, shamefully, during domestic altercations, I have even insulted my wife about her being fat — a not uncommon technique known as "the cheap shot."

About fifteen years ago, however, my antifat attitude gradually began to crumble. A lot of the dissipation, I'm sure was due to the fat people I knew. They did not fit the negatively stereotyped mold. They were as capable, ambitious, intelligent, friendly, warm-hearted, etc. as people of any other body type. The role of all of these people in starting me to question society's massive denigration of fat people must be acknowledged. In particular, though, there was a young, female opera singer, whose name I have long forgotten. She was a student in one of my health classes. One day I made what she perceived to be an antifat comment and she immediately reprimanded me for it. Although I apologized, at the time I did not really think I was guilty. But her words haunted me for years. That incident did not open my eyes to fatism but it was the first to jiggle my eyelids.

As far as fat people being unattractive, well, my wife was in a bathing suit the first time I ever saw her, and before I ever said a word to her, my hormones started bubbling. And most people in our culture would have considered her to be fat. Of course, I thought she was very pleasingly plump. After nearly thirty years of marriage she has gained weight and I still think she's very pleasingly plump.

Eventually it occurred to me that the only problem with being fat is that it is unhealthy. Even that belief gradually eroded, however, as I gradually became aware of the gross inaccuracy of most antifat reports. In response, I started studying more carefully the conclusions of "fat" research. All research has delimitations, but some of the conclusions I saw were clearly unfounded. It almost seemed as if there was an antifat conspiracy. I have too much respect for researchers, however, to believe that. The real villains are the self-serving people in the massive antifat industry who report the research in misleading ways. I began to realize that while true obesity does have associated health problems, the vast majority of people who are thought to be fat are not any more unhealthy than people of lighter weights. In fact, they are often healthier.

Eight years ago, almost like a religious experience, the words, "fat is NOT a four-letter word," flashed into my consciousness. I recognized the words as being as being an interesting and meaningful book title. That did not result in my putting my typing finger to a word processor, but I became even more aware of antifat attitudes and the reasons for them.

Then on Columbus's birthday, October, 1988, I suffered an illness that almost pulled my plug; THAT is what spurred me into action. I figured I had better get this book written before it was too late. Vanity led me to think if I did not write it no one else would. Maybe vanity was right. At any rate, a month later I was pronounced as good as ever (whatever that meant) and I immediately started serious library research for *Fat is NOT a Four-Letter Word.*

Writing a manuscript is almost as much fun as having a root canal done by a sadistic dentist, but the pain was ameliorated by the advisory assistance of several of my colleagues at Memphis State University. The term "mentor" means "wise and trusted advisor," and that describes precisely how I view Dr. Joseph K. Davis, former Chairman of the English Department and two-time Fulbright Scholar. Another former chairman, Dr. David Williams of the Music Department, is well deserving of the title, "the terminator of the split infinitive." We spent innumerable lunch periods together while he ripped the book apart. Yet, he did it with such sensitivity I always walked away feeling encouraged. Also gratefully acknowledged is the contribution of a eagle-eyed, pencil-wielding librarian by the name of Janelle Rudolph. I would send a "perfect" manuscript to her and she would send it back looking like a Christmas tree with all of her red marks. Due to the input of this distinguished and candid trio, this book is immeasurably better than it would otherwise have been. I would like to say they should also be blamed for any weaknesses in the book, but in truth I cannot. Besides, it is traditional for the author to modestly assume that responsibility.

While the sources of permissions are listed throughout the text and in the CREDITS, permission directors are also being thanked here as an indication of my appreciation. Andrew Humphreys too is recognized for doing the computer artwork (graphs and normal curves) that appear in this book.

Only a man who has been happily married for several decades can fully appreciate the value of a loving wife in any kind of difficult undertaking. In addition to excusing me from washing dishes for a few years, my Judy was extremely helpful in every aspect of preparing this book but particularly in those areas which are so distasteful, frustrating, and time-consuming—such as getting permissions for the use of relevant quotes, artwork, photographs, and cartoons. Words cannot express my heartfelt appreciation for her assistance — and for being my wife.

All of the above named people helped get the manuscript to the publisher's doorstep. There, the Chromimed staff took my "offspring" and skillfully "cleaned her up" and dressed her for presentation to the public. I am particularly indebted to David Wexler, associate publisher; Donna Hoel, editor; and Pat Richter, copy editor.

Before moving on, I must acknowledge the support and encouragement of the dean of my college, Nathan Essex. He's the rare educational leader who inspires effort and creativity.

These people all *cared* about the finished product. For that I am very thankful.

PREFACE

If the title of this book does not make sense to you, walk up to a woman and tell her you think she's fat. But be prepared to make a hasty retreat. Typically, she will react as if you have called her one of those four-lettered Anglo-Saxon words associated with body wastes, private body parts, and S-E-X. "Fat" is even more of an insult, though, since a variety of negative traits have come to be associated with people who are fat. They include gluttony, laziness, stupidity, and clumsiness. In other words, to be fat is to be immoral. These beliefs are, of course, absolutely ridiculous.

Of the two sexes women are especially scorned if they are fat. This circumstance is particularly unfair since women as a rule are genetically programmed to have a higher percentage of body fat than are men. Indeed, throughout most of history women, who would be considered fat or obese by today's standards, were highly regarded in terms of beauty and sexuality — as documented in this book with art ranging from 40,000 B.C. to the twentieth century. Even today in spite of current fashion dictates, many men, perhaps most, find voluptuous women more attractive than thin ones. The saying, "thin is in, but fat is where it's at," may be closer to the truth than is commonly realized.

Only since 1920 has thinness been in style, and the historical, social, and philosophical reasons for this unique situation are discussed. After 1920, and for decades thereafter, however, fat women were not ridiculed. Only after about 1960 did "fat" become a *de facto* four-letter word. This book exposes the powerful antifat industry that for purely monetary gain has propagandized the public into believing that fatness is not only ugly but unhealthy. Many of the industry's worthless weight reduction gadgets, pills and potions are also exposed along with the industry's gross misinterpretation of research that it uses to support its advertising lies and deceptions. The industry is so influential it has even duped the overwhelming majority of health professionals into believing fat is a four-letter word. Other professionals stick their heads in the sand, are frightened to speak out, or have been "bought."

There is nothing inherently evil in making money, but the industry has prospered by instilling in countless millions of fat women such feelings as guilt, worthlessness, and self-loathing. Because these feelings erode their self-esteem, and therefore their chances for happiness, the lives of vast numbers of women thereby have been shattered. As might be expected, hordes of people with weak and cowardly character have sensed the current vulnerability of fat women and have descended into bigotry and intolerance—or more precisely, they have become FATISTS.

There is absolutely no reason why fat women should have diminished self-respect — even if they *are* fat — even if they are *very* fat. In Chapter Fifteen it is pointed out that people have the right to be fat, for whatever reason, without being vilified by a fatist society. But the book shows that multitudes of so-called fat women are not excessively fat, anyway, in terms of either appearance or health. Many women who believe they are fat are actually too thin, often morbidly so. Although the public has been bamboozled into thinking that less body fat is always healthier, this thinking is erroneous. Contrary to common misinformation, there is not even an ideal body fat percentage that applies to everyone. In spite of arbitrarily conceived percentages, such as 20%, ideal fatness may in reality range from 5% or less to 40% or more. Much depends upon inherited body types, which is an *individual* matter. Although there is no formula for determining a person's ideal percentage of body fat, this book reveals a very practical, healthy, and enjoyable way for everyone to achieve his or her ideal body fat percentage.

A far more important objective, however, is to help alleviate the sad and grossly unfair denigration of fat people that is rampant in our culture. Since fatness has become primarily a women's problem, the thrust of this book is naturally directed toward them.

LIST OF ILLUSTRATIONS

6 Cartoon, courtesy NEA

16 *Venus of Willendorf*, 30,000-10,000 B.C.
Natural History Museum, Vienna

24 Turkish Goddess, 6,000 B.C.
Archaeological Museum, Ankara

24 Greek Goddess, 4th Century B.C.
Ny Carlsberg Glyptotch, Copenhagen

24 Wall Painting (Pompeii). Reign of Nero.
National Archaeological Museum, Naples

25 Albrecht Durer. *Adam and Eve*. 1504
Metropolitan Museum of Art, New York

25 Peter Paul Rubens. *Venus and Adonis*. 1635
Metropolitan Museum of Art, New York

26 Louis Elisabeth LeBrun Vegee-LeBrun. *Madame Vegee-LeBrun and Her Daughter*. 1789.
Louvre Museum, Paris

26 Francois Boucher. *The Toilet of Venus*. 1751.
The Metropolitan Museum of Art

26 Pierre Auguste Renoir. *Seated Bather*. 1906.
Founders Society, Detroit Institute of Arts, Detroit

31 Hans Memling. *St. Ursula*. 1489.
Memling Museum-SintJans Hospitaal, Bruges

31 Jean Auguste Dominique Ingres. *Madame Reiset and Her Daughter*. 1844.
Museum Bogmans-van Beuningen, Rotterdam

32 Hieronymous Bosch. *The Garden of Earthly Delights* (detail from center panel). 1505-1510.
Prado Museum, Madrid

32 Grant Wood. *American Gothic*. 1930.
The Art Institute of Chicago, Chicago

33 Pablo Picasso. *Seated Nude*. 1905
Museum of Modern Art, Paris

34 Pieter Bruegel, the elder. *Wedding Dance*. 1566.
Founders Society, Detroit Insititute of Arts, Detroit

35 Michelangelo. *The Fall.* About 1515.
(Detail from the Sistine Chapel, Vatican City)

36 Cartoon, by permission *Playboy* magazine. 1958.

44 Jan Van Eyck. *Giovanni Arnolfini and his Wife*. 1434.
National Gallery, London

46 Illustration of pannier

46 Illustration of bustle

50 Ad for Grover's Tasteless Chill Tonic. 1880.

52 Ad for Coca Cola from 1923.

53 A 1920 fashion

57 Bev Francis. The Ultimate Hard Body. (photo)

60 A 1902 "Bust Developer"
(From the 1902 edition of the Sears, Roebuck Catalog)

71 Development of a fat cell (cross-sectional view)

82 Cartoon from *American Scientist* magazine, 1979, by
Sidney Harris

88 Cartoon from *Flaws and Fallacies in Statistical Thinking,*
Stephen K. Campbell, 1974. Prentice-Hall, Inc., Englewood
Cliffs, N.J.

90 Normal Distribution of Scores

90 Percentages of Scores Found within the Standard
Deviations

101 An Arbitrary Range of Ideal Body Fat Percentages

107 Variations in Ideal Body Fat Percentages
(Three body types: Ectomorph, Mesomorph, Endomorph)

108 Drawn from Photographs in *The Varieties of Human Physique,*
William H. Sheldon Trust, A 711, 171, and 117

109 Drawn from Photographs in *The Varieties of Human Physique,*
William H. Sheldon Trust, A 343

110 An Extended Range of Ideal Body Fat Percentages
(assuming seventeen body types)

124 Cartoon, courtesy Johnny Hart and NAS, Inc.

149 Diet product cartoon, from *Playboy* magazine, July 1988Obesivac-10^6

172 Mortality Rates Table (Metropolitan Life Insurance)

213 The Eating Right Pyramid. USDA, 1991

218 Cartoon from *Minneapolis Star Tribune*

225 Comparisons of Dietary Fats and Oils

229 Cartoon, *Health Care News*, 1990

230 Comparison of Turkey Products

244 Cartoon, permission of North American Syndicate

247 Neck (Carotid) Pulse and Wrist (Radial) Pulse locations

253 Four Layers of Abdominal Muscles

254 Cross Section of the Abdomen

254 A "Crunch"

256 Prime Movers for Curl-Ups and Sit-Ups

257 Bent-leg Raises

257 Trunk Twisting Exercise for the Abdominal Oblique Muscles

274 Cartoon, Johnny Hart and Creators Syndicate, Inc.

294 Cartoon, Cathy Guisewite, Universal Press Syndicate

296 Lingerie Offering from V-Fashions

About the Cover Painting

Flora

"It is not a portrait, but rather the ideal type of feminine beauty as Titian conceived it: a woman ripely formed, with golden hair, and clear rosy flesh."

Filippo Rossi
Director of the Museums of Florence, Arezzo, and Pistoia

TABLE OF CONTENTS

Acknowledgements . . . . *iv*

Preface . . . . *vii*

List of Illustrations . . . . *ix*

1. Four-Letter Words 1
2. Fatness and Gender 9
3. Fatness and Attractiveness 21
4. Fatness and Visual Beauty 39
5. The Goodness of Fat 67
6. Fatness and Statistics 81
7. Fatness and Body Types 101
8. The Antifat Industry 115
9. Antifat Pills and Potions 137
10. Antifat Gadgets and Lotions 155
11. Fatness and Health 171
12. Thinness and Health 189
13. Diet and Health 205
14. Exercise and Health 239
15. The Right to be Fat 267
16. Summary, Conclusions, and Outlook for Fatness 285

Credits 301

Footnotes 305

Selected Bibliography 307

Index 311

1

FOUR-LETTER WORDS

Four-letter words — those nasty and socially unacceptable words that are used to refer to such things as certain body parts, sexual activities, and body wastes — we all know them. Most of us use them. Some of us use them frequently. But, for fear of offending someone, I will not list them here. In spite of their common use, when most of us use the four-letter words we tend to feel at least a little unclean, immoral, and guilty. Our sense of self-respect, of self-worth, diminishes.

Of course, the degree of these feelings depends upon the situation in which we use the words. For example, I never felt bad about using four-letter words while conversing with my moss-back buddies in the United States Marine Corps. And practically every sentence contained at least one such expression. At that point in my life the words were so habitual that they did not seem obscene or vulgar.

As anyone knows, whose language has similarly degenerated, such usage can lead to some exceedingly uncomfortable situations. My landmark incident occurred one Thanksgiving day when I was on military leave to have dinner at my grandmother's house. All of my very conservative relatives, old and young alike, were present and in their "Sunday" clothes. We were a large but closely knit clan and Thanksgiving was always the special day of the year. Having been overseas for the few previous years this occasion was an especially joyous one for me.

The clamor of the happy reunion began to subside, though, when tantalizing fragrances from the kitchen wafted over the gathering and gave rise to gnawing hunger pangs. When the call to dinner finally arrived, a second call was not necessary. The aromas emanating from the mounds of food were indescribably enticing and were surpassed only by their delicious tastes. Midway through the meal, amidst the cheerful buzz of conversation, I smiled sweetly across the table and, with suitable reverence to our beloved matriarch, asked, "Grandma, will you please pass the f—ing potatoes?"

The marvelous gustatory respite from military chow had captured most of my attention, but still I was vaguely aware of some discomfort on the part of the people sitting nearest me. Maybe the sudden and drastic improvement in their posture was the clue, or perhaps their mouths had merely stopped in mid-chew. Grandma's wrinkled, benignly smiling face suddenly looked stricken and even paler than usual. I quickly ascertained it must have been something I had said — or had not said. I smiled fondly as I realized I must have forgotten to say, "Please." Grandma, bless her gentle heart, was always a stickler for politeness.

But I knew I had said, "Please." I had concentrated on using it. Maybe she had not heard me. "Boy!" I thought, "From the look on her face it's even more important to her than I had figured." The conversation in the room and around most of my table had maintained its enthusiastic volume. "Maybe she didn't heard me," I surmised, and with a booming voice I repeated my request. "Grandma, will you pass the f—ing potatoes, PLEASE?" At the precise period during which I was concluding my request a hush fell on the conversation. No, I will never believe it was coincidental. Someone "up there" was trying to make a point — and was immensely successful.

This time the entire room lapsed into silence and the gaiety never really recovered its full bloom that day. Uncle Bill quickly reached over and got the potatoes for me. After resuming my assault on the turkey and trimmings, I glanced at my still immobile grandmother and thought she was looking kind of poorly, but dismissed any undo concern because she was, after all, getting up in years.

Later my uncle took me aside and with solemn demeanor said simply, "Roy, you shouldn't talk that way in front of Grandma."

"What do you mean? I said 'please,' Uncle Bill. Maybe not the first time, but I really stressed it the second time."

"That's not what I'm talking about."

"Well, gosh, all I asked for were the . . . oh, sh-t!" He just turned and walked away shaking his head in dismay. My parents had been sitting at another table at the fateful moment, but surely must have either heard or been told of my *faux pas*. Gratefully they never mentioned the incident. Like the time when I was thirteen years old and my mother found a partially empty package of condoms in my wallet — some things are just better left unsaid. No one needed to reinforce Uncle Bill's chastisement, anyway. Incidentally, I had used the missing condoms for water bombs fights, a circumstance that had filled me with chagrin at the time since my friends were beguiling me with wonderful stories of their multitudinous conquests — episodes almost as titillating as the purely imaginative ones I had been telling.

I have used four-letter words since that unforgettable Thanksgiving outburst, more than a few times. But I have never deluded myself into thinking they were anything but low-class, degenerate terms.

Since that shameful day, I've done some study on the origins of words in general — and on four-letter ones in particular. I first began to wonder why four-letter words are considered by polite society to be so detestable, although such terms as *feces* or *urine* are quite acceptable. Even on television a person can look Phil Donahue right in the eye and say *coitus* or *fornicate*. True, Phil may squirm a bit, but the censor will not even blink. Oprah may giggle nervously but infectiously, while Geraldo would probably say, "Hey, man, you can use the 'real word.' We're all adults here."

Although four-letter-words now belong to the world, literally — they originally were Anglo-Saxon terms. This language, once the official written and spoken language of England, was remarkable for its time. It was developed centuries before the other European "state" languages and is claimed by modern linguists to have had a very rich vocabulary and a special kind of dignity. Much of this Old English is preserved in a rich literature of which the remarkable epic *Beowulf* is the most well-known.

The four-letter words were quite acceptable at the time because they were the only words those early Englishman had for body wastes and sexual matters. Then, in 1066, the Normans, under William the Conqueror, defeated the Anglo-Saxons in the Battle of Hastings. These Normans were actually Vikings, who generations earlier, had settled in northwestern France and had adopted that country's culture and language.

In England the victorious Normans immediately became the noblemen and the vanquished Anglo-Saxons became the peasant-laborers. These poverty stricken unfortunates were considered by their masters to be little more than animals — disgusting animals at that. It is difficult to treat fellow human beings in a harsh, demeaning manner unless they are first dehumanized. It's tough on the conscience. A verbal method of brutalizing, for example, is to refer to people with such demeaning names as "gooks, niggers, or kikes." The list is endless and includes every person on Earth. Once a group is sufficiently dehumanized, its land and property can be taken and its members can even be killed without arousing such bothersome feelings as remorse or guilt.

Fraternizing with a socially inferior class is the supreme "no-no" since it greatly interferes with the dehumanizing process. The Normans accordingly kept their distance from the Anglo-Saxons; two cultures and two languages thus co-existed in England. Of course, the Normans wearing fine, clean clothes and residing in their impressive castles, felt far superior to the peasants who lived like animals in dirty rags and hovels. Everything about the Anglo-Saxons was considered to be "common" in its most pejorative sense. In fact, the Latin word for common is "vulgar" — a term that came to mean disgusting and revolting — and this included the Anglo-Saxon's language itself.

The peasants raised cattle, for instance, but, when a cow was butchered and appeared on Norman tables, it was called by its French name "boeuf" (beef). Similarly, the meat of the Anglo-Saxon pigs was called "porc" (pork) by the Normans. And that is why even today, more than nine hundred years later, it's considered *trés gauche* to order a serving of cow or pig at a restaurant. And whoever heard of a person eating snails when he or she could have escargot?

About a hundred and fifty years after the Battle of Hastings, the Normans were driven out of their base in France. Since they were then confined to England, they began to think of the country as their homeland. The Anglo-Saxon language was gradually reaccepted for general use, although considerable Norman French influence remained along with bits of Latin and other European languages. The four-letter Anglo-Saxon words, however, retained their vulgar aura.

Considering the persistent stigma of using Anglo-Saxon words for such mundane stuff as meat, it is not hard to imagine the revulsion coefficient of Anglo-Saxon words having to do with body wastes and sex. In English-speaking countries, the literal meanings of the four-letter words are exactly the same as the socially acceptable ones. The connotations, however, have tremendous variations as far as their emotional impacts are concerned.

This disparity is true for many words that have nothing to do with sex or body wastes. But there is no more dramatic, or illogical, example than the word — fat. Fat is simply a type of oily substance formed in the tissue of animals, including man, and some plants. Yet, today, the word "fat" has a powerful, negative connotation for most of the people in the United States, as well as in many other other parts of the western world.

If you need convincing, walk up to a woman you have not seen for awhile, stick out your hand, and say, "Gosh, I hardly recognized you. You've gotten so fat." You may find that outstretched hand crammed up one of your orifices. If you're lucky, it will be your mouth. Conversely, if you say, "Gosh, I hardly recognized you. You've gotten so thin," you'll probably get a hug and be in her prayers for the rest of your life.

In other words, fat has become a four-letter word. More correctly, it has become a *de facto* four-letter word. In our society, calling people fat implies they lack self-respect and self-control, that they are gluttonous and lazy. Since these traits are often perceived as sins, it follows that such people are immoral. Research, however, has shown that there is absolutely no relationship between these traits and fatness. Thin people, for instance, are just as likely to be gluttonous and lazy as fat people. Still, the demeaning beliefs about fat people persist, even among those who should be expected to know better — fat people themselves!

The tenacity of negative myths surrounding fatness should not be too surprising. It merely gives additional credence to the long-held realization that many people need a scapegoat to enhance their own feelings of inadequacy. And who better to choose as targets than people who as a group are weak and vulnerable? Fatism is merely another form of bigotry and, as with the other "isms," it feeds upon ignorance and cowardice — of which, apparently, there is no shortage.

FATISTS, a term that is used throughout this book, is capitalized since it is not only analogous to such terms as racists and sexists, it is an acronym for: Fat Abhorring, Terribly Insulting, Sadistic Tormentors. FATISTS, by persistently badgering and ridiculing fat people, have managed to destroy their spirits and ruin many of their lives. It is difficult to imagine a greater sin.

To add insult to injury, fat has become virtually synonymous with ugly. Indeed, the phrase "fat and ugly" has practically become a single word for many people. Like the Anglo-Saxon four-letter words, fat has clearly acquired the connotation of disgust and revulsion.

ARLO 'N' JANIS By Jimmy Johnson

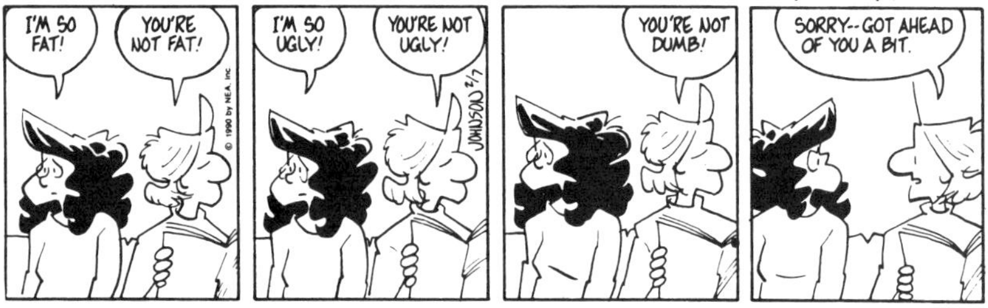

Reprinted by permission of NEA, Inc.

Fat, however, is not precisely in the same class as the other four-letter words. With the traditional four-letter words, the acts themselves are not so awful. We all defecate, urinate, indulge in coitus, and "break wind" — though not necessarily in that order and preferably at appropriate moments. Indeed, restricting these activities is not only unnatural, it can be most unpleasant and even result in serious medical problems. We have to do those things; they are *natural*, healthy functions. We just are not supposed to refer to the acts with socially unacceptable terms.

With fat a far more complex situation exists. Not only is the word offensive when used to describe a person, the term has come to be a reflection of a "nasty, disgusting, and socially unacceptable" *unnatural* condition — one which most genetically thin people feel is quite avoidable and easily remedied. Therefore, when a person gets fat, it is considered to be clear evidence of a personality flaw, at the least — and probably even of a basically immoral character.

If the general society has this view of fat people, it is not difficult to imagine how people who *are* fat, or who *believe* themselves to be fat, must feel about themselves. If they are sensitive at all, they're going to have deep feelings of shame and guilt about their condition. This leads to low-esteem and ultimately to self-loathing. In other words, being fat gives people feelings about themselves that are very similar to those experienced when people use four-letter words.

But fat is a great deal worse. A person can apologize for saying a "bad" word and the incident is over — it is done with. People will usually give the transgressor the benefit of the doubt and accept an apology as being sincere. What good does it do to apologize for being fat, though? The offending tissue is still there. Fat critics are left thinking, "If fat people were really sincere about being sorry, they would lose the fat."

The denigration of fat people must be especially difficult for people who have fat friends or loved ones. Can you imagine the psychological dilemma of thinking of a sainted grandmother or beloved mother who is fat, as being repulsive and immoral? Fortunately, a host of euphemisms come to the rescue. "Grandma is stout," "Mom is heavy-set," "My wife is plump," "Uncle Joe is portly," "My daughter is big-boned," and "Junior is hefty."

On the other hand, did you ever notice how satisfying it is to describe fat people you do not care for? You may use such terms as *obese*, *corpulent*, or *porky*. And a particularly odious person may be described as a *lard ass*. Connotations can be delightfully useful tools. No matter what term is used, though, being fat is a stigma.

It is of utmost importance for the reader to know what the term "fat people" means in this book. An extremely general term, it refers to anyone who is thought by other people to be fat — and it also refers to anybody who personally thinks he, or she, is fat. Please keep in mind that it does not mean all of these people actually are excessively fat. In fact, as shown later in this book, many "fat" people, in reality, are excessively or even morbidly thin.

Usually when referring to fat people, a number of words, such as "large" and "overweight" are often used in place of "fat" since those words are not thought to be as offensive. In this book, diverse terms are used strictly because variety in terminology is interesting to readers.

"Fat" is used most often, however, with the expressed intent to desensitize the reader to that currently derogatory term. The term "fat people" should not be anymore offensive than "thin people." Fat, after all, is NOT a four-letter word!

2

FATNESS AND GENDER

Women tend to be fatter than men; it's a genetic difference. This dissimilarity exists in all racial and ethnic groups, although the degree does appear to vary. In fact, males and females tend to be dissimilar in a great many ways, particularly after puberty. Differences manifest themselves in a variety of ways — anatomical, physiological, biochemical, behavioral, and psychological.

These statements are fighting words in some quarters but they are nevertheless true . Exceptional intellect is not required for a person to be aware of the basic differences. The most obvious physical contrasts are in the pelvic region, but they exist in all parts of the body from the head to the feet. For instance, men tend to have thicker bones in their skulls, which should surprise no female with an ounce of experience. And females have daintier feet — usually. It is because of such differences that a medical forensic expert can look at a skeleton, or often just a part of a bone, and be able to determine the sex of the original owner. This skill can even be applied to the remains of prehistoric humans.

The information which follows, based upon *averages*, is far from being complete or exact but it gives some indication of the differences between males and females. Structurally, men are five to six inches taller than women and their bones are heavier and more dense. Men also have more muscle fibers per muscle and each fiber is larger. As a result, 40% of an average man's body weight consists of muscle, compared to 23% in an average women. Men have longer arms, broader shoulders, and larger chest circumferences. Men also have relatively larger hearts.

Women have a wider pelvic bone structure with a larger, more circular central opening (pelvic brim), for which babies and mothers are no doubt most grateful. The sockets in the sides of the pelvis (acetabulum) that hold the heads of the thigh bones are located a bit more toward the front in women. That gives their hips that distinctive side-to-side gait that most men find so fetching. Women also have a relatively larger abdomen.

In all cultures adults females have 10% to 15% more body fat than do their male counterparts. At twenty years of age the *average* healthy female has about 29% body fat. The percentage gradually increases; at middle age, a healthy female will have about 38% body fat. Most of the fat is subcutaneous with extra thick pads on the hips, thighs, and breasts. These energy deposits come in handy since a woman requires about 80,000 extra calories to sustain her and her fetus through a successful pregnancy.

There are also functional (physiological) differences between the sexes. Men burn calories at a faster rate because they have more muscle tissue and a higher basal metabolic rate. This difference means women are more efficient in burning their energy stores, that is, they require less food to survive. Men have about 500,000 more red blood cells in *each* cubic centimeter of blood. Which means the average man has a total of about twenty billion more red blood cells to carry oxygen than the average woman. Whereas men tend to sweat in excess, women sweat just enough to cool their bodies. When they say they just "glow," they are not lying. Because they sweat less, women are less likely to become dehydrated than men.

Fingernails, which protect the ends of fingers from injury, grow faster in men than in women. Men produce about thirty times more testosterone (male hormone) than women — which makes males more aggressive. Women have more "female hormones" which results in a more nurturing nature. The hormones also make it easier for women to convert food into fat for storage. Women have more pliable blood vessels which serve to accommodate the larger blood volume during pregnancy — and which, incidentally, along with their hormones, decreases their chances for hardening of the arteries.

The brains of men and women are different as well — relative to cell size and neural connections. That may explain why men are more analytical in their approach toward problems that confront them whereas women are more intuitive. Females also have superior verbal abilities, manual dexterity, and more precise small motor coordination while men tend to excel in mathematical and visual-spatial skills, and do better at large movement activities. Put simply, men and women think differently — which should be absolutely no surprise to anyone. This concept is not a new one nor should it be viewed negatively — as the French have long declared, "Vive la difference!"

The information above is much abbreviated; the list of differences could go on and on. Instead of memorizing all of them, however, merely remember that men are designed for running, jumping, grappling, and dealing with situations of an aggressive nature while women are designed to have babies. Or even more succinctly, women are built to bring forth life while men are built to protect it. When making this point before a room full of women, I try to make sure there's an exit close-by. Some listeners react with ill-concealed hostility before I can hastily add that this does not mean women cannot, or should not, have the right to function in a myriad of other ways, of their own choosing, in and out of the home.

Hastening on, it is important to remember that humans evolved over many millions of years. Females developed into creatures who were increasingly better designed to carry fetuses successfully. For example, their relatively heavier weight, shorter legs, and lower weight distribution, particularly when pregnant, gave them a lower center of gravity. This meant they naturally had better balance and were less likely to fall and injure themselves or their precious cargo.

With the short life spans and dangers that abounded in prehistoric times you can be sure the "intra-abdominal cargo" was indeed extremely precious — as was its carrier. There can be little doubt that females were considered the important sex. They were the ones who gave birth — who enabled each primitive clan to retain its frail and tenuous hold on this planet. Since these early people surely had no concept of sperm and ovum, the "miracle of life" must have seemed particularly magical to them.

Cartoons of cave people sometimes depict a man clubbing a woman and dragging her home by the hair. Such scenes are amusing only because they are so unlikely to have occurred. Cave men may have been primitive but they couldn't have been that stupid. Common sense alone would suggest that prehistoric people had to be very perceptive and intelligent to survive the perils of the time. Lending credence to their mental abilities are the skulls of the ape-like Neanderthals which show they had brains that were about 10% *larger* than our own. They apparently also had sophisticated emotions such as sentiment, religious beliefs, and an appreciation of beauty as indicated by grave contents. Fossil pollens, for instance, revealed that flowers had been placed upon the bodies of the dead.

The modern looking Cro-Magnon men, who appeared on Earth about 40,000 years ago, had brains that were even larger than than their predecessors; they were about a pint larger than ours. No, being intelligent, our early ancestors were not about to abuse their women. On the contrary, the highest priority would have been to protect them. That means keeping them in a safe place, such as in (or near) a cave or tribal compound.

When a cave woman's belly started to swell, she became even more precious. The entire tribe knew she was on the verge of creating life. Either she was "god-like" herself, or the gods had bestowed their blessings on her in a very visible and tangible way. It is difficult to imagine the reverence men must have felt for a woman, and women in general, when they actually witnessed life emerging from her body. It is little wonder that most anthropologists now believe that the principal deity of early humans was a woman and that the first servants of gods were *priestesses*.

As mankind's numbers multiplied and it appeared as if the species was here to stay, women became less valued. Social structures became more patriarchal, and religions became more oriented toward males and masculine values. I have a haunting feeling that civilization at this point, except for the superficialities of technology, started going downhill. However, the attitude of putting women on a pedestal did persist until well into the twentieth century. It still lurks, to some degree, in the minds of many men, whether they admit it or not, in spite of the drastic sociopolitical changes that have recently occurred.

When prehistoric women gave birth, their status in the tribe certainly could not be expected to diminish. As nurturers of valuable offspring, women were the keepers of the "family jewels" — an expression which in those days would have had a far less macho meaning than it does today. After all, a man certainly could not successfully breast-feed "God's gift" to the tribe.

The tremendous responsibility of raising an infant to a healthy child required a cave woman to stay close to the hearth. It does not require a Pavlov to understand that "home" and "women" became closely associated in the human psyche. Women became the anchor of the family. Although the world eventually became a safer place in which to reside — in most regions — this anchorage was a valid rationale, until quite recently, for requiring women to stay close to home.

The social structure of the cave dwellers had the effect over millennia of causing male and female physical structures to become even more differentiated than merely in the reproductive areas of the body. The men who were larger, stronger, and had a lot of the hormone that made them aggressive tended to survive to bring home the mammoth steaks — and to father more children.

Women would naturally be attracted to those dominant men because they were good providers and protectors. Women are still attracted to good providers. Virtually every modern questionnaire shows this characteristic to be at the top of the list of desirable traits in a husband. Now, however, a provider brings home the *bacon* and that allows, or perhaps requires, him to be a different kind of man. Instead of being a club-swinging cave man he can even be sensitive, or a wimp, depending upon one's perspective.

Oftentimes cave men took a long time to get back home. Some of them, even the fittest and most skillful, never returned. Back then it literally was "a jungle out there." Fat women would have survived much longer during these and other lean times than thin women. This fact would not have gone unnoticed among the males. They would also have noticed that when a person lost his or her appetite and started losing weight, it was a sure sign of illness. Fatness — the modern concept of fatness — therefore, assuredly would have been equated with glowing good health as it still is in many parts of the world.

A cave man must have realized that his own relative leanness was due not to illness but to his more strenuous lifestyle. All it would take to increase his fatness would be an event, such as an injury, that forced him to be inactive for an extended period. Upon returning to the active list, though, he would have realized quickly that leanness was an advantage in both tracking and attacking prey — and to retreat discreetly and hastily when circumstances warranted it. Indeed, lean men were more likely to survive the hunt and produce sons with the tendency to be lean.

Cave men — the smart ones — must have surmised that fat women with their visible energy reserves were good breeding stock and were very desirable as mates. Indeed, modern scientific investigation has revealed that the risk of having underweight babies is doubled in underweight women. If a man's mate became fat with only a small amount of food, he could consider himself really blessed. The selection of amply endowed females (by early man) as producers of off-spring would of course lead to the propensity for fatness being increasingly more prevalent in the genetic make-up of females.

This desirability of fatness in females could also be expected to become closely associated with deeply ingrained feelings of sexuality in general. The fact that lush, voluptuous women are mighty nice to snuggle up with on cold nights surely would not have detracted from their allure. That they provide more shade in the summer as is sometimes alleged by modern aficionados, however, is probably of insignificant practical value.

The male leader of a tribe would be in the position to choose one of the fattest women from his, or another, tribe as a mate. Then, because of her position as "first lady" of the tribe, she could be expected to receive the largest and choicest portions of food at meals. In addition, she would not have to work as hard, or at all, at menial chores such as food gathering, cooking, and animal skin preparation. So while the working women stayed merely fat, the leader's mate blossomed into obesity. By showing that she didn't have to work, her fatness became a symbol of superior status. Extreme fatness would thereby quite likely become the ideal condition for women in general to strive toward.

Such a scenario is not without modern parallels. The most extreme case is the Polynesian culture — before its people were subjugated by western adventurers and "civilized" by missionaries. The Polynesian queens were massaged, kept virtually immobile, and were constantly being stuffed with fattening foods so they would get as fat as possible. Some achieved monumental proportions. Her social and authoritative stature depended largely upon physical stature. The fatter the queen got, the more royal and revered a figure she became, and this reflected most favorably upon the prestige of the tribe as a whole. On state occasions she was carried out on a pallet to impress visiting dignitaries.

Obesity is still a favored trait in many parts of the world. The Banyankole of East Africa even restrict the physical activity of their girls from the age of eight to fatten them in preparation for marriage. A man's status is enhanced if his wife is fat. This is true for many tribes in East and Central Africa.

The bodies of men and women obviously have much in common. In accordance with the laws of the survival of the fittest, though, it is easy to see how each gender would have developed into beings with different, but complementary, body structures and functions. It's not a bad arrangement, either, if one thinks about it.

The desirability of fat women in prehistoric times is mere conjecture — logical and probable, yes — but it cannot be stated as fact. Supporting the theory, however, is hard evidence. It exists in the form of small, stone statues, and evidence does not get much harder than that. Practically all of the many ancient statuettes that have been found were of fat women, whimsically referred to as "Venuses." They have been found in locations ranging from France and Italy to Siberia. The most famous neolithic statuette is the limestone "Venus of Willendorf" which was unearthed near Willendorf, Austria. Statuettes with large buttocks, abdomen, and breasts were also common among the prehistoric Greeks, Babylonians, and Egyptians.

The charming Venus of Willendorf is thought to have been a fertility symbol or goddess. No one really knows for sure. Perhaps a hunter carried it on long trips to remind him of his "woman," or of women in general, which would make it a stone age version of a girlie magazine. At any rate, only those areas having to do with childbearing are accentuated — the breasts, abdomen, and pubic region. Her sturdy legs taper off to feetlessness, her arms across her breasts are barely visible, and her facial features are nonexistent.

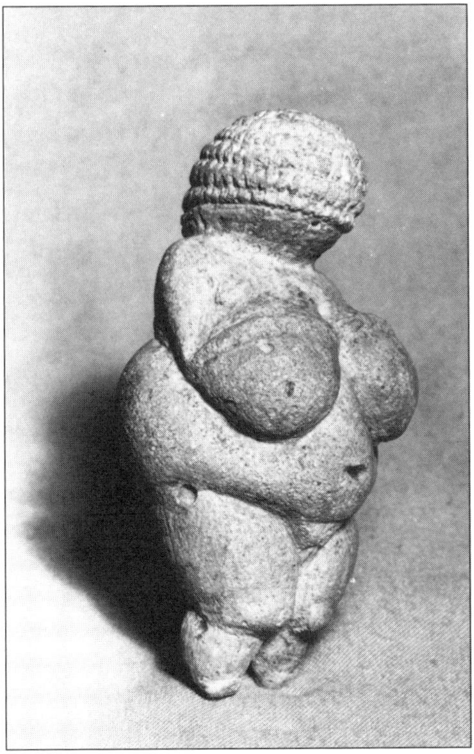

***Venus of Willendorf*. 30,000 -10,000 B. C.**

(Natural History Museum, Vienna)

The *Venus* most likely represents the ideal woman of her time. The lack of detail on the face, or even an attempt at it, suggests that facial beauty was not of the slightest importance in a woman. The sculptor certainly had the carving skill to include facial features if he had wished. This is revealed in the detail seen in the hair style and pubic region. Because she was obviously good breeding stock, she surely must have been considered sexually attractive.

The sculptor, incidentally, also must have sensed and appreciated the inner beauty of women. The *Venus* with her slightly bowed head and hands over her breasts clearly exudes a shyness, a sweetness. Indeed, the more she is studied the more one senses an inner charm radiating from her — a warm, gentle, loving nature captured in stone — characteristics not strikingly evident in the extremely thin models that appear on the pages of today's glamour magazines.

Even if the people of the time thought of women only as breeding stock, the fact that it was a consideration at all certainly speaks well of their intelligence. Today a farmer would be considered a fool if he did not attempt to improve his breeding stock. Currently, we are using the science of genetics to improve many animal species to better serve our needs. This includes horses, cattle, hogs, sheep, chickens, and turkeys. Many plants such as corn, soy beans, and wheat are also being changed with selective breeding and genetic engineering.

While humans are quick to practice eugenics on other living organisms, they are reluctant to practice it on themselves. This is not to imply that genetics should used in determining who should be allowed to have children. The opposite of eugenics, called cacogenics, however, has been practiced for many years. Though cacogenics may be a fascinating word, it is an asinine policy. Yet that's exactly what the nations of the world do when they send their healthiest and most intelligent young adults off to battlefields to be slaughtered while the remainder stay home to breed. Maybe, this explains why the human brain has shrunk in size since 40,000 B.C. A person has to wonder about the direction civilization is taking. It should be no surprise that mankind has "progressed" to the point where a single individual can press a button and destroy all life on Earth many times over.

The point of this discussion of prehistoric times is to show that what we are today, relative to our anatomy and physiology, is based upon millions of years of evolution. During this time women have evolved into creatures with a far greater tendency to be fat, according to current standards, than are males. It is a legacy of distant ancestors that is carried in their genes. In spite of this natural tendency, however, modern fashion has arbitrarily dictated that women must be thin to be desirable. This dilemma, to quote some forgotten bard, has served to put the average woman "between a rock and a hard place." It's no wonder she is plagued with feelings of frustration, guilt, and a lack of self-esteem, all the result of blaming herself for being fat.

Men, on the other hand, typically do not blame themselves when they are fat — even though they are genetically programmed to be thinner than women. Perhaps a major reason for fat men having a more accepting attitude toward their condition is that they suffer relatively minuscule amounts of "fat bashing" from society. They are not constantly being pushed into a defensive position.

Fat men do not generally picture themselves as being fat, but rather as robust, stocky, or big-fellows. Indeed, some men proudly display their spectacular "beer bellies." Why else would they wear their belts down in front near the pubic bone? You've seen them pat the prodigious protuberance with paternal pride and proclaim, "Yep, it took many years and many barrels of Budweiser to develop this here belly." When people suggest they should lose weight, these men look at the advisers as if they were daft. On the other hand, have you ever seen a fat woman swagger into into a room with her slacks low in front and her thumbs hooked in her belt? And I will, tastefully, not even bring up the subject of buttock cleavage.

The intense social pressure exerted on women to be lean is clearly inappropriate. Particularly so since it has been estimated that 40% of American men are medically too fat while only 32% of American women are in the same category! But the most insidious aspect of the social pressure is that it is the women themselves who are probably the most guilty of applying it to themselves. Their efforts are incredibly inconsistent in an age when females are striving for liberation. Even as women are being exhorted to take pride in their gender, they are urging one another to reject their own genetically programmed body shapes. In their attempts to defy nature, their physical and emotional health is adversely affected — and along with it, their hope for happiness. Sadly, their attempts to change their nature body types are rarely, if ever, successful over the long haul anyway.

A revealing picture of gender differences regarding fat acceptance appeared in *Playboy*, October, 1990. This is a magazine with an interesting menu of important interviews, feature articles, and fiction — in addition to its well-known frothy photographic hor d'oeuvres. In her column, "Women," Cynthia Heimel wrote about a barbecue party she attended in Malibu, California:

> There were a bunch of women there eating nothing. The men were happily tucking into ribs and potato salad. Some of them looked good, but some had big pot bellies. I don't know what goes on in a man's darkest, deepest soul, but even the fat fellows looked enormously, richly pleased with themselves.
>
> The women looked wary and skinny with stringy muscles and questionable breasts. Their faces were disturbing . . .
>
> There was another woman, a major celebrity, who looked just plain skeletal . . .

Societal roles are accentuated in the glitzsy world of Hollywood, and that makes it easier to see the social truths that exist in general. One axiom is that men are judged far more by their successes in life than by the shape or fatness of their bodies. A woman, however, can achieve at the very highest levels of her profession and still be expected by society to have a thin and (presumably) beautiful body. And if the woman does not have a perfect body, the "failure" causes her to feel worthless and depressed in spite of all her other achievements. A perfect example of this is Eleanor Roosevelt, a woman with vast accomplishments and one of the most acclaimed women of her time. When asked what her number one wish would be, she replied, "To be beautiful."

One of the chief objectives of this book is to help alleviate the sad and grossly unfair denigration of fat people that is rampant in our western culture. Since fatness has unfairly become primarily a women's problem, the thrust of this book is naturally directed toward them.

3

FATNESS AND ATTRACTIVENESS

It can be assumed there have always been people on Earth who have been relatively thin, or muscular, or fat. The percentage of each of these types within a group would depend chiefly upon genetic, environmental, and cultural factors. Some body types are better designed for certain environmental conditions than are others. For instance, the more spherical a person's body is the less surface area it will have for a given body weight. This physique is ideal for helping the body to conserve its heat. In addition, the fat that helps to make a person round is an excellent insulator against cold. Therefore, in regions that are perennially cold, such as Alaska, northern Asia, and Canada, a short, round, fat body type could be expected to have evolved—and this seems to have been the case, as exemplified by Eskimos and Mongolians. It is probably not coincidental that the most rotund of the prehistoric "Venus" figurines were found in regions with the coldest climates.

In hot, dry climates a tall, lean type of body would be most suitable. It would produce less heat and its relatively large surface area would be ideal for dissipating heat. Such a body could be expected to evolve in hot, dry regions such as the eastern Sudan in Africa and this too has occurred. Not surprisingly in temperate regions such as Europe, an intermediate physique is the genetic norm.

Upon the genetic predispositions, local environmental factors exert their effect upon a group's fatness. Chief among these are the availability of food and the amount of energy required to secure the food. Hunters, for instance, would logically expend considerable energy in acquiring food, especially if game were scarce. Farmers with a more reliable and plentiful food supply close at hand would typically expend less energy. Therefore, people in a farming environment could be expected to be fatter in general than those in a hunting one. And studies do confirm that to be the case.

When food is generally abundant within a society, cultural factors have a lot to do with determining if its people will tend to be fat, thin, or somewhere in between. Currently, in the U.S. and much of Western Europe thinness is "in," particularly among the upper socioeconomic classes. But throughout most of history, and in many parts of the world today, fatness was the fashion. Thinness was a sign of poor health or at least a weak constitution. Fatness, conversely, was an indication of contentment, happiness, and a lack of worry. As stated in the Shirburn Ballads of 1585:

> Let care kill a cat,
> We'll laugh and grow fat.

Twenty years latter Thomas Wright was more specific. In *Passions of the Mind* he observed:

> Fat and merry,
> Lean and sad

A man with substantial bulk commanded respect. He possessed what was called a "noble" waistline. If a lot of the weight was fat, so much the better. It was tangible proof that he could not only acquire enough food to stay alive, he could acquire *more* than enough. In Chaucer's Prologue to the *Canterbury Tales* the monk was described as being, " . . . a fine, fat lord, and in good shape." More recently, Walt Whitman wrote, "I find no fat sweeter than my own." Being fat meant a man was successful. And tangible evidence of success, just as it currently does, virtually guarantees a man social acceptance.

If none of these quotes impresses you, perhaps a message from the Bible will. In Proverbs XXVIII, 25, (c. 350 B.C.) it is written:

> He that putteth his trust in the Lord shall be made fat.

Now, that has got to make a believer stop and think a bit! Until quite recently, a man's fatness was of no great significance as far as his personal appearance was concerned, except in extreme cases of a deficiency or excess of fat. Other men did not especially care how he looked. If anything, bulk gave the impression of power and sexual vigor even if much of size consisted of fat. The opposite sex was more interested in a man's ability to be a provider than anything else. And, remember, a fat man had conspicuous evidence that he was an able provider.

As discussed previously, women have a natural tendency to be fatter than men. Still, like men, and for the same reasons, they can range from being morbidly thin to morbidly obese — and without a doubt always have. During prehistoric times the relative numbers of any body type in a particular geographic region probably would not have changed very much except in relation to food supply. Again, the fatter women would probably have made up the largest group by far if sufficient food was available since fat women were most highly prized.

Because men wanted fat women, women strove to be fat — at least the smart ones did. This presumption may sound simplistic in today's social atmosphere in which many women are disclaiming the need to have a man, but there was no question about a woman requiring a man in those early times. She needed a man for protection, and especially to provide for her when she was "with child." Acquiring the right man, or any man, could be a matter of life or death. This dependency upon men explains why a woman's physical appearance traditionally has been so important. It may also explain why men have been so cocksure of themselves — at least on the surface.

From the beginning of historic times to the early part of the twentieth century, as revealed in visual art, the most desired female body was the fat one. Or perhaps "plump" is a better term since this word means to be fat in an attractive way. Of course, plump is itself a subjective term. What is considered "plump" by one person, may be thought of as "fat" or even "obese" by another.

To corroborate the perennial attractiveness of plumpness, or fatness, a representative series of pictures of paintings and sculpture follow. When including the *Venus of Willendorf*, they range from prehistoric times to the twentieth century.

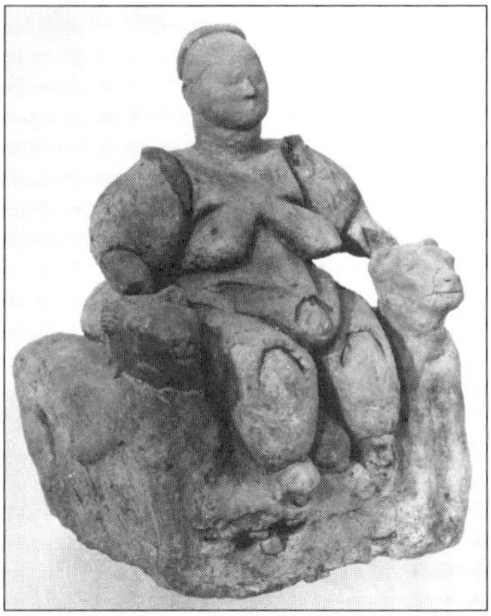

***Turkish Goddess*. 6,000 B.C.**

(Archaeological Museum, Ankara)

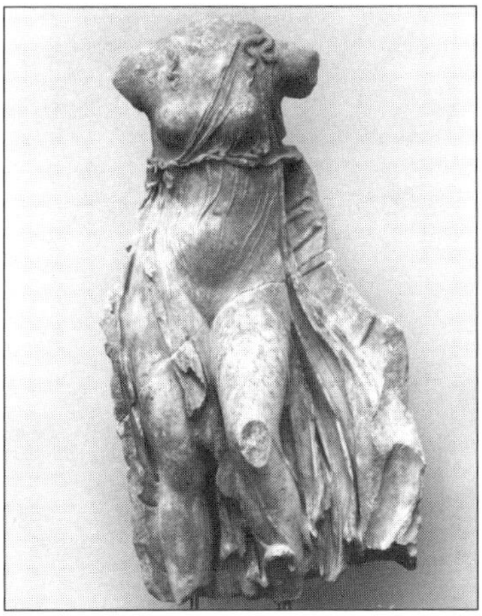

***Greek Goddess*. 4th Century B.C.**

(Ny Carlsberg Glyptotch, Copenhagen)

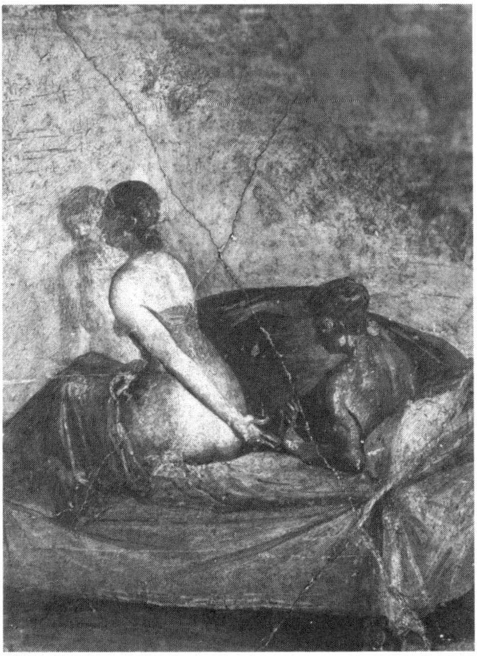

***Wall Painting* (Pompeii). Reign of Nero.**

(National Archaeology Museum, Naples)

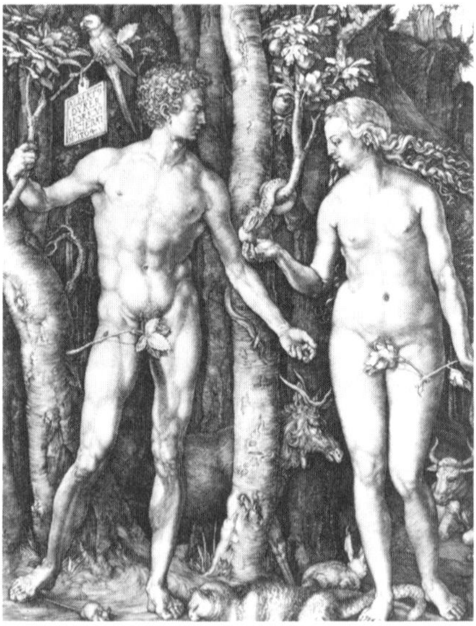

Albrecht Dürer. *Adam and Eve*. 1504.

(Metropolitan Museum of Art, New York)

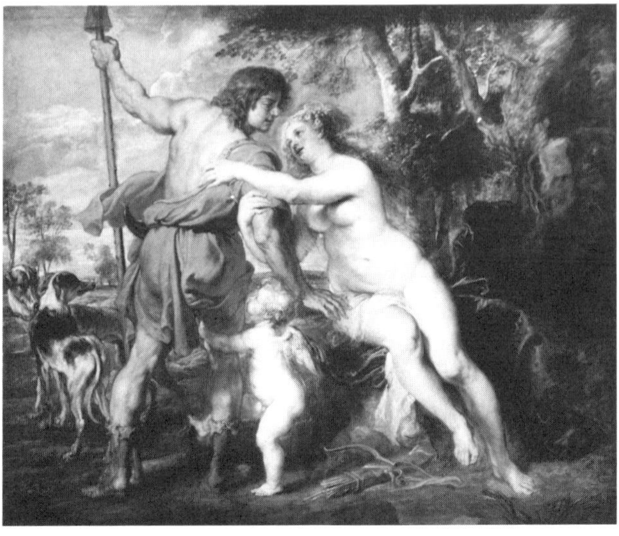

Peter Paul Rubens. *Venus and Adonis*. 1635.

(Metropolitan Museum of Art, New York)

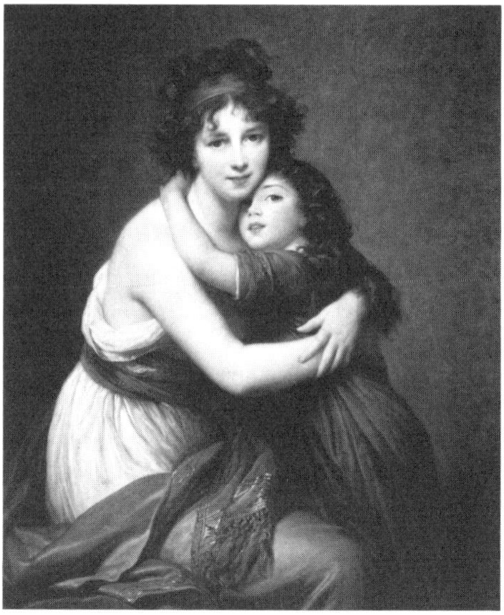

Louis Elisabeth LeBrun Vegée-LeBrun.

***Madame Vegée-LeBrun and Her Daughter*. 1789.**

(Louvre Museum, Paris)

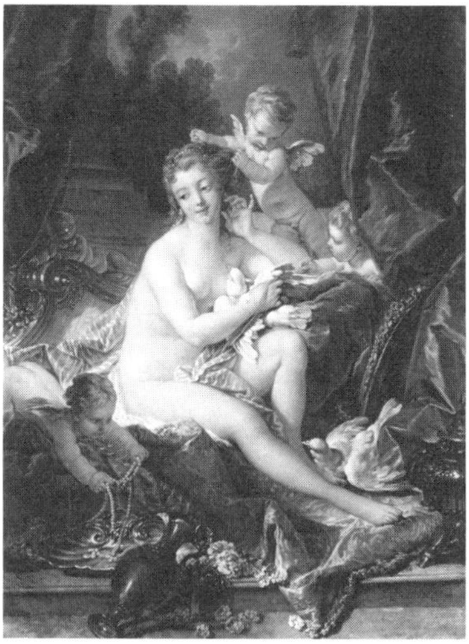

François Boucher.

***The Toilet of Venus.* 1751.**

(The Metropolitan Museum of Art)

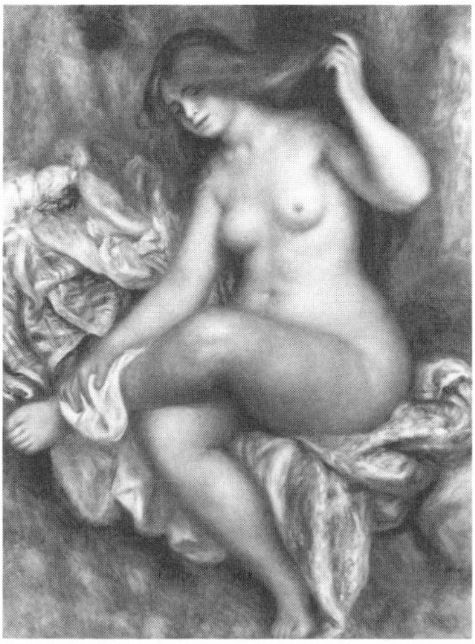

Pierre Auguste Renoir.

***Seated Bather*. 1906.**

(Founders Society, Detroit Institute of Arts,)

Most of the art shown above is from Europe because that is where most of our American cultural background originates. Comparisons with modern concepts of physical attractiveness therefore have more significance. The appreciation of women with more than a little fat on their bodies was not limited to Europe, though. It was the rule in practically every region of the world — and in many places it still is.

Because of the inherent subjectivity, not everyone will think of all the women in the artwork as being fat. It must be agreed, however, that the women are all heavier than what is considered by today's western culture to be fashionable.

Are the bodies of the women in the pictures attractive? That, too, depends upon the tastes of the viewer. It is very likely that the artists, all of whom were male, thought so. Since it is inconceivable that every woman in a particular period and locality had the same physical proportions, the artist probably chose those women who he and his society, in general, thought were most appealing — when he wanted to paint a picture of an attractive woman. This hint of feminine perfection is often revealed by the subject matter of the artwork such as "love" and "romance"; names such as "Eve," "Venus," or "bather" in the titles; and by the use of famous beauties, noblewomen, or consorts of kings as models. Dürer's *Adam and Eve* is almost identical to his drawing of the *Idealistic Male and Female*.

The historical appreciation of feminine fatness has also been revealed in literature through the ages. In the first century A.D. the Roman poet Ovid wrote in *Amores:*

> Stark naked as she stood before mine eye,
> Not one wen on her body could I spy.
> What arms and shoulders did I touch and see,
> How apt her breasts were to be press'd by me!
> How smooth a belly under her waist saw I!
> How large a leg, and what a lusty thigh!
> (Translated from the Latin in 1585 by Christopher Marlowe)

In 12th century England, Chaucer wrote:

> The daughter was stout and well-developed, with a pug nose, blue eyes, broad buttocks, and round, high breasts . . . Because she was pretty, the town parson planned to make her his heir.

As shown in the paintings and sculptures, largeness in the abdomen, hips, and thighs, was most desired. Large breasts can only be defined as a modern fashion that has become a fetish.

In the 17th century a diet specialist, Jean-Anthelme Brillat-Savarin, wrote a book entitled *The Philosopher in the Kitchen*. In it he said:

> Every thin woman wishes to put on weight; this is an ambition that has been confided to us a thousand times.

This statement is a far cry from the current allegation that "inside every fat woman is a thin woman screaming to get out." Brillat-Savarin went on to recommend fattening diets since society expected women to be full-bodied, and thin figures could not be disguised by fashionable dresses. Such an attitude still prevails in many parts of the world today. In the June, 1979 issue of National Geographic Magazine a Russian woman gently admonishes a young American exchange student to eat so she will gain weight and be more attractive.

A passage from Guy De Maupassant's short story *Boule de Suef (Ball-of-Fat)* shows that in France of the 1700's even extremely fat women could be considered desirable:

> The woman, one of the so-called ladies of the night, was famous for a precocious rotundity and it earned her the nickname Boule de Suef. She was short, round and soft as goose fat, her fingers were pudgy and squeezed at the joints like strings of little pork sausages; her skin was taut and shiny and she had enormous breasts that threatened to burst through her dress, but she was very appetizing and much sought after because her youthful freshness gave men such pleasure. Her face was a round apple, a peony bud ready to pop into bloom, and inside that

> opened two great black eyes shaded with thick brows that cast a shadow within; and a charming mouth, humid for kissing, furnished with shining, microscopic baby teeth. She was, it was said, full of admirable qualities.

In his 1797 play, *Irish Minnie*, John O'keeffe described his heroine in a similar though more succinct fashion.

> . . . fat , fair, and forty was all the toast of the young men.

The earliest successful settlers in the U.S., the pilgrims, had a saying that revealed how they felt about women of substance:

> A fat wife and a full barn
> never did any man harm.

The sentiment persisted for a long time. Katrina Van Tassel, in Washington Irving's *Legend of Sleepy Hollow* was described as being:

> . . . a blooming lass of eighteen; plump as a partridge; ripe and melting and rosy cheeked as one of her father's peaches, and universally famed not only for her beauty, but her vast expectations.

This passage introduces "beauty," a term which thus far has been purposefully avoided. The attribute refers to a pleasing of the senses — the visual sense, when one is talking about visual beauty. When considering attractiveness, however, far more than appearances are involved; a strong emotional reaction is implied. Dictionary definitions of "attractive" usually include such words as "alluring and charming" and such phrases as "winning attention and liking," and "to tempt very strongly."

When attractiveness is considered in this manner, it certainly is not synonymous with beauty. A man may find a woman extraordinarily beautiful and yet not *feel* an emotional response toward her. He may neither "like her" nor "be strongly tempted" by her appearance. On the other hand, it is quite common for a man to speak of seeing a woman (perhaps for only a few seconds), who he claims was, "not all that good-looking but she made my head spin," " . . . took my breath away," or " . . . made my stomach do flip-flops." Sometimes the effect on a even lower organ provides a visually unmistakable confirmation of the woman's impact.

The concept of attractiveness is definitely more complex than that of beauty. A women's attractiveness to a man is usually difficult or impossible to explain. It seems to be based upon something primeval — something deep within a male. Probably the best way of describing the feeling, though it may be a bit crude, is that it's an appeal that occurs at the "gut level."

Women also report this phenomenon in their reactions toward the physical appearances of certain men. Even, a homely man can be quite attractive. Some people would say rock star Mick Jagger is a prime illustration of this. A more extreme example was seen in the television series, *The Beauty and the Beas*t. The series owed its popularity almost exclusively to the attraction of female viewers toward the beast — who had distinctly bizarre features.

In *The Beauty Myth: How Images of Beauty Are Used Against Wom*en, Naomi Wolf delves deeply into the topic of beauty. She contends that attraction depends upon *unique* qualities, memories, and patterns of desire between two people — while beauty is a *generi*c quality. Wolf says the myth of what passes for beauty is based almost exclusively upon the visual sense — and that this sensory limitation actually undermines sexual attractiveness. She is obviously correct. Sight is primarily an information-gathering sense, while those of touch, smell, and taste are the sensual ones. Ironically, the latter senses are ignored in the current myth of beauty.

Anyone with even a mild familiarity with art is going to realize that not all of the women portrayed in works of art throughout history were fat. As shown below, there were also thin women, but they were far fewer in number.

If there is one common aspect in the portrayal of the thin women in these pictures it is a lack of sensuality — a characteristic that pictures of

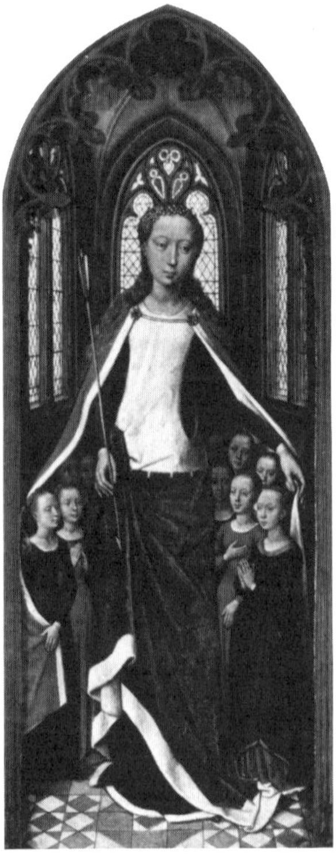

Hans Memling. ***St. Ursula*****. 1489.**

(Memling Museum

SintJans Hôspitaal, Bruges)

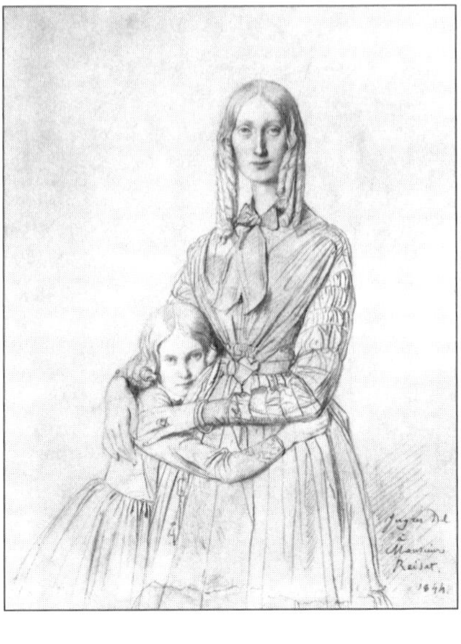

Jean Auguste Dominique Ingres.

Madame Reiset and her Daughter**. 1844.**

(Museum Bogmans-van Beuningen, Rotterdam)

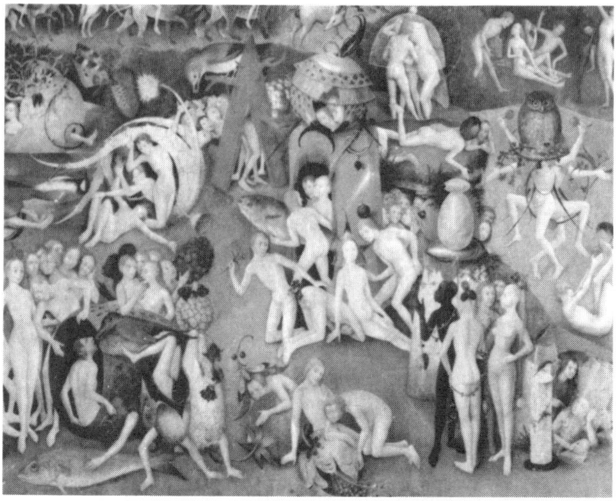

Hieronymous Bosch. ***The Garden of Earthly delights***
(detail from center panel). 1505-10.
(Prado Museum, Madrid)

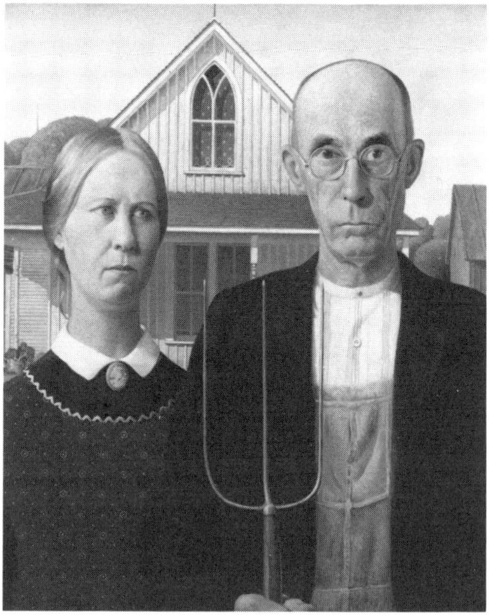

Grant Wood. ***American Gothic.*** **1930.**
(The Art Institute of Chicago, Chicago)

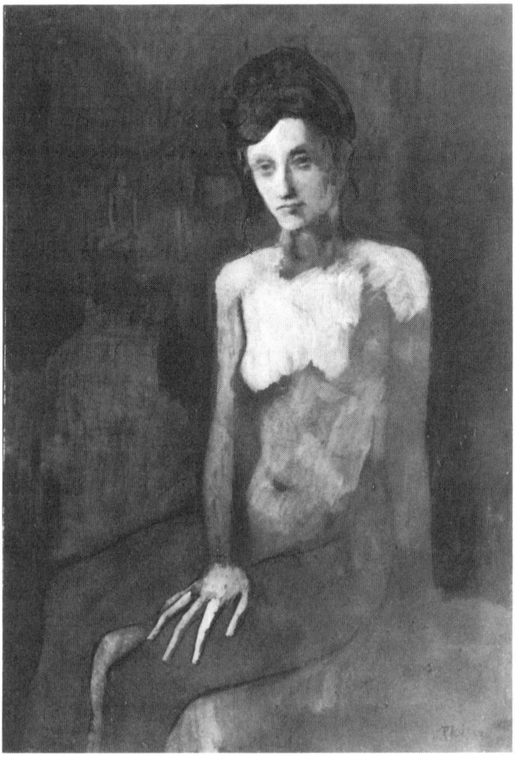

Pablo Picasso. *Seated Nude*. 1905.

(Museum of Modern Art, Paris)

plump women nearly always have in voluptuous abundance. It would appear as if a well-padded female figure is just naturally more sensuous to the human mind than a thin one is. This would lead an artist to choose a plump woman when sensuality is desired in a painting. Conversely, a thin model would most likely be chosen for a work where sensuality was inappropriate, such as spiritualistic art.

In a painting entitled *The Garden Of Earthly Delights* one would expect boundless sensuality. This trait, however, is clearly not portrayed in Bosch's strange work. Nor could the slender figures be considered all that erotic even though the painting would be classified by some viewers as an X-rated work.

The thinnest figures of women, as well as of men, appeared in Medieval art — most of which was associated with the Roman Catholic Church. With the human spirit being all important during that period, physical realism reached rock-bottom. The bodies of females, so reminiscent of the Woman who caused the downfall of Man (Hey, it's a religion created by men. Who would *you* blame?), most assuredly was not to be displayed in a desirable form. Poor mortal Man with his natural sexual sweet tooth was tempted enough as it was by living seductresses. It did not make sense to further stimulate man's "weak flesh" with sensuous images in stone and paint. On the contrary, female bodies were shown in the most undelectable way the Church could imagine — in straight, vertical lines. No soft, rounded curves in their women. Oh, no. Sensuality was almost paranoiacally avoided.

Of course, most of the real women in medieval life did not have thin, linear shapes. A product of millions of years cannot be changed within a few years or generations even by Papal decree. It is inconceivable, too, that church art had any effect on changing the tastes of men when it came

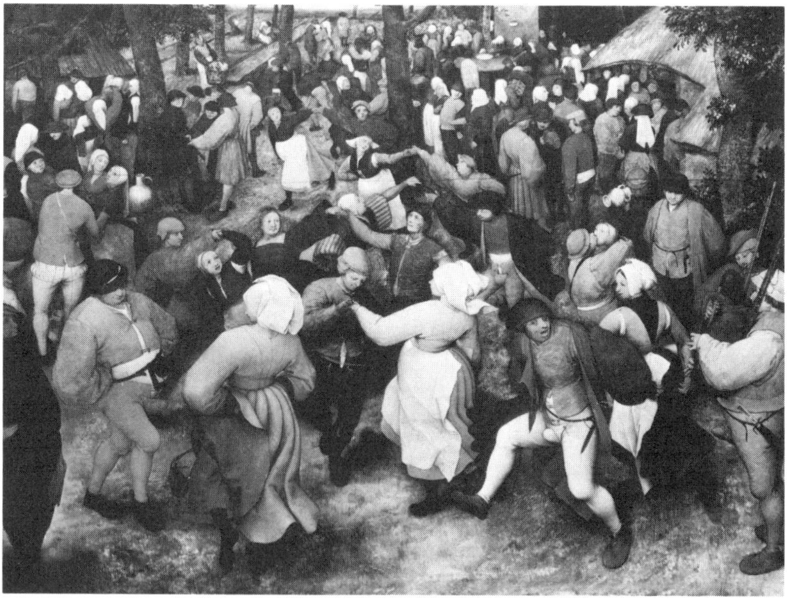

Pieter Bruegel, the elder. *Wedding Dance*. 1566.

(Founders Society, Detroit Institute of Arts, Detroit)

to women's bodies. If anything, the cold, spare church figures probably gave men an even greater appreciation of their own warm, huggable, stout women. This appreciation is certainly evident in Bruegel's Medieval painting entitled *Wedding Dance.* All of the women are fat (by today's standards) and the men, as evidenced by the three "dandies" in the foreground, obviously and unabashedly find them more than a little appealing. None of the men, of course, are fat; they are "robust."

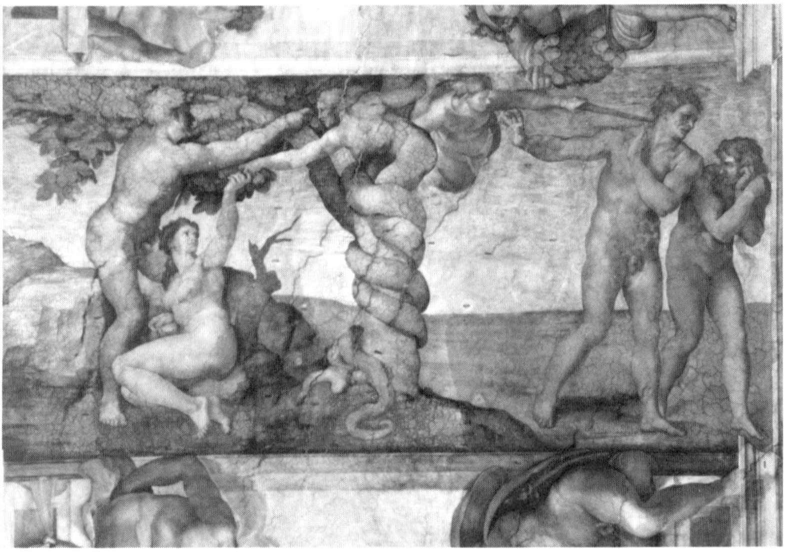

Michelangelo. *The Fall.* About 1515.

(Detail from the Sistine Chapel, Vatican City)

With the flowering of the Renaissance, and relative freedom from church control, there was a dramatic shift in the portrayal of humans even in church art. Linear, "spiritual" bodies were passé; massively muscled men and voluptuous women were back in style. Nowhere is this more evident than in Michelangelo's work in the Sistine Chapel. (Incidentally, the apparent discrepancy in dates relative to Medieval and Renaissance art is due to the fact that the cultural rebirth began in Italy and slowly progressed to other parts of Europe.)

With increased fleshiness being portrayed in religious art, it is not surprising that women in worldly art were fatter than they had ever been.

Happy days were back again and the good times rolled. With unleashed fervor Renaissance artists gave full vent to their seemingly instinctual preference for fat women.

Seemingly instinctual? Perhaps the desire for fatness in women actually *is* instinctual. Maybe there is a race memory in the minds of men that links their feminine preferences to those of their ancient ancestors and makes fleshy women attractive to men. As Robert Brain wrote in his fascinating book, *The Decorated Body*:

> Obesity has always been associated with ideas of maternal abundance and erotic desire, and this state was often produced by artificial means — by fattening processes. Fat, particularly on the buttocks, was considered a sign of well-being . . .

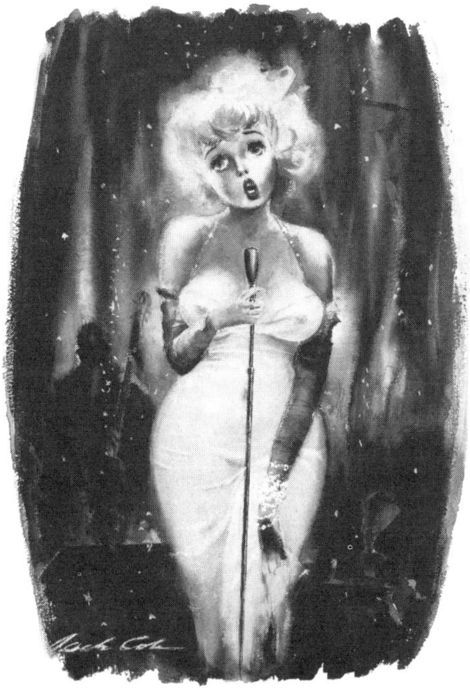

"I ain't got no bod-eee . . "

Playboy has, for several decades, been a strong force in shaping the tastes of American men in regards to the female form. Although its nude centerfolds certainly would not be considered excessively fat by most people, the women in their cartoons often *are* portrayed as being extremely voluptuous. The body of the woman in the cartoon below, in fact, is clearly reminiscent of women in many of the old masters

The use of cartoons in this book, by the way, is more than an embellishment. Cartoons have been chosen on the assumption that conceptual points are usually best made with a touch of humor. Besides, there is truth in cartoons. Long ago, I learned there is more truth in the comic sections of newspapers than on the rest of the pages—particularly the editorial sections.

On a 1989 segment of a highly rated TV comedy series, *Night Court*, a circus fat lady fell on the prosecuting attorney, the inveterate womanizer of the show. When she was removed, the man had a pop-eyed stare of disbelief and said, with awe in his voice, that he had just been covered with 400 pounds of cellulite. As the audience chuckled, one of the actors asked him, "What's the matter, Dan? She's off now."

With a whimsical smile he replied, " . . . I liked it!" The audience of course, exploded in laughter. It was an hilarious scene to be sure, to be sure, but Dan's reaction was probably a lot closer to the truth than some men will ever allow themselves to know — or admit. Indeed, on a Sally Jessy Raphael show (September, 1991) devoted to the subject of fatness, a middle-aged man in the audience said to the host, "Once you've been in a relationship with a fat woman, there's no going back to thin women. Fat women have special qualities."

That preference apparently inspired the Roman poet, Martial (first century A.D.), to write:

> I do not want, O Flaccus, a threadlike
> lover on whose arms you could slip a ring,
> with sharpened buttocks and pointed knees . . .

There are males who occasionally "sleep with" obese women and then crow to their friends that they are merely doing "charity work."

Anyone who falls for that line is gullible enough to believe these insecure, insensitive jerks are gentlemen. Besides, males are not likely to produce erections for "charity work." The only favors these "men" are doing are for themselves. They just do not have the strength of character to stand up to society's narrow dictates. When a *man* is attracted to a fat woman, his attitude is, "You guys may think she's fat, but I think she's a luscious fox — and I'm going for it."

In addition to succumbing to an innate attraction to "fat" women, such men may have learned through experience what modern science has recently confirmed — namely, that fat women are "sexier" than skinny ones. Oh yes! For example, studies conducted at a number of research centers around the world have shown that fat women have more sexual fantasies and desire sex more often than thin ones. Fat women also scored twice as high as thin women on scales of erotic excitability and readiness. Not surprisingly, men are very likely to find such characteristics sexually arousing.

In general, a modern layer of cultural influence has largely suppressed the historical attraction of males to fat women. In many men, though, the primal attraction to lush women has burst through the veneer and into their consciousness — and they openly admit it. To these men fat certainly is NOT a four-letter word.

4

FATNESS AND VISUAL BEAUTY

Whereas a person's attractiveness is "in the gut of the beholder," beauty is often said to "lie in the eye of the beholder." Actually, since concepts of beauty are acquired through learning, it is more accurate to say that "beauty lies in the *mind* of the beholder."

Beauty learned? Certainly. No one can be so naive as to believe humans are born with a specific concept of beauty. One of the most memorable episodes of the *Twilight Zone* television series dealt powerfully with this issue.

The story revolved around a woman with a hideously deformed face. Her only hope for a normal life was through corrective surgery. During the first part of the program, surgeons had attempted to correct the condition and her head was completely swathed in bandages during most of the show. The surgeons were not at all hopeful due to the severity of her deformity. Interestingly, through skillful stage direction, *none* of the actors' faces was shown on the screen until near the end of the program. At that time the patient's bandages were removed and she looked into a mirror. The television audience saw her face at the same time. She shrieked in disappointment at the results and cried hysterically as the medical personnel recoiled in revulsion at the sight of her face.

Viewers were taken aback because her face was absolutely beautiful. Then the television cameras panned to show, for the first time, the faces of the doctors and nurses. They all had grotesquely ugly faces — according to our standards. But their faces were obviously the norm in their society and the woman varied so far from it that *she* was considered a freak. Not surprisingly, the episode was entitled, "Eye of the Beholder."

In our world, different standards of beauty have prevailed during different historical periods. That these standards change from time to time, often dramatically, is proof that concepts of beauty are not innate but are acquired according to the fashions of the day.

Fashion, incidentally, refers to the preference of the majority of people within a society toward virtually anything. It may be clothing, hair styles, social mannerisms, or a concept of feminine beauty. Unfortunately, not everyone can expect to be fashionable in spite of the desire to be so. Primary limiting factors are genetics and finances.

Fashions do not necessarily have anything to do with basic, instinctual attractions. The fact that a society can learn to prefer one type of female body over another is evidence of this. Body hair is another example. Some societies prefer their women to have body hair while others demand that it be shaved, plucked, hot-waxed, depilatoried, or electrolysized.

This variation in preference is not limited to the visual sense. Recently, for instance, it has been discovered by scientists that humans, as do many other animals, exude distinctive scents called pheromones. In humans they are secreted from tiny glands at the base of hair follicles. The glands are especially common in the armpits. The underarm odors are currently thought to be quite objectionable in our "squeaky-clean" culture. Yet, scientists believe the scents have an attractive role in sexual behavior since they are not secreted until puberty. In addition, it has been shown that when the underarm "essence" of men is sprayed into the air of a room, women tend to react more positively to a man in the room. The pheromone's effect is not merely subjective. When a pad that has been tucked in a man's armpit for awhile is removed and wiped across the lips of a woman's mouth, it effects her menstrual cycle and also makes her more fertile. The women volunteers were not aware of the pads' exotic origins — and I'd hate to be the one to enlighten them. Women produce only about one-third as much of the pheromones but their's also acts as an aphrodisiac.

Perceptive swains have probably used the pheromone phenomenon to their advantage throughout the ages. At least it is known that roguish Frenchmen during the reign of Louis XIV would tuck handkerchiefs in their armpits — to be retrieved upon appropriate occasions. When a lady swooned (dresses were very restrictive in those days) one of these cads would surreptitiously whip out his "loaded" hanky to revive her. It got her immediate attention as one might imagine, and it also reputedly got her hormones bubbling. American counterparts of the period were themselves not above engaging in this hanky-panky. Women who exuded pungent, musky odors were similarly thought to be "foxy" — as opposed to those who smelled like roses.

The likelihood of such obvious pheromone ploys being successful today is remote. By using the same tactics as the antifat industry, the public has been brainwashed by the perfume-cologne industry into believing that body smells are no longer sexual turn-ons but are actually repugnant. Defying nature, women odorize their bodies with relatively mild olfactory bait. To make up for the loss of "zing," manufacturers resort to such names as Passion, Seduction, and My Sin.

Men, too, are now expected to smell as sweet as women. Wisely, the industry counters "sissy" connotations by giving these men's perfumes such macho names as Brut, Sweat, Hai Karate, and Iron. The typical claim is that the products drive women wild. Before long, the industry can be expected to stop "pussyfootin'" around and put an Erection on the market. A product so named would sell like suntan lotion in a Swedish nudist colony. The makers could really ravish the marketplace a few years later with a "new improved formula" called Blue Steel — an appellation that would make "Iron" seem as manly as rose-scented toilet water.

Of all sensory experiences, the variations in visual standards of beauty are easiest to document. Clothing fashions are a prime example since a clear and vast record has been captured by artists in stone, paintings, and photographs. Even though the foundations for clothing fashions in a particular region are determined chiefly by practical considerations, which include the climate and materials that are available, there is tremendous flexibility within these boundaries. Fashion in a hot climate, for instance, ranges from the wearing of a string necklace and nothing else — as demonstrated by early Australian Aborigines as well as by African, Philippine, and Amazon tribes, and modern nudists — to the wearing of fur coats by tourists during balmy summer evenings in Miami Beach. The latter custom may make the tourists seem a tad balmy, too. But fur is actually very practical if a person's prime objective is to impress other people with wealth, even at the expense of the wearer's good taste, or sanity, being questioned.

It is not at all unusual for people to select clothing to impress others. Throughout history one of clothing's chief functions is to provide conspicuous and immediate distinction between the "haves" and the "have-nots." The practice probably started when the chief of a cave dwelling tribe claimed the finest furs for himself and his mate.

In early historical cultures it was sometimes against the law for commoners to wear upper class styles even if they could afford them. In ancient Rome, for instance, only royalty could wear clothes dyed purple. Violation of the law carried a death penalty. This ultimate in snob appeal no doubt created an intense desire among some of the citizenry to wear the color.

In addition to revealing one's social position, men who wish to improve their prestige — and therefore, power — usually feel an ostentatious image is mandatory to impress other men. At one time that was achieved with brightly colored silks, laces, and embroidered jackets. Today more subdued designer clothes are "in," along with accessories that include outrageously expensive cars, houses, and jewelry. Books are even available to instruct people on the wearing of Power Clothes to Power Meetings and Power Lunches. Besides impressing other men, such grandiose displays also serve as a very effective lure for a certain, common, type of female.

Only rarely, until recently, was a woman able to drape herself with expensive garb without the financial assistance of a male. Of course, a husband was duty-bound to see that his wife was dressed according to his station in life. This rationale also applied to the father of a young, unmarried woman. Besides, it was smart for him to package his daughter as well as possible to increase her chances of marrying well. Marriage was, after all, practically the only career open to a respectable woman until recent times. Her task was to run the household and to assist her husband in any way she could. This function was prescribed either by custom, law, or religion.

Men who feel compelled to impress other people have always sought appropriate women. Whereas most women use make-up and dangle ornaments from various parts of their bodies to enhance their appearance, a status-seeking man typically adorns himself by having a *woman* dangling from his arm. She is his chief fashion accessory. For this ploy to be effective she, of course, has to be physically beautiful.

Women, gentle souls that they are, tend to be accommodating by doing what they can to enhance their beauty — according to the style of the times. Judging from the incredibly stretched necks and ears, grossly elongated skulls, saucer-sized lips, scarification, skull and feet deformation, and tattoos of women in various cultures, it seems as if their capacity for accommodation is virtually boundless.

Modern women of the western world may shudder when thinking of the barbarous techniques primitive women had to go through (and some still do) in the interest of capturing an illusion called beauty. Of course, the primitive women would do their own share of shuddering if they witnessed a modern woman having rhinoplasty, breast enhancement surgery (reduction or enlargement), or liposuction. The latter, particularly, has to be seen for the bizarre nature of the procedure to be appreciated; it would scare the daylights out of any sensible primitive woman.

Since over time there have been extreme variations in styles of clothing and body tamperings, it can be assumed that the prevailing tastes relative to female body types have also varied considerably. Although it's unlikely that the percentages of the various body types have really changed much throughout history, within any racial group the *desirability* of a particular type could be expected to vary. In some periods, for instance, women who were quite fat could be expected to be the most highly prized, while at other times thinner women would be in fashion.

Again, a perusal of art reveals this to be true. Not only were there variations in terms of overall body fatness, different body parts took turns in being in or out of vogue. The large abdomen on Arnolfini's bride in Van Eyck's painting, for instance, is due to the fashion of the day. Padding and folds of clothing account for most of the abdominal bulk. Some art experts believe that a small part of the swelling, however, may be the result of the couple's sexual activity prior to the ceremony. Such a practice, after all, is not solely a modern phenomenon.

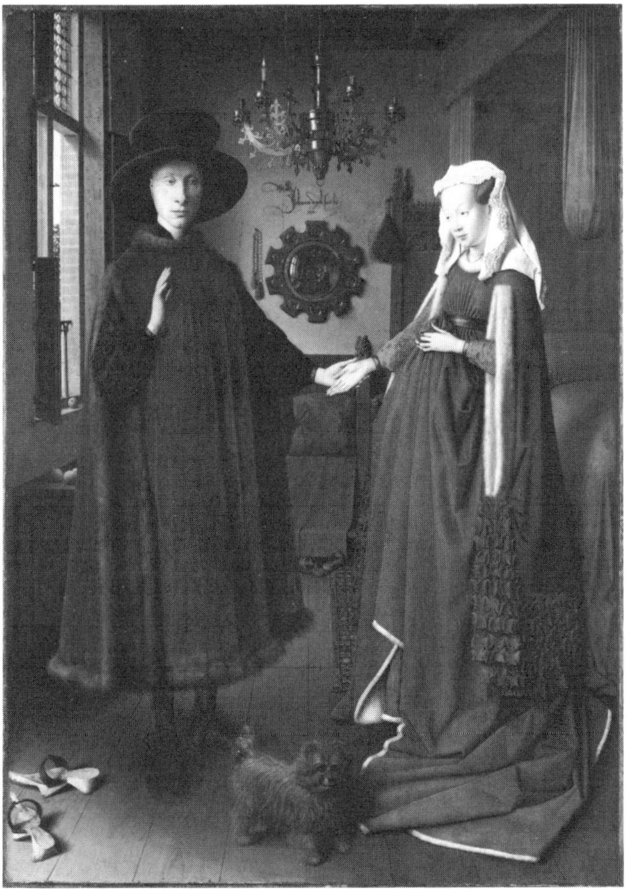

Jan Van Eyck. *Giovanni Arnolfini and His Wife*. 1434.

(National Gallery, London)

One needs not be an especially keen observer of the current scene to sense that female breasts are now particularly popular. This is true for both the natural and artificial varieties, though not with equal enthusiasm on the part of mammary-crazed males. A person might be surprised, though, to learn that breasts have not always been the focus of fascination in the western world. During the Elizabethan era, for instance, breasts were so out of style that women wore tight bodices to make the breasts seem nonexistent. Large hips, on the other hand, were the rage. As Papp and Kirkland wrote in *Shakespeare Alive*!:

> Indeed, the softer the body, the greater the beauty. Ivory skin, rosy cheeks, a round face, rounder hips, and yielding flesh were all requirements for the beautiful woman. Modern concepts of womanly beauty — thin and tan — would have struck a female Elizabethan fashion plate as very odd indeed.

If milady were slim-hipped — not to worry — she could add a few petticoats. This little subterfuge may have fooled the menfolk, but other women were not so easily deceived. All the practice did was force other women, even those who were already amply blessed by nature, to resort to wearing more petticoats themselves. Not to be outdone, the underblessed then reacted by wearing hip pads or wire hoops. Of course, the naturally padded beauties merely followed suit. This cycle progressed and eventually culminated in farthingales — a flat, oval-shaped structure that extended several feet laterally from each side of the wearer's waist. Variations of the farthingale, such as the moderate example of the pannier shown below, were popular in much of Europe from the 1500s to the end of the nineteenth century among the middle and upper classes. Such extremes in body proportions, of course, fooled no one but they were fashionable nonetheless.

A few decades later, breasts were back in fashion as objects of masculine appreciation and low-cut, push-up bodices were the style. Farthingales disappeared but, like all fashions, variations popped up periodically and, though it may at present seem quite unlikely, will probably appear again.

Buttocks, too, had their periods of prominence. With the appearance of the bustle, however, which reached its extreme size in the 1880s, the gals with gargantuan gluteals were in their glory. These magnificent structures — bustles, that is — consisted of padding or ingenious frames that sometimes extended rearward for more than two feet. Although bustles gave women a rather centaurian appearance, the effect was thought to be so sexy at the time that schoolmarms were not allowed to wear any that jutted out more than ten inches. The truth is, bustles do tend to accentuate the rather fetching side-to-side hip motion that is so characteristic of the female gender and which so rivets most astonishing fashion turnabouts, however, occurred in England in 1649. For a quarter of a century before that date, Charles I reigned according to the belief in his Divine Right, with the support of a privileged, frivolous minority of Cavaliers. Their haughtiness was mirrored in their luxuriously curled wigs and elegantly extravagant clothing.

The arrogance of Charles eventually severed him from power, as well as from his head. Oliver Cromwell and his Roundheads took over the country. They represented a large, industrious middle class, new ideas of power to the people, and puritanism. The latter was the key factor. No dancing was allowed, theaters were closed, and laughter was officially frowned upon. The statement, "A puritan is a person who lives in mortal anxiety that someone, somewhere, may be having a good time," captures their rigid spirit precisely.

Dark, drab, simple clothes with white accents were the style. This was an instance where beauty definitely was not an objective in determining fashion — displaying one's piety was. Paradoxically, while the celestial sphere is often ablaze with a dizzying variety of magnificent hues, black and white have been chosen in the Christian world as colors for the religious raiment of priests, nuns, and preachers.

The traditionally fun-loving English endured this grim state of affairs for eleven years before they coaxed Charles II to come out of exile and ascend the throne. As might be expected, with his return there was an immediate explosion of gaiety. Clothing styles were dazzling with an abundance of curls, puffs, ribbons, and feathers. To the delight of gallants, young and old, the high tight necklines on women's dresses plummeted to expose generous portions of conspicuously ripe bosoms.

Fashions can change quickly or slowly. Knee breeches, for instance, were the vogue for men for two hundred years from about 1600 to 1800. The twentieth century fashion scene, on the other hand, has been a unique roller coaster affair. Not only have styles changed often and quickly, many of them have been completely original. Most fascinating, though, has been the drastic change in the style of the female form itself as totally new standards of physical beauty have emerged. And body styles reflect cultural philosophies even more dramatically than clothing styles.

Before the early 1900's the fashion for women's bodies ranged from a bit fleshy to downright obese — according to today's standards. Yes, around 1830 Harriet Beecher Stowe complained, "Our willowy girls are afraid of nothing so much as growing stout . . . We in America have got so far out of the way of a womanhood that has any vigor of outline or opulence of physical proportions, that, when we see a woman made as a woman ought to be, she strikes us as a monster." But the willowy women Stowe was referring to was described by Lois Banner, author of *American Beauty* as, " . . . rounded and curved. Her shoulders slope; her arms are rounded; a small waist lies between a rounded bosom and a bell-shaped lower torso . . ."

At the same time much fleshier women were admired in Europe. That preference was soon readopted in America. More than appearance was considered. By the 1870s doctors were advising plumpness to improve the health of women and their personalities. Thin women were said by some neurologists to be invariably querulous and discontented.

Ten years later the epitome of feminine pulchritude was Lillian Russell. Known as "the American Beauty," she was hailed by one journalist of the 1880s as being, "fleshly arresting" with "all the undulations of the prima donna's figure moulded graciously in ripples that were so many sonnets of motion." What a wonderfully poetic way of saying she "jiggled."

Toward the end of her twenty-year reign of fame Miss Russell was forced to lose some weight due to the shifting of fashion. The women of the gay nineties still carried plenty of fat but their waists were torturously laced-in to accentuate their upper and lower attributes. The standard measurement of their hour-glass figures with corset in place was 36"-22"-40", but many women with ample upper and lower measurements were able to endure lacings that reduced their waist measurements to an agonizing eighteen inches.

The Gibson girl, created in 1890 by artist Charles Dana Gibson, for *Life* magazine became the most admired body type for more then a decade. It was considered a more athletic build, but it was a far-cry from "hard bodies" of today.

By 1902 the full figure was still admired even though the new corsets forced women's bodies into elegant, though uncomfortable "kangaroo bends." The low slung bosom was thrust forward, the flat abdomen slanted rearward, and the buttocks extended opulently to the rear — thereby accentuating both the bust and the buttocks. There is obviously nothing new about the "T and A" emphasis, so plaintively acknowledged in the popular 1970s musical *Chorus Line*. In fact, the standard figure in 1902 was 36-26-43 1/2.

Until the twentieth century thin was never "in." Far more than simply lacking in vitality and eroticism, thinness was sign of frailty or illness. As late as 1904, newspapers and magazines carried many articles on the dangers of being thin along with advertisements for products that helped people gain weight. The 1880 advertisement for Grover's Tasteless Chill Tonic, is funny today, but in its time it was not meant to be a joke. If the ad can be believed, the elixir was not a minor, fly-by-night product.

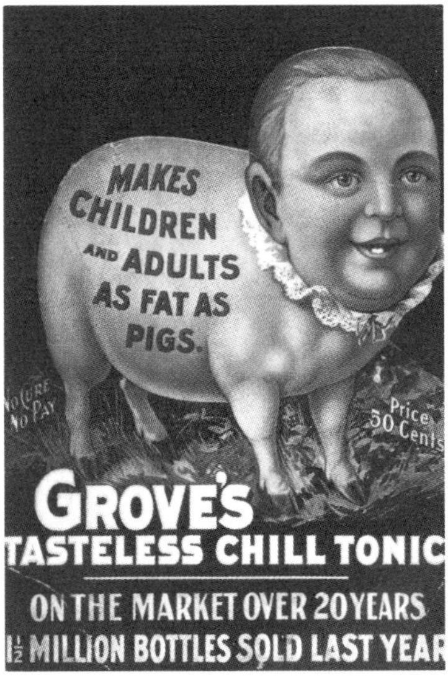

A young woman of those times was as ecstatic over gaining ten or twenty pounds as her modern counterpart is over losing a like amount. Infant's, too, were supposed to be fat. In the July, 1887 issue of *Godey's Ladies Book* there appeared a baby food ad that promised, "To the mother of any baby born this year, we will send on application a Cabinet Photo of the 'sweetest, fattest, healthiest baby in the country.' It is a beautiful picture, and will do any mother's heart good."

A review of magazines such as *Godey's*, *Vogue*, and the *Ladies' Home Journal* from about 1800 to 1903 shows that ads for losing weight were quite rare. Even up to 1950 there were very few articles dealing with weight reduction according to the *Readers' Guide to Periodic Literature* (an index of articles published in major magazines). Between 1937 and

1945 there were fewer than two per year! Compare that to todays's deluge.

There were even fewer antifat advertisements. Of course, "snake oil" for weight reduction occasionally bubbled to the surface because there have been some massively obese people in every era due to severe hormonal and neurological disorders.

It was in the second decade of the twentieth century that a drastic, mind-boggling change in the standard female form began to appear. A new sheath corset permitted a woman's *waist* to assume its normal girth but her *bust and hips* were now compressed with undergarments. The result was to give women a bosomless, hipless silhouette. This form was an historic first in the fashion realm, relative to both clothing and body shape. Thin women were finally in fashion and they reveled in their ascendance! The period has been called by some, the "revenge of the thin women."

A few years later the upper portion of the corset was shortened, but busts were still flattened with a tight brassiere-like undergarment. Fashionable women adopted a hollow-chested stance and managed to stand so their rear ends were flat also. The resulting body type seemed to be a repudiation of all that had previously passed for femininity.

A number of factors accounted for this rejection, but the political basis was a revolution that was taking place. The upheaval was not one of armed combat; it was a women's suffrage movement that had started before the turn of the century. By 1908 the movement had gathered considerable strength and was expanding into a more general concept of women's liberation. Apparently, to many women, throwing off the bonds of tradition included throwing off their traditional physical forms as well. If men could be bosomless and hipless, so could they.

At least this linearity was the style among women who put great stock in being fashionable. Unfortunately, the average women was unable to look linear, which is why pictures in fashion magazines of the day usually consisted of drawings instead of photographs.

The picture of the woman in the 1923 Coca-Cola ad, below, suggests that the more traditional female form was not completely unappreciated by middle America. And to quote Goodrum and

Dalrymple in *Advertising in America*:

> Coca-Cola associated its product with fashionable, beautiful women from the very start. The wholesome American look became so tied to the Coca-Cola women's image that scholars are still trying to decide whether the mid-century woman worked to look like the Coca-Cola girl, or the Coca-Cola image was simply the perfect reflection of the ideal "mid-American" woman.

Coinciding with the women's movement, stunning technological advances, such as the telephone, radio, electricity, movies, and automobiles, swept the nation. The inventions were no longer curiosities; many lay within reach of the masses. Flying machines even existed! The huge lighter-than-air Zeppelin airships had regularly scheduled runs in Europe. In America, "aeroplanes" were barnstorming all over the country leaving spectators shaking their heads in awe.

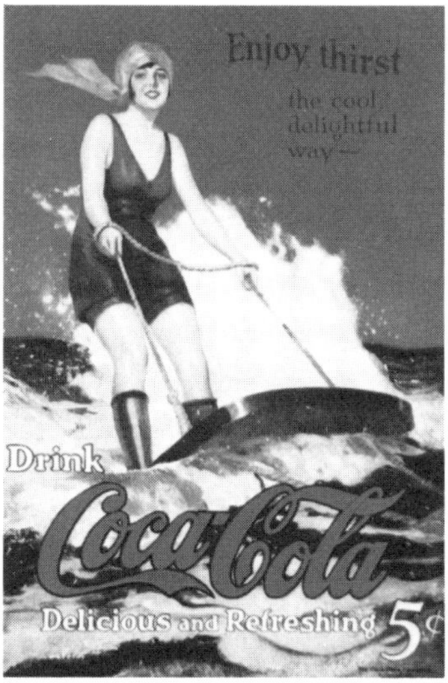

In more stable times it is very doubtful that the women's drive for rights and their new fashions would even have been envisioned — much less tolerated. As it was, some bills were introduced in state legislatures to regulate women's styles of dress. But "the times they were achangin'" in practically every aspect of the American culture. The prevailing attitude of "anything is possible" further stimulated the growth of innovative ideas and made acceptance of everything much easier, including women's rights.

Most of the major new inventions were the kind that made the nation, and the world, seem smaller. Happenings in one part of the country could be spread across the nation in hours through the cooperation of telegraph and newspapers. Motion pictures of events could be splashed, within days, across the immensely popular and ubiquitous cinema screens. It was easy for new ideas to rapidly sweep the nation, including fashions in women's clothes and women's body types.

In spite of the women's liberation movement and linear clothing fashions, the glorification of full-figured women persisted to a large degree until around 1920. Since that time, however, the general trend in women's fashions, both clothing styles and body types, has been one of increasing leanness and masculinization. Apparently women felt, and understandably so, that they had to look manly to be taken serious enough to be allowed by men to enter their world of work.

In the "roaring twenties" the boyish look was adopted. Short, bobbed hair was the fashion. Dresses were perfectly straight and unfitted with no suggestion of a waistline. They also ended above the knee which was yet another fashion first, and there would be many more to come. Some lawmakers again tried to regulate women's dress styles and again they failed. Women even adopted the bad habits of men. Many women took to smoking cigarettes, drinking booze, and "carrying on." I'm not sure what the latter means, but it sounds like fun — which means it's probably sinful. Since alcohol was illegal, women adopted the wrinkle of carrying flasks in the tops of their stockings. (This was before the "full body" search that today is practiced with such zeal by the nation's finest.)

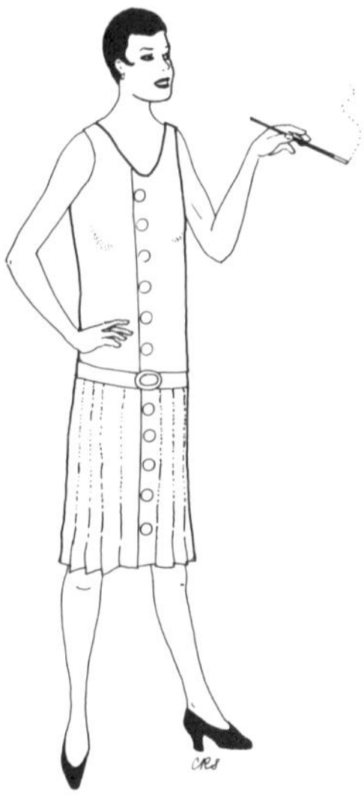
A 1920 fashion.

The excerpt below from a 1920 publication entitled *Equal Rights* compares the dress styles of 1848 to those of 1920. It clearly shows that the styles of dress reflected the thinking of females of the times, whereas previously the styles were more of a reflection of the male's thinking.

> The hoop-skirt, the small waist and the general impracticability of the clothes worn at the first Seneca convention interpret far more graphi-

> cally than words can phrase the position of women seventy-five years ago. The artificial helplessness, the wretched discomfort, the denial of nature, all are emblazoned in sartorial terms. The absolute dependence of woman upon man was blazoned forth in her clothes . . . The frailty and incompetence inherent in an eighteen-inch waist and a hoop-skirt stimulated the male ego to an unconscionable extent. It was not difficult to feel superior to that. Probably there was no more wholesome encouraging symptom of the times than is to be found in women's clothes. They indicate that women are no longer doomed to live on sex, that men are no longer such impossible egoists as they were, and they predict the girls of the future will enter life booted and spurred for the fray as they never have been before.

These were prophetic words. In the thirties the boyish look grew up. The thinness craze had moderated. Women began wearing slacks, culottes, and shorts. Tailored suits with padded shoulders also came into fashion.

During the forties, World War II was the dominant influence on clothing for women. Since women necessarily assumed traditionally masculine roles in industry, they also got used to wearing, and seeing other women wear, men's work uniforms. Today, blue jeans, once worn only by "working men," are as popular among women as they are among men. And even the most confirmed male chauvinist has to admit that females have given an entirely new dimension to the way jeans look on the human form. Actually, chauvinists might be the first to admit it.

The dates stated for the fashions described above are not precise for every region of the country. Some areas are traditionally more conservative than others and are slower to adopt new styles. In addition, throughout the entire nation there have been periodic shifts back to more "feminine" styles such as peasant blouses, long skirts, and crinolines. The fashion industry, naturally, is eager to encourage and create fashion fluctuations so they can sell more clothes, shoes, accessories, cosmetics, magazines, and whatever. Of course, there have also been fashion flashbacks relative to body types. Marilyn Monroe, in the fifties was a classic case of the reemergence of the "fuller" figure.

Ironically, it was shortly after 1950 that the "fat hit the fan." The real push to be thin began. And it continued with increasing fervor into the nineties, for reasons discussed in Chapter Eleven.

Overall, the shift of the fashionable female form since 1910 toward what has traditionally been masculine has been spiraling upward like the rate of inflation. This applies to behavior as well as to appearance. The use of what genteel folks would call coarse language is being used increasingly by women. Also, they are engaging in sports in ever greater numbers. Many of the activities are ones that were previously reserved solely for men, including such extremes as football, boxing, and serious amateur wrestling along with the more theatrical mud and professional wrestling. And to be completely objective and fair there is no reason why women should not have the right to engage in these or any other activities including military combat.

In the 1980s women successfully scaled one of the few remaining bastions of masculinity — bodybuilding. Legions of women are now avidly seeking "hard" bodies — eschewing shoulder pads for the real thing. The ultimate women bodybuilders, those most respected and idolized by their sister athletes, enter the fray of physique contests. To achieve success in that arena requires much more than pumping iron for several hours a day — no mean task in itself. Closely monitored nutritional programs must also be followed. Indeed, for many weeks preceding a contest, females (as well as male contestants) must literally starve themselves if they want to walk on stage with highly defined, "ripped" muscles. Not surprisingly, they have to apply make-up to cover the facial signs of exhaustion. Diane Rutkowski was quoted in *Women's Physique World* (Fall, 1991) as saying she didn't seem to have time for anything after bodybuilding since she devoted her time to lifting and aerobics, shopping for and preparing food, and practicing posing. This regimen is typical for serious contestants.

When a woman bodybuilder achieves a "contest level" body, what does she have? Even today, with the emphasis on health and fitness, most people do not know what to think about about her extreme muscularity. As the authors, Charles Gaines and George Butler, of the most revealing book on women's Bodybuilding, *Pumping Iron II: The Unprecedented*

Woman, wrote:

> Most of us, male or female, can appreciate a female body viscerally and visually as a female body only up to a certain point of modification; beyond that point, modification registers as distortion and we feel that we are looking at something disturbingly *other than* the original thing. This may be particularly true of the female body, loaded as it is with visual biological symbolism. Strip a woman's curves of its breasts and hips, of all its nurturing curves, and replace it with enough stringy, sinewy muscle, and a lot of people will simply not know what to make of what you have left. They may say it looks like a man; what they really mean is that, in no longer looking like a woman, it has become visually, existentially, strange: unknowable.

As revealed in, *Muscle: Confessions of an Unlikely Bodybuilder*, at least some female bodybuilders are aware that something strange is taking place in their bodies. The author, Samuel Fussell, in an eye-popping, inside look the sport, quotes a female bodybuilding friend as proudly proclaiming in a foghorn voice (and punctuated with the currently ubiquitous "F" word) that she had reversed the course of nature.

The above passages are merely brief views of the hard body look of today for females. None are meant to be a "put down" of women bodybuilding competitors. True, many people think today's ultimate in the hard body look for females is a bit too much. But what they think, or what I think, is totally irrelevant. These women are doing *their* thing. People have different priorities. Besides, it is difficult to have anything but respect for anyone who is so committed to achieving such a difficult personal objective. It is doubtful that anyone is as dedicated as the consistently highly ranked professional competitor, Bev Francis, the 1991 and 1992 runner-up in the Ms Olympia contest.

To increase their chances for winning bodybuilding contests, many women (and men) take anabolic steroids to help them build larger, stronger muscles. Now, that *is* bad; it's unethical as well as being very dangerous to health. Nearly all commercial anabolic steroids are artificial compounds, but, in essence, they are male hormones. More research needs to be done, but the preponderance of evidence shows that,

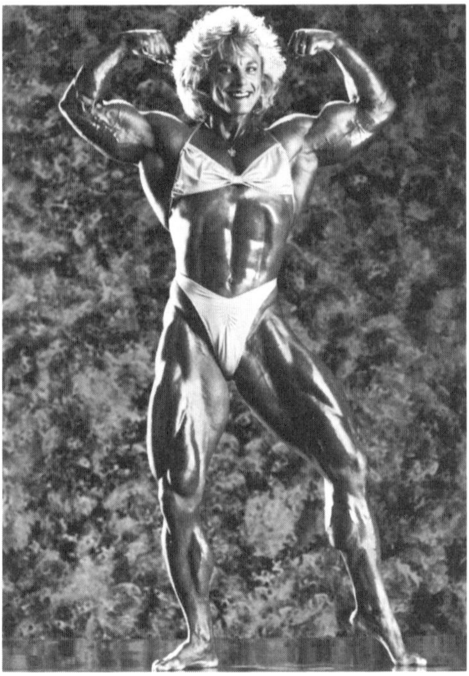

Bev Francis, The Ultimate "Hard Body"

although steroids can help to build muscles, long term use presents many serious dangers to a *male* user's health.

There is even less, far less, research regarding the taking of male hormones by *female*s, but many of the harmful physiological and psychological changes that occur in males are believed to also occur in females. Steroids clearly do have a masculinizing effect on females which can be permanent. Changes include a deepening of the voice, extremely combative behavior, acne, increased growth and coarseness of facial and body hair, male pattern baldness, reduction of the breasts, amenorrhea, shrinkage of the ovaries, enlargement of the clitoris, coarsening and yellowing of the skin, internal organ problems, and changes in the shape of the face and skull — such as a larger, more squared jaw due to increased collagen deposits. Collagen is the supportive protein found in skin, bone, and connective tissue.

An article in the largest selling bodybuilding magazine, *Muscle and Fitness* (December, 1988) entitled "Chemical Corner: Let's Stop Kidding Ourselves," gives a flesh and blood picture to the problem of anabolic steroid use by women. Its author, Sir Dominic Certo, a vice-president of the International Federation of Bodybuilders, described a 23 year-old woman who, in two years of steroid use, had the skin of a 35 year-old laborer, a baritone voice, and a five o'clock shadow. She had come to Certo in tears because of the changes that steroids had produced.

Tina Plakinger, 1982 Ms America winner (the top amateur women's body building contest in the world), took steroids and became increasingly concerned over their side effects. In an *American Health* (September '87) article entitled, "Steroids: The Rambo Drug," she told of her thoughts before the 1986 Ms Olympia contest, the top professional competition. After giving herself an injection with a two-inch needle, she looked in a mirror and was extremely unhappy with her bloated, "zit covered" body. The change in her behavior, though, was most disturbing because she had gone from being a sweet, gentle person to a "raging bull." Although she stopped taking the drug at that point, her marriage had already been a victim of her steroid use.

Logic cries out that male hormones must have powerfully adverse effects on the functions of the female body. It is already well-established that when females take *female* hormones they are exposing themselves to a long list of risks. Some are severe to the extent of being fatal. For confirmation one merely has to refer to the *Physician's Desk Reference* (PDR) which is available at any library.

The promoters of most bodybuilding contests claim their contestants are drug-free because they are tested for steroid use. But savvy contestants know it is easy to avoid detection — by "cycling down" and using masking drugs. Only the "dumbies" are caught. One of the more ingenious tricks involves urinating just before a steroid test and then refilling the bladder with "clean" urine (with a catheter). Another method is to conceal in the crotch a rubber bulb (and thin tube) filled with clean urine. A sneaky squeeze at the appropriate time and the bulbist is home-free. Also, the ingestion of sugar and carbohydrate supplements in appropriate amounts has a 98% masking effect on steroids.

The former Duchess of Windsor, Wallis Simpson, spoke for a lot of women when she reputedly stated, "You can't be too rich or too thin." Of course, even without the taking of male hormones, when fat is lost from the body it also disappears from the breasts, too, since a large proportion of the breasts consists of fat tissue. In other words, it is unrealistic to want a hard body and expect to retain discernible breasts as well.

Apparently, most women desperately do want Venus's pectoral twins, however, and they have found a way to "have their cake and eat it, too." More breast augmentation surgery is now being performed than ever before. Next to liposuction it is the most common type of cosmetic surgery and the procedure is expected to rise sharply in the '90s.

Measures for achieving more attractive breasts, which usually means larger, are not a recent phenomenon. Attempts have probably been around since time immemorial. In the late nineteenth century the advertising for a patent medicine, named Peruna, suggested that its chief effect was to enlarge the bust. The alcohol content of the drink was about nineteen percent. That's 38 proof! It could be that after a few healthy swigs, a woman just thought her breasts were larger. I never read the directions; maybe she was supposed to slip the stuff to a man she wished to impress.

To ladies who wanted a more rapid response, an advertisement by Nature's Rival Company (*Woman's Home Companion*, September, 1908) asks:

> ARE YOU TOO THIN?
> Does your form lack normal development, wholly or partly? You can display a perfect figure, showing the natural, well-rounded bust form of a beautifully developed woman, by using Nature's Rival, an AIR FORM CORSET WAIST inflated to any desired size — a perfect bust.

The ad, below, from the 1902 Sears, Roebuck catalog features a suction cup device with a "positive guarantee." Alas, in spite of the guarantee, it did not do what it promised — but at least it would appear

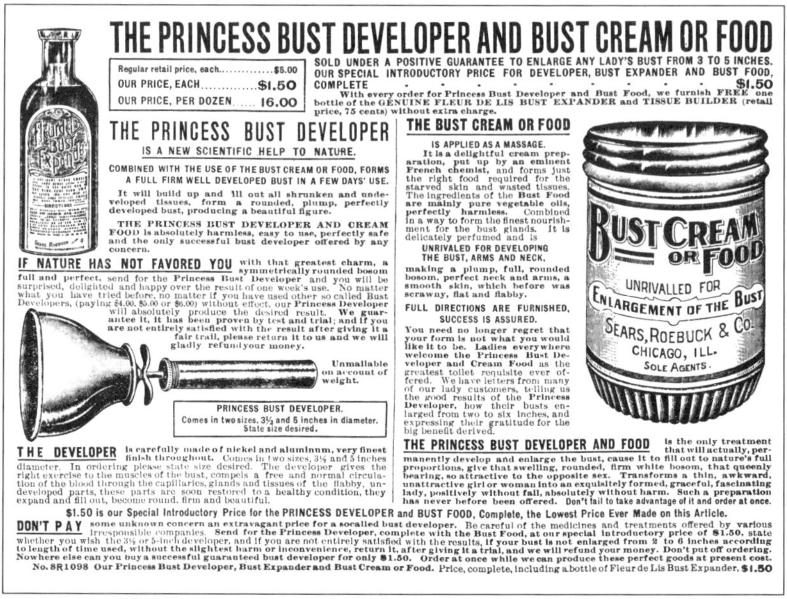

A 1902 "Bust Developer."

(From the 1902 Edition of *The Sears Roebuck Catalog*).

to have had some recreational potential.

For readers who may feel that consumers must have been incredibly gullible in those presumably more innocent days, it must be added that these suction cup and "breast food" scams have been periodically resurrected to harvest a new crop of suckers. The modern gunk does not work any better than the 1902 Sears product. It is not unusual to see several "breast Creme" ads on a single page of a modern women's magazine.

Incidentally, should males look condescendingly at the the breast suction device, it might be added that there are similar devices for penis enlargement — with somewhat different shape and dimensions, of course. They do not produce positive results either. That's obvious since there haven't been any riots in stores that sell them.

Of course, the breast enlargers have "European" entries. The ads for one announces, "Change from flat to FABULOUS! . . . Your search is over! . . . "NO phony exercises . . . NO painful surgery . . . No costly hormone creams." And it offers a "raw glandular concentrate." Unfortunately, its foreign pedigree does not make it any more effective than domestic offerings.

As far as names are concerned, my favorite product is Mammrae-900™. Its marketing people were obviously striving for a "classy" approach! Promising that "FULL, ROUND, EYE-CATCHING BREASTS WILL MAKE YOU PROUD!" the ad revealed a three-step application that involved "vigorous massage" and holding a hot water-soaked towel firmly against the breasts. I don't know if the model would catch the eye of a typical woman, but I was rather impressed. The displayed procedure, even without the product, will result in a temporary swelling of the skin due to an increase in blood flow, but a woman certainly should not build her hopes on the ad's promise that "the entire breast EXPANDS to magnificent proportions right before your eyes . . . According to one testimonial, one "proud" user even got larger nipples — to her "delight."

At the risk of breaking many a heart it must be added that not even the much advertised Mark Eden Bust Developer will increase the size of breasts, no matter how much a woman uses the exercise device. If pectoral exercises stimulated the growth of breast tissue, female body builders would have massive breasts. As it is, the opposite extreme is the case — unless they have breast implants.

Lest the last phrase be construed as encouragement to dash off to a cosmetic surgeon, consider the following. In many of the operations there is subsequent hardening of scar tissue around the silicone gel implants. The "exciting" part occurs when the doctor has to lean on the lumps with his full weight to reduce their size with his hands. In other cases, the breasts have to be reopened and the implants removed. Silicone gel leakage is linked with infections, inflammation of the joints, and toxic shock syndrome. According to the FDA, leakage may cause the body's immune system to make antibodies that attack a woman's own healthy tissue. That's not good.

An alternative is the saline (salt water) implants, although they do not feel as natural as the silicone variety and tend to make sloshing sounds. Saline implants are much safer when they leak but, unfortunately, they are much more likely to leak — which could be a deflating experience, especially should it occur during an intimate moment.

Any surgery to the breast can result in a loss of erotic feeling in the nipple; that has to be a "downer." It is minor, though, when compared to the fact that implants interfere with the X-ray detection of breast cancer.

About 80 percent of the implants are for cosmetic purposes — as necessary as lipstick. A friend recently told me his wife had breast implants because,"she could not resist the two-for-one coupon." That was meant to be an amusing comment — I think — but the fact that she had the procedure done should not be taken so lightly. The FDA, in fact, early in 1992 issued a moratorium against the silicone gel implants due to evidence of associated disorders. Later the FDA permitted the device to be worn by breast cancer victims, but there are severe restrictions for other women desiring them. The silicone implants had not been scutinized by the FDA for nearly thirty years; when they came on the market in 1963 they did not need government approval to be legally sold. Now there are just too many reports of serious problems for them to be overlooked. Many critics are lobbying for a permanent ban on silicone implants and, of course, powerful (that means, wealthy) forces are lobbying for legalization of the devices. In the meantime, all the one to two million women with implants can do is cross their fingers.

The risks to obtain larger breasts are generally quite unnecessary. Except for those who have had mastectomies, most women who want larger breasts merely have to allow their body fat to increase — usually to the *individual's* natural level. Stringent dieting to attain and maintain a fashionably thin body is hardly natural. Yes, some women are destined to have small breasts no matter how much weight they gain. So? As with fatness, breast size has nothing to do with a woman's femininity, sexuality, intelligence, or value as a person. Hopefully, women with small breasts would think enough of themselves to reject the idea of breast surgery. But don't hold your breath until that occurs. There is too much money to be made by trying to mold women into impossible standards.

Clearly, the standard of female beauty relative to body type has made a complete turnabout in the past seventy years. It is not that the structure and function of women's bodies has changed during this brief period of time; evolution does not work that fast. The modern "ideal" body type that our culture has adopted is based upon a historically unique set of philosophical, social, and technological factors—not upon genetics.

The luxuriously curvaceous bodies with bulging bosoms and prodigious derriéres that were highly admired as late as the second decade of this century, were replaced on center stage within just a few years by thin, angular bodies. At present, the muscular, low-fat body is the "in" fashion. Which body type is the most beautiful? It is, of course, impossible to say since there are no fixed, absolute standards. What is beautiful depends upon the era, and even within each era there is a wide variety of individual preferences that are in contrast with the majority view.

There were surely men in the 1880s and 1890s who in opposition to prevailing opinions thought thin girls had the most attractive bodies. Just as certainly, there are men today who feel that plump women are the most desirable. In fact, there are men who state on network television shows, such the Phil Donahue Show, and in magazines that they find fat women (400 pounds or more!) most appealing. Whether they are referring to beauty or an innate attraction is not clear, and the difference may not be important anyway. But when considering the innate aspect of attractiveness and the learned concept of beauty, perhaps the adage, "Thin is in — but fat is where it's at," has some basis in fact.

There is massive contradiction in the fact that today's idea of a beautiful and *healthy* female body requires a woman to devote practically her entire existence to exhaustive hours of physical labor, periodic starvation, dangerous exposure to skin damaging sun or ultra-violet lamps, and the taking of various drugs including male hormones. Indeed, in *Muscle: Confessions of an Unlikely Bodybuilder*, it is brought out that competitive bodybuilding has nothing to do with health; the activity "is about *looking* good, not *feeling* good."

The hard body concept of a beautiful, healthy woman can hardly be considered normal or natural, and brings to mind a statement written by

Mary Wood-Allen in 1905 in her widely read book entitled, *What a Young Woman Ought to Know*. Her comment was in reference to the corsets of the time but it is no less applicable today.

> The reason we admire the tapering waist is because we have been wrongly educated. We have acquired wrong ideas of beauty. We have accepted the ideals of the fashion-plate rather than those of the Creator.

In 1987 this statement was recently echoed by Dr. Susan C. Wooley, Co-director, Eating Disorder Clinic, Psychiatry Dept., University of Cincinnati Medical College. She said, "The time has arrived for women to take a hard look at the mania for thinness that is so prevalent in this country and to reclaim their right to an authentically female body."

It is ironic that when today's women finally achieve hard bodies, they often have to hire a surgeon to tack on a pair of breasts. It would not be surprising if fashion eventually dictates the implanting of three or more of the silicone pads — just as earrings are now commonly worn in multiple groupings. Maybe some women will select several sizes just for variety. Some might even have two or three pairs implanted on their chest and maybe a pair on their backs — circumstances that offer some intriguing scenarios.

The discussion above is not meant to imply that bony, angular, or hard female bodies are necessarily lacking in beauty. There is no reason why these body types should not be accepted and appreciated — for women who are genetically able to develop them. But to expect all women to conform to the "hard body" look is unreasonable to the extent of being asinine.

It is an irony of monumental proportions that most of our society now consider lush, naturally padded women to be abnormal and unnatural — and even ugly and unhealthy. Now, that *is* difficult to accept! What is infinitely more disturbing is that the constant condemnation and harassment by FATISTS, even though their methods are sometimes subtle, has coerced multitudes of "fat" women into feeling guilty, unattractive, unsexy, immoral, and lacking in worth in general.

These negative feelings are totally irrational since most of these so-called fat women are not *excessively* fat!

With such depreciation society loses, also. Anytime it allows the disparagement of a group of people for whatever reason — religion, nationality, color, age, sex, or fatness — a society as a whole is itself reduced. Further, when any such group is injured — emotionally, physically, or economically — a society is guilty of a highly significant crime. And, by diminishing itself in the moral sense, society diminishes the quality of life for *every* individual residing within it—even the bigots.

From the standpoint of esthetics, finding delight in only one female body type makes as much sense as appreciating only one type of voice, personality, painting, music, or food. Diversity in a culture is enriching. It is a blessing. After all, variety is the spice of life. And *acceptance* is the greatest virtue.

How exciting it would be to live in a society peopled by beings who range in size from dwarfs to giants and whose skin varies in color from alabaster to ebony, with all colors of hair in textures ranging from straight to kinky; with noses varying from long and pointy to wide and flattened; with a wide range of clothing fashions, with a variety of distinct subcultures — and, yes, with people who range from very thin to very fat. How wonderful that would be. And that is precisely the situation that exists in America. We just have to learn to see the beauty in each group. When that time arrives, there will be no thought of belittling those who do not fit a narrow standard. The acceptance and appreciation, of the diverse appearance of others—and of oneself—will be *the* fashion. That really will be beautiful!

5

THE GOODNESS OF FAT

Fat has always been a subject of considerable interest when its distribution on the female form is under scrutiny. When studied merely as a substance, fat is even more fascinating. Okay, that's a matter of opinion. It is true, however, that fat is considered to be a villain by most people in our culture — and villains are always fascinating. For instance, there are many times more books, movies, and television shows dealing with Adolf Hitler than with his democratic counterpart, Franklin Roosevelt.

Fat has become the Nazi equivalent in the world of nutrition and body composition. At any given time, practically every magazine on the stands has at least one article on the "evil" nature of fat. Every form of media, broadcast and print, is peppered with commercials for products that promise to get rid of "that ugly, horrible stuff" on our bodies.

If indeed fat is so harmful, doesn't it make sense to know a bit about your "enemy?" And if perchance it is *not* a villain, that too would be nice to know, wouldn't it? Well, you're going to learn a lot about fat in this chapter. Perhaps more than you care to know. The main idea is that fat is not all bad — not by a long shot. To begin, it is a marvelous source of energy. That energy is necessary for all of our cells to do "their thing." Without energy our bodies come to a standstill; we die.

Although fat is our main source of energy, that fact alone does not even begin to do justice to the complicated ways in which our bodies produce energy. ATP (adenosine triphosphate) is the *immediate* source of energy in our bodies. In fact, it is the immediate source of energy in all living cells of every animal and every plant — "from cabbages to Kings." When the ATP in cells breaks down, energy is released and used by the cells to stay alive and to carry out their functions.

There is only enough ATP in our bodies, however, to keep us going for a few minutes, at most, before it is completely used up. This is where the fat and carbohydrates in our bodies become invaluable. Each of these foodstuffs combine with oxygen to produce energy, a process called metabolism. That energy is used to rebuild the broken down ATP molecules. In other words, the manufacture of ATP is a continual recycling process. The waste products of metabolism, ultimately, are carbon dioxide and water — which are passed from the body every time a person exhales.

Much of our energy comes from the breakdown of carbohydrates. Foods rich in carbohydrates are grains, vegetables, fruits, milk, and concentrated sweets such as candy and soft drinks. Consumed carbohydrates are broken down into a very simple sugar called glucose. Glucose enters the blood stream and is carried to our muscles and other cells. Some of the glucose that enters cells is immediately used to rebuild ATP while some is stored in the cells (particularly muscle fibers) in a concentrated form, called glycogen, for later use. About half a pound of glycogen can also be stored in the liver of an average-sized man; proportionately less is stored in an average-sized woman.

When a muscle cell, or any other cell, uses up its glycogen, the liver converts some its stored glycogen back to glucose and sends it by way of the bloodstream to the muscle cell. This is a very fine arrangement except for one thing. Only about 454 grams (one pound) of glucose can be stored in the entire body. Since each gram of glucose provides approximately 4 calories (C.), a person has a total store of about 1800 calories. This is enough to sustain the average man for about thirteen hours. Because a woman typically has a lower metabolic rate, she could be expected to endure for about twenty-two hours. That time is reduced, though, because she has a smaller storage of glycogen.

Our body's sugar stores are enough to keep us alive until the next meal, and even overnight, but they certainly were not enough to sustain our early ancestors for long periods of unsuccessful hunting or food gathering. And there are plenty of people in the world today, including the United States of America, who have periodic lean times during which their sugar reserves will not meet their energy needs. This circumstance is especially disturbing since glucose is the *sole* source of energy for nearly all of the cells in the nervous system, including brain cells.

If the body did not have another readily available energy source, upon depletion of its sugar stores it would have to break down its protein into amino acids to produce more glucose for energy. Proteins can provide about 4 calories per gram but only a few types of amino acids are capable of being converted into glucose. The remaining amino acids are filtered from the blood by the kidneys and passed from the body in the urine. Because amino acid molecules are rather large, they tend to damage the delicate filter system in the kidneys.

Besides being very wasteful and inefficient, when the body uses protein for energy it does so by consuming its own muscle tissue. This self-cannibalism not only includes skeletal muscles but structural protein in the various organs, such as those of the circulatory, respiratory, reproductive, and digestive systems. Certainly, protein is not a desirable source of energy from the standpoint of health.

This is where fat comes charging to the rescue. Yes, fat is a biological hero, though not ostentatiously like muscles; fat is far more modest and unassuming. Because our bodies are able to store large quantities of fat and then use it for energy, our protein is spared. If our ancestors had not had the capacity to store fat, humans (as well as most other animal species) would have been extinct a long time ago.

Though it may not seem very significant at first thought, a gram of fat provides about 2.25 times as much energy as a gram of carbohydrate. It's difficult to be precise because the results of research vary a bit. Usually the energy figures are reported as 9.0 C. for fat and 4.0 C. for carbohydrates. Based upon this 2.25 times difference, it seems logical to assume that fat storage would only take up about 45% as much space as a glycogen deposit of equal potential energy. But fat is even more economical in terms of space because its constituent parts are more flexible than the rigid glycogen structure and can be squeezed into a more compact space.

Also, fat does not attract water — as does glycogen. For each gram of stored glycogen there will be three to four grams of water accompanying it. When the weight of this water is taken into account, fat deposits provide about *nine* times as much energy, gram for gram, as do glycogen stores. To give more meaning to this figure, consider a 120 lb. woman who has a basic weight of 90 lb. — plus 30 lb. of fat. This means 25%

of her body consists of fat which is nearly average for women in their early twenties in the U.S. If all of this energy were stored as glycogen instead of fat, the woman's sugar deposits (plus its associated water) would weigh 9 x 30 lb, or 270 lb. In other words that 120 lb woman would weigh 270 + 90 or 360 pounds! So, people who complain about being fat should be very thankful their energy is stored in the form of this golden liquid instead of as sugar.

Where does the stored fat in our bodies come from? From the food we eat, naturally, and not only from dietary fats but from carbohydrates and protein as well. If we eat more of either of the latter two than is needed to produce energy or build tissue, the liver converts the excess to fat. The body also throws off some of the excess sugar and protein (amino acids) in the urine — a process known among more earthy members of the nutritional community as "pissing away good food." And another four-letter word rears its ugly head.

All of the meat we eat contains some fat, and many of the plants do also, particularly nuts and seeds. None of the many kinds of fat are identical to the kind we have in our bodies, but they are similar. All of these fats, including ours, are called *triglycerides* since each of their molecules consists of three fatty acids that are attached to a single glycerol (glycerine) molecule. Triglycerides are also called neutral fat, yellow fat, or just plain fat.

Ingested fat is emulsified in the small intestine by a liver secretion called bile. The tiny droplets of fat, called chylomicrons, then enter the bloodstream (via the lymphatic system). If fat were to remain in this form, it would coalesce into large, deadly clumps of fat. Fortunately, the chylomicrons break down into glycerol and fatty acids. Some of the glycerol is used for energy in much the same way as glucose. The fatty acids, however, are immediately surrounded by a layer consisting of protein and cholesterol. These minuscule packages of fat and protein are called lipoproteins.

The lipoproteins are carried in the bloodstream to the "working" cells of the body such as nerve, muscle, and bone cells. Once inside the cells, some of the fatty acids immediately combine with oxygen to provide energy while others are stored for later use. The production of energy actually occurs inside elongated structures called mitochondria.

After the working cells are filled, the lipoproteins head for the adipose tissue. There they temporarily accumulate on the walls of the blood vessels while the remaining fatty acids (with the help of the enzyme lipoprotein lipase) are transferred to the interior of fat cells. Scientists, with their knack for fancy names, call these cells "adipocytes." Inside the adipocytes, the fatty acids are recombined with glycerol to form triglycerides.

An empty fat cell consists solely of living tissue and has an irregular-shape with many thin projections emanating from its main body. When droplets of fat enter the cell, it begins to expand. Eventually the droplets coalesce and stretch the living part of the cell into a thin layer that completely surrounds a drop of fat. When the cells are full of fat, they are usually yellowish in color and roughly spherical in shape — unless squeezed tightly together. Fat cells are among the largest cells in the body and according to one's genetics, the cells under the skin and in some parts of the body are larger than those in other parts.

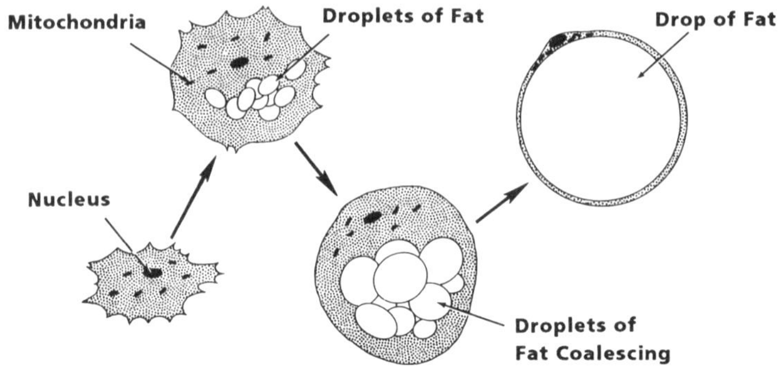

The Development of a Fat Cell (cross-sectional views)

Some fat is brownish in color and is, therefore, called brown adipose tissue (BAT). It is stored in cells that are smaller than those of yellow fat. Newborn babies have a lot of brown fat. Since BAT has a very high metabolic rate, it burns large amounts of calories and produces a lot of heat. This is beneficial to an infant since heat is generated at a time when the baby's temperature control system is not well-developed. Adults have relatively small amounts of BAT although the amount varies between individuals.

When the level of glucose in the blood decreases, the fat in adipose cells breaks down to glycerol and fatty acids. The fatty acids pass into the bloodstream and are carried to the body's working cells for energy. Some of the glycerol follows the same path, but most of it stays in the fat cells and is used there for energy.

Although the average number of fat cells in the body is about 30 billion, the number varies tremendously between individuals. At one time it was believed that the total number of fat cells adults had was determined mainly by how fat they were *before* birth — along with how fat they became during their first year. That is, as infants got fatter, more fat cells were created to hold the fat. This obviously would affect their potential for fatness during adulthood. Later research showed early adolescence to be another significant age for increasing the number of fat cells. For women, pregnancy is another time when fat cells tend to proliferate.

The latest evidence reveals that the number of fat cells can actually increase at any period in a person's entire life. When all of the body's existing fat cells fill to a certain critical level with fat (about 85%), new cells are created. Although the number of fat cells never decrease, they may get smaller in size.

Most of the fat cells are enmeshed in loose connective tissue. This tissue, as the name implies, is a loose, random weave of several kinds of fibers. It's the most widespread tissue in the body and serves to hold the various parts of the body together into one functional unit. The loose connective tissue, with its trapped fat cells, blood vessels, and nerves is called *adipose tissue.*

Adipose tissue is not evenly distributed over a person's body. The pattern depends upon a person's heredity and the activity level of lipoprotein lipase in the different areas of the body. Most women, for instance, store fat primarily on their thighs, hips, and buttocks because their lipoprotein lipase is about five times more active in those areas.

Men, on the other hand, tend to store fat primarily on and inside the abdomen—particularly on the front and sides. Even within each gender, though, there is much variation.

Probably the most distinctive example of adipose distribution is seen in the Hottentot and Bushmen tribes of Southern Africa. The women store their fat almost exclusively on their buttocks. While their upper bodies and legs remain slender, their rear-ends can swell to extraordinary proportions. They do not bemoan that propensity, however, since the men of the tribe find the characteristic quite attractive. In fact, that's probably the reason the characteristic evolved in the first place.

Hereditary fat patterns do not mean that each fat cell is destined to remain permanently in one place. On the contrary, the cells slowly move about, but the proportion of total body fat stays the same in any part of the body (for each individual). Fat cells are also active in the sense that their contents are constantly being used for energy and are constantly being replaced. Not all of the fat molecules stored in your body today are the same ones that were there yesterday.

Some regions of the body do not contain fat. They include the skin of the eyelids, the penis and scrotum, and the labia minor of the female vulva. Internally, there is no fat in or on the lungs or within the skull. So, while it may be difficult to believe, the term "fat head" really has no basis in fact — no literal basis.

There is generally a lot of loose connective tissue under the skin. It contains variable amounts of fat, called subcutaneous fat. Because fat is a poor conductor of heat, the subcutaneous layer serves as insulation to reduce the loss of valuable body heat. It helps to keep us warm, which comes in handy since we do not have enough body hair to do the job. If it were not for that fat, we would have to bundle up when the air temperature dipped into the seventies. Since fat is such an effective insulator, a fat person can survive many times longer in cold weather than a thin person. That is why long distance swimmers fatten-up for a race. Besides helping to prevent the loss of body heat, the blanket of fat provides a swimmer with a large amount of energy. Fat also makes a swimmer more buoyant so he or she can swim more efficiently.

Subcutaneous fat also cushions blows. Skin and muscles are highly vascularized, damage to them would rupture underlying vessels. Adipose tissue, on the other hand, has relatively few blood vessels. Since fat is liquid at body temperature, a force applied at any point of adipose tissue is spread over a larger area, thereby reducing the pressure of contact. The palms of the hands and the soles of the feet also have fatty pads that serve as shock absorbers.

Due to their higher levels of female hormones, women tend to have a thicker layer of subcutaneous fat. It softens their contours in a most delightful way and, of course, the extra thick pads of fat that accumulate in the breasts, buttocks, hips, and thighs are not without their own special allure to most members of the opposite sex. Blood capillaries in females, compared to those in males, have thinner, more delicate walls which is why women tend to bruise more easily. Therefore, their thicker layer of subcutaneous fat is especially valuable as protection.

In both men and women there are also pads of fat near, and even at, the skeletal joints. Since adipose tissue is capable of assuming any shape within wide limits when under pressure, it serves to facilitate joint movements.

Our skin also has a very thin layer of fat (oil) on its *outer* surface. Each hair follicle (cavity) on our bodies has a sebaceous oil gland associated with it, and every time a hair moves a bit of oil is squeezed from the gland. Of course if the hair is shaved off or plucked completely out of its follicles, as some of the new devices do, not much oil can subsequently be squeezed out.

Sebaceous oil, which is somewhat anti-bacterial, serves to waterproof the hair. The fatty substance also coats the skin and keeps it soft and pliable — and nice to touch. The oil is a natural "moisturizer." The only reason many people have to slather on so many commercial moisturizers is because they remove the body hair, and take too many baths and showers with oil-dispersing soaps. The daily cleansings also slaughter the beneficial bacteria on our skin.

The natural layer of "skin oil" was especially useful to our early ancestors. By making their skin slippery, it allowed them to escape the clutches of an enemy — which, of course, is lucky for us, too, or we would not be here today. The oily surface also reduced the effect of blows by causing them to slip sideways, and if a blow did land squarely, the "moist" skin would not tear nearly as easily as dry skin. The last two factors help explain why boxers have petroleum jelly smeared on their faces, particularly around the eyes, where ridges of bone lie closely under the surface. The protective aspects of the surface fat is not only beneficial to pugilists, it greatly reduces the chances of skin tearing every time a person bumps or rubs against something. The surface fat, by the way, does not turn rancid, nor is it so anti-bacterial that it completely eliminates the beneficial bacteria on our skin.

Adipose tissue is not located only beneath our skin. About half of it is distributed throughout the interior of our bodies. Our organs are held in place by various kinds of tissue, but adipose tissue on and between most of the organs acts as a firm and resilient packing and keeps the organs from bouncing about excessively. Fat also acts as lubrication where organs and tissues rub against each other, as they are almost constantly doing.

Much of the internal adipose tissue is located in the abdomen, particularly in a doublefold of tissue that hangs like an apron from the stomach and upper part of the large intestine. Called the greater omentum, this fatty apron lies between the abdominal organs and the muscular front wall, and extends nearly to the pubic region. This structure helps to cushion the abdominal organs from blows to the front of the abdomen.

Kidneys are especially well-padded by adipose tissue. This is advantageous since there isn't much muscle tissue between the kidneys and the outside of the body. Any person who has ever been struck in the lower back will immediately appreciate the benefits of fat in that area. It does not offer perfect protection but it's a lot better than nothing. The adipose tissue also keeps the kidneys in place. When a person gets very thin, this fat padding also gets thin and allows the kidneys to shift about. The "floating kidneys" can cause the tube (ureter) that carries urine from a kidney to the bladder to become kinked. When this happens, urine "backs up" and the kidney becomes infected. These organs, incidentally, should be treated with respect. About 20,000,000 Americans suffered from kidney diseases in 1990 and about 80,000 died from them. The healthiest display of respect for your kidneys would be to drink a toast to them with a glass of water at least six to eight times a day, or more — depending upon a person's sex, environment, size, and activity level.

Another pad of adipose tissue is located directly behind each eyeball. The function of the pads is to serve as shock absorbers to those delicate jewels that give us so much information and pleasure. Besides, when the fat pads are reduced, as in morbidly thin people, the eyeballs sink rather deeply into their sockets and all the eye-make-up in the world is not going to eliminate the haunted, cadaverous look that results.

The term "lipid" is often used interchangeably with "fat," but they are not synonymous. It is true that the neutral fat (triglycerides) discussed so far is a kind of lipid — and the other kinds of lipids do have physical properties similar to fat in that they are greasy to the touch and will not dissolve in water. Other lipids, however, do not have fatty acids and glycerol in their chemical formulae.

In addition to the neutral fat, which makes-up about 95% of the fat in our bodies, the other major lipids are the phospholipids and steroids. These are even more important than the neutral fat. Phospholipids, for instance, are yellowish, greasy solids that play a vital part of the structure of cell membranes. These "skins" surround each cell, and inside the cells other membranes surround such structures as the nuclei.

Although membranes are not identical, about 40% of all membranes consist of phospholipids. The fattiness of the membranes is highly desirable since lipids will not dissolve in water. Since every living cell in our bodies is surrounded by a thin layer of water, it would be disastrous if the cell membranes *were* soluble in water. Without the membranes the protoplasm in our cells would all intermix and our bodies would resemble, and be as useful as, giant globs of jelly on the floor. Some people may claim that is a good description of at least one of their in-laws, but in most cases they are probably exaggerating.

One of the myriad hazards of cigarette smoke is that it contains molecules that interact with the fat portions of the cell membranes. The damage that is inflicted can result in lung cancer and other kinds of cancer.

In addition to its role in the structure of membranes, phospholipids have other functions. Some are essential components of blood plasma and nerve fibers. Another phospholipid, called lecithin, is a key ingredient in bile.

Other types of lipids are called steroids. Cholesterol is the one people have heard most about. Although technically a kind of alcohol, its central structure does consist of particles that come from broken down molecules of fatty acids. This structure gives cholesterol the pearly look and oily feel that resembles fat.

People can get cholesterol in their bodies by eating foods that contain cholesterol, such as egg yolks, butter, cheese, and red meats. A person's liver stores a bit of the cholesterol, but normally the large majority of it is secreted in the bile. This bitter, yellowish-brown juice is stored in the gall bladder and after a meal that contains fat, the bile is squirted into the small intestine to emulsify the fat. The remainder of the cholesterol is sent via the blood to all the cells in the body.

Even if you were on a 100% cholesterol-free diet, you would still have enough to meet your needs. Typically, about 75% of the body's cholesterol is manufactured by its own cells, including those that line the walls of arteries. They do so mainly by using some of the particles from fatty acids, but they can also make cholesterol from the broken down products of carbohydrates and proteins.

The liver is the main producer of cholesterol. As might be expected, when more cholesterol is ingested, the body makes less — and when less is ingested, the body makes more. If the level of cholesterol gets too high in the body, the liver even excretes some. For this reason, *dietary* cholesterol levels are not nearly as important in the control of *blood* cholesterol as most people are led to believe. The real villain is saturated fat in the diet.

In addition to chemical similarities, cholesterol also has many functions in common with the phospholipids. For instance, cholesterol is found in the membrane of every cell in the body. In red blood cells about 25% of the membrane (dry weight) consists of cholesterol. It is also a primary component of the myelin sheaths found on nerve cells. These sheaths serve to increase greatly the speed of nerve impulses.

Cholesterol also settles into spaces in the outer layer of skin which helps to prevent many harmful chemicals from penetrating the skin. The oily sediment is especially important since it also provides a barrier to the loss of water. Because the skin is essentially watertight, a body loses only about a pint and a half of water through it each day. If it were not watertight, it would lose about thirty pints through evaporation! Since about 70% of the weight of a healthy body consists of water, its easy to see that a person would not want to lose very much of it. In addition, some of the cholesterol in the skin is used as an ingredient in the manufacture of Vitamin D.

Sex hormones, both male and female, are also steroids. As are several other hormones, sex hormones are formed from cholesterol. Hormones control a great number of the body's functions. Clearly, while cholesterol is generally portrayed as an archvillain to good health, it is actually a vital component of the body. Like anything else, though, too much of a good thing can be harmful.

Since our bodies can manufacture fat from ingested carbohydrates and protein, it may seem as if fat is not all that necessary in our diets. In reality, dietary fat is vitally important because some vitamins will only dissolve in fat. These are vitamins A, D, E, and K. If there were no fat in a person's diet, these vitamins would pass right on through the body. The fat soluble vitamins are also distributed throughout the body by fat molecules.

Although carbohydrates can be converted to fat, we would have to eat about two and a half times as many carbohydrates as fats, relative to weight, to get the same number of calories. The reason for this is that plants, the source of carbohydrates, contain a lot of cellulose and our bodies cannot digest and release the energy contained in cellulose. In fact, most animals cannot digest it—which is why herbivorous animals, such as horses, have to eat practically nonstop to get enough calories to stay alive. Cattle, sheep, and goats are special grazers because they can quickly eat grass and other plants and swallow it into a special "pre-stomach" pouch called a rumen. Bacteria in the rumen help to digest the cellulose. Later, these ruminate animals regurgitate the "cud" and chew it again at their leisure. The process allows them to "eat and run." When there are predators lurking about, that ability is a distinct advantage.

Carnivorous animals, who eat the herbivorous animals, do not have to ingest nearly as much food because the fat in their prey provides them with an abundance of calories.

Fat also makes food palatable, especially meats and bakery goods. This may not be of life-saving significance, but eating a hamburger that did not have a speck of fat in it would be almost like eating sawdust.

Although most people in our society speak of fat as if it were our body's mortal enemy, it obviously is not. The substance has been taking a increasingly bad rap for about seventy years, particularly the last thirty, but it should clear by now that if it were not for the fats in our bodies and in our diets, we could not possibly survive. Fat, from the standpoint of good health, most certainly does NOT deserve to be considered a four-letter word!

6

FATNESS AND STATISTICS

In light of the information in the previous chapter it must be conceded that fat is wonderful stuff — practically a miracle substance. At the same time it must also be admitted that an excessive amount of fat on our bodies is unwelcome. That is only logical since "excessive," by definition, means too much. Of course, as discussed previously, the term "too much fat" does not have much meaning relative to appearance since "too much" depends strictly upon an observer's opinion. On the other hand, excessive fat as it relates to a person's health and longevity is definitely undesirable.

The concept of excessiveness is hardly unique to fat. Too much of practically anything is detrimental to a person's health. Too high a percentage of oxygen in the air we breathe is poisonous. Too much exercise leads to a wide variety of physical problems such as shin splints, stress fractures, joint disorders, heatstroke, and heart attacks. Other things commonly associated with good health and longevity — including water, vitamins and minerals, medicine, and sleep — can also be harmful to health if they are taken in excess.

Having established that a person can have too much of a good thing, including fat, the question that immediately arises is, "How can I tell if I'm too fat?" When my older daughter was seven years old she gave me an answer she had heard at school, "You know you're too fat when you're standing on a street corner dressed in a red, white, and blue outfit, and a little old lady comes up, forces your lips open, and shoves a letter into your mouth" (mailboxes were much larger then). That was an example of second grade humor and the answer was undeniably true. In reality, though, the question is an extremely difficult one to answer. If there was an easy answer, this chapter and the following one would be very short.

Oh yes, there are many techniques for *measuring* body fat. The findings are usually expressed as a percentage of total body weight. It is often written that the ideal amount of fat on a man's body is about 13% of his total weight, and the ideal amount on a young woman's body is about 18%. The figures vary according to the source but typically they range anywhere from 8% to 15% for men (under forty) and from 15% to 25% for women under forty. The ideal percentages are usually said to be about 4% higher for people over forty. For comparison, a typical professional female ballet dancer has about 17% body fat.

It is not always clear what "ideal" means, but it usually implies a positive relationship with health and longevity. The implication is that scientists have discovered a fairly precise percentage of body fat that healthy men and women should have on their bodies. And if they have more than that amount, it is excessive. Further, if people have more than s*ome arbitra*rily assigned level of fat, they are classified as being — horrors—*f*at! The numbers are usually stated as above 15% for men and above 25% for young women. And when a male's body fat exceeds 20% and a female's exceeds 30%, they are — horror of horrors — obese!

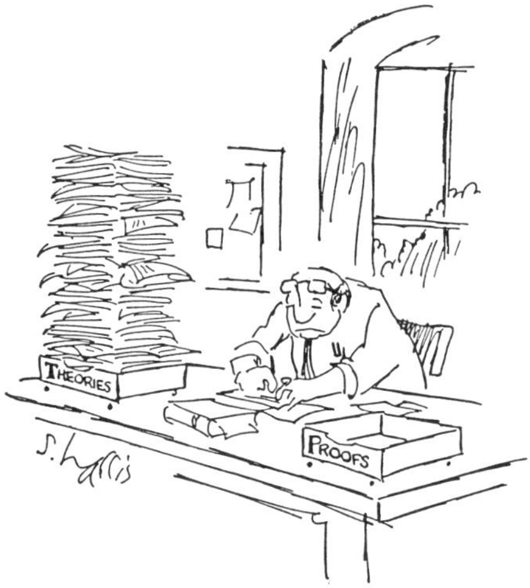

©1979 by Sidney Harris - *American Scientist Magazine*

Well, the simple fact is that no one knows what the ideal percentage of body fat is for any individual. "B-but, b-but!" I can almost hear the fitness gurus stuttering, "these figures are based upon research!" Ah yes, RESEARCH — a god that has ascended the highest throne in our technological pantheon. Research, however, is a tainted deity; it is far from being infallible. As the cartoon above from *American Scientist* indicates, research provides theories, at best — rarely proof. Indeed, nearly all studies are inconclusive and/or contradictory.

False and misleading results of research occur even in studies conducted by the brightest and most ethical of scientists. Because there is such pressure to publish in order to advance — relative to salaries, promotions, professional status, and to acquire research grants — some scientists rush through research, make errors, and publish prematurely.

The problem is exacerbated by administrators who evaluate researchers on the quantity of their research as opposed to quality. This has led unscrupulous researchers to intentionally juggle their figures or plagiarize data to hurriedly publish "original work." Occasionally these deceivers are exposed and disciplined within their professions, but transgressions are difficult to prove. Only rarely will a researcher admit to cheating on research, and then only after being caught "red handed." Significantly, though, most researchers know of colleagues who have falsified research data. A book entitled *Betrayers of the Truth: Fraud and Deceit in the Halls of Science* gives an interesting historical account of science gone awry. Data falsification has gotten so bad it has been given its own name, "lab-scam." In the late 1980s Congress began investigating the problem and the National Institute of Health has established a new office of Scientific Integrity.

Even without fraud, researchers rarely agree as to findings. Experts claim the truth will eventually surface. That may be true, but in the meantime what is the public to believe?

Many fatness studies have been conducted using various species of lower animals and the findings are assumed to also apply to humans. While it is true that all animals have a few things in common, and some closely related species have many things in common, it is erroneous to assume that different species are biologically identical. For example, the red blood cells of pigs, unlike those of humans, are impermeable to glucose — and pigs are not too different, physiologically, from humans. As Benjamin Franklin once said, "Dogs look up to humans, cats look down at humans, but pigs accept humans as equals."

In spite of Ben's sage observation, however, the findings of research done with lab animals, even pigs, cannot be assumed nonchalantly to pertain to humans. One of the reasons the National Anti-vivisection Society is so incensed about the use of animals for research is their claim that studies have shown animals to be totally inadequate as models for the study of human disease. Further, Dr. Neal Barnard, 1991 president of the Physician's Committee for Responsible Medicine has stated that animal tests are so slow they are part of the problem, not the solution — and that testing with human cells is not only faster and cheaper, the correct species is being studied. This position is strengthened by a 1972 report in *Lancet*, the leading British medical journal which stated that since no animal tumor is closely related to a cancer in human beings, an agent which is active in the laboratory may well prove useless clinically.

There is a rumor that researchers would rather perform laboratory experiments on lawyers than rats because (1) there are more of them, (2) technicians don't get so attached to them, and (3) there are *some* things rats just won't do. That's just a rumor, mind you.

Even *within* species there are vast differences between individuals' anatomy and physiology. The proteins, for example, in each person's body tissue are different from all others (except for identical twins). Because of this difference, tissue from one person cannot be transplanted to another without the recipient having to take anti-rejection drugs. Because of individual differences, no medicine affects all patients in exactly the same way.

Research done with human males, logically, cannot always be applied to females (and vice versa) due to differences in body chemistry, particularly hormones. These differences, incidentally, explain why leaders of women's equality are so incensed over the exclusion of women as subjects in most federally funded research projects. The new director of the National Institutes of Health, Bernadine P. Healy, however, has vowed to eliminate that sexism — and has created the Office of Research on Women's Health. Until the present, men were studied and it was assumed cavalierly that the findings also applied to women. Further weakening the validity of research findings is the use of male rats (a term some women might find redundant) in nearly all research, including that dealing with medicine and health practices.

When women *are* used as subjects in research dealing exclusively with feminine concerns, the findings are still extremely difficult to evaluate. Female birth control pills are an excellent example of the confusion that can exist even when research involves the use of many millions of human subjects. Since "the pill" became popular several decades ago, there has been a persistent vacillation within the medical research community as to its safety. Currently, thirteen million women are taking the pill, yet experts admit they still do not know whether a link exists between it and breast cancer (the rate of which, incidentally, continues to climb). Information relative to other medical problems is even more nebulous; there is just too much contradiction between studies. Oliver Wendell Holmes once stated, "Certainty is an illusion." This is certainly true as far as research is concerned.

The use of simple common sense would help, but as Gertrude Stein wrote in the 1920s, "Everybody gets so much information all day long that they lose their common sense." At that time in history there were no television, computers, or communication satellites. What would Gertrude say if she were around today? The truth of her statement has only intensified with the explosive proliferation of technology. Today we are being deluged with information and misinformation, much of which originates from research.

I am not against research. On the contrary, being an exercise physiologist for more than a quarter of a century, I place great value on that investigative process. The problem is not that too much research is being done; it's that not enough is being done. Far too many uncertainties exist. Scientists do not know nearly as much, in any field, as the public is led to believe. So, until more truths are established, we *have* to use some common sense. And that is the approach advocated in this book — research findings tempered with common sense.

This dual approach requires people to have at least a rudimentary understanding of research and its limitations. To begin, all experimental investigation involves the collection of data — usually individual measurements (or scores), such as the percent of fat on a person's body. The data are then analyzed through the use of STATISTICS. This is done for several reasons: (1) to summarize, organize, and simplify data, (2) to allow generalizations about an entire population to be made from a small sample of that population, and (3) to permit researchers to compare one variable (such as body fatness) with another (such as longevity) and determine it there is a relationship between the two.

Each of these three uses of statistics has intrinsic shortcomings which effect the validity, or truth, of research. But the most basic imperfection of statistics, one that can never be corrected, is that statistics, at best, merely reveals generalizations and probabilities. As a result every *individual* measurement, or person, is completely obscured.

This situation is not surprising at all when considering we live in a bureaucratic society. Because a strict adherence to rigid rules and routines is the established policy in such institutions as government, business, and education, there is naturally a suppression of individualism. How many times have you tried to have the simplest, most clear-cut, grievance or unfairness rectified and been told curtly or with a barely suppressed yawn, "I'm sorry, we can't do a thing about it. That would violate Policy." The "P" in policy is capitalized, of course, because it is another deity. This bureaucratic approach does help institutions run more easily, but it does so at the expense of common sense and justice — and the individual.

In a bureaucratic society statistics is the perfect scientific tool. Statistics is, simply, a bureaucracy in mathematical form. If statistics show you are heavier than average, then by Jove you had better lose some weight. It may be that you have the perfect amount of fat for your body type, or perhaps your extra weight is muscle. That is beside the point; the populace must bow before the alter of statistical Policy!

A reader with keen perception may by now suspect that I do not hold statistics in great reverence. That is true, but I'm just being realistic. For those who may believe me to be a "wild-eyed" renegade in this respect, though, I offer the passage below. It is from the Preface of a very informative book, *Flaws and Fallacies in Statistical Thinking*, by Stephen Campbell.

> When a person loves something, he hates to see it abused. Such is my feeling toward statistics. Hardly a day goes by that I fail to see the subject I love put to use in faulty and misleading ways in newspapers, books, speeches, and, especially, advertising. . . This book was written with two purposes in mind — the first, less important, purpose being that of getting something off my chest. For many years I have been distressed by the frequency with which (1) relatively simple statistical tools such as percents, graphs, and averages are misused and (2) faulty conclusions are drawn from, perhaps, faulty data in our news media simply because the purveyors of the information don't know any better. Moreover, I have been annoyed — indeed, made damned mad — by the frequency with which bogus statistical evidence is used intentionally by some unconscionable people to sell their products or pet ideas to others.

The distrust of statistics is hardly a modern revelation. The British prime minister Benjamin Disraeli has often been quoted as saying, "There are three kinds of lies: lies, damned lies, and statistics." It is doubtful that he was the first the make such an observation — or the last.

In unscrupulous hands, even with the best of collection of data, statistics can be misused to completely distort and subvert research conclusions. A classic, and not far-fetched, example would be a weight-loss company's claim that 90% of its customers lose a large amount of weight. That seems quite impressive. But what constitutes a large weight loss? For how long did the people keep the weight off? How many people dropped out of the program due to lack of success? The drop-out rate of one major Australian weight-loss firm was 98% within the first year! Assuming the success rate of their remaining customers was 90%, the success rate of the entire original group would be less then two out of a hundred — hardly a figure to brag about, but one which is consistent with the success rate in general of weight reduction schemes. It is easy to see how a company, by selectively choosing its data, can make lofty claims for its product even though it is a miserable failure. This kind of chicanery, which pervades the business world, lends credence to the often expressed belief that statistics can be used to make numbers say anything a person or company wants them to say.

The public is constantly being fed information about such topics as crime rates, economic trends, and health — matters that affect us all. Because of the common use of statistics to present this information, it is important to understand the inherent flaws in this mathematical science. Such understanding is particularly necessary when it comes to determining what constitutes excessive fatness since statistics are used so often to portray the condition as a health hazard.

The simplest function of statistics is to summarize, organize, and simplify data (measurements). These procedures allow a person to acquire some understanding of a mass of confusing data at just a glance. The most commonly used statistic is the measure of central tendency — commonly called the *average*. Although this seems simple enough, there are many kinds of average. The three most often used ones are the "mean," "median," and "mode." Of all the definitions I've ever seen of these three, the cartoon below provides the clearest differentiation. The cartoon also shows that the "average" that a person chooses can be drastically misleading.

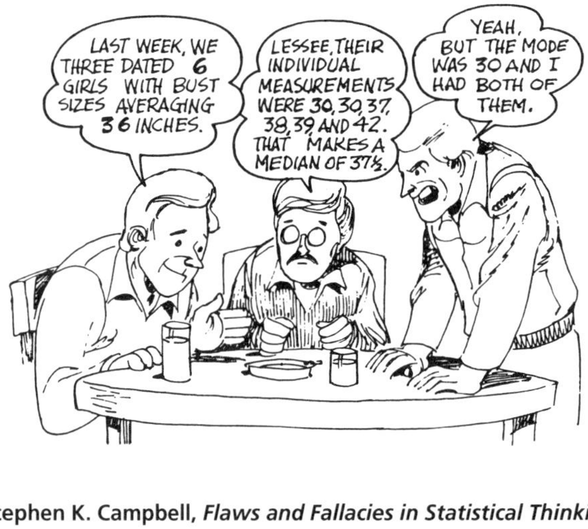

Stephen K. Campbell, *Flaws and Fallacies in Statistical Thinking*

Of all the measures of central tendency, the arithmetical average, or *mean* is used most often. This figure is obtained by adding together all the individual scores in a group and then dividing that sum by the total number of scores.

Imagine being told that the heights of forty-six people in a group, expressed in inches, are 68, 70, 66, 71, 69, 70, 72, 68, 71, 73, 69, 61, 71, 69, 71, 67, 74, 72, 70, 73, 76, 74, 67, 71, 66, 70, 72, 69, 64, 68, 70, 81, 65, 72, 68, 70, 73, 70, 67, 71, 75, 69, 68, 70, 69, and 72. Kind of confusing, right? It would help if at least the heights were organized from short to tall: 61, 64, 65, 66, 66, 67, 67, 67, 68, 68, 68, 68, 68, 69, 69, 69, 69, 69, 69, 70, 70, 70, 70, 70, 70, 70, 70, 71, 71, 71, 71, 71, 71, 72, 72, 72, 72, 73, 73, 73, 74, 74, 75, 76, and 81. A few moments study would reveal some pattern to the numbers. Namely, that the heights range from 61 to 81 inches and most of the people are between 68 and 72 inches tall. It would be a lot simpler, though, if it were reported that the average height of the people was 70 inches or 5'10".

Like a bureaucratic policy, the arithmetical average makes things easier. Knowing that figure alone, however, would not reveal anything about any particular *individual*'s score. Further, from the average a reader would not know if everyone in the group was exactly 70 inches tall — or if half were about 60 inches tall and the other half were around 80 inches tall. Impossible? Not if the group consisted of jockeys and professional basketball players. Since the average reveals nothing about the height of any particular individual in the group, a person might be less than 4 feet tall or more than 8 feet tall. Again, as in any bureaucracy, mathematical or otherwise, the individual is "lost in the shuffle."

For a dramatic example of how an average, or mean, figure can be misleading, imagine standing with each of your feet in a separate bucket of water. Imagine the temperature of one being a freezing 30°F and the temperature of the other being a scalding 130°F. The average temperature would be a comfortable 80°F, but knowing that would not make the situation any more pleasant, would it?

If each height measurement of all the people in a given population was placed on a graph in the form of a dot, the dots could be expected to be distributed around the average height in the shape of a bell. That is, the largest number of height "scores" would cluster about the average score — with the numbers of scores tapering off the further they were from the average (in both directions). A line drawn along the top of the dots would produce a bell-shaped curve. Since most measurements are normally distributed in this shape, the curve is usually called the *normal curve.*

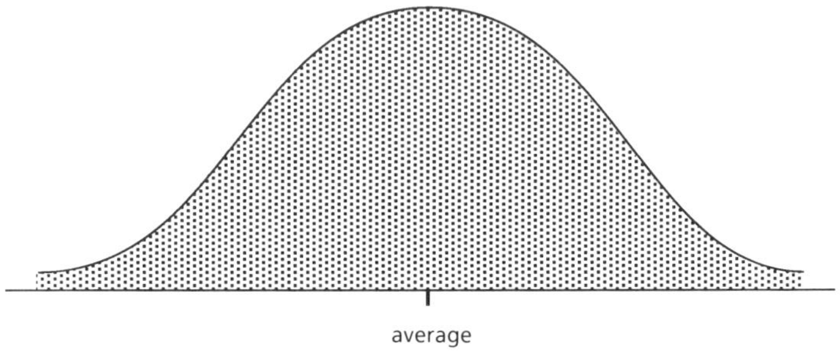

A Normal Distribution of Scores (showing the normal curve).

There is a statistical term called the standard deviation (whose symbol is "σ") which gives a numerical description of the way scores tend to be distributed around an average. In a normal distribution about 68% of the scores could be expected to fall within one standard deviation (plus and minus) of the average. About 95% of the scores could be expected to fall between -2σ and $+2\sigma$, with about 99% falling between -3σ and $+3\sigma$. The likelihood of scores below and above -3σ and $+3\sigma$ are slim, but there could be some.

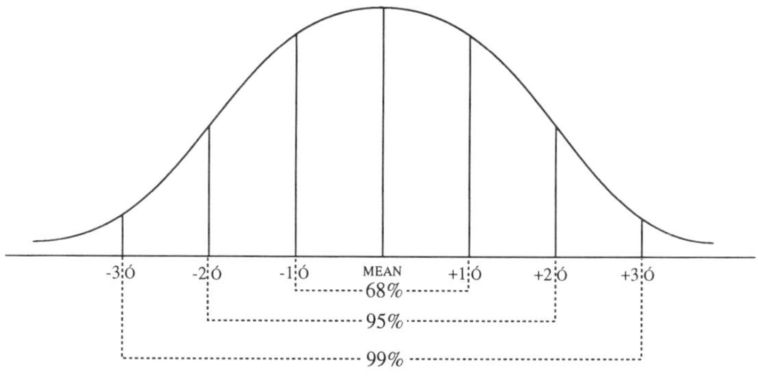

Percentages of Scores Found within the Standard Deviations.

Most people do not find the subject of statistics to be especially scintillating, but please "hang in there" in this discussion of the normal curve; it is necessary to understand the concept before addressing the issue of excessive fatness. It is also important to realize that virtually every human characteristic, *genetic or acquired*, varies according to the normal curve. This distribution pattern applies to every aspect of our anatomy, such as height, bone density, and number of muscles fibers within each muscle. It applies to every physiological aspect such as heart rate, visual acuity, and maximal speed of muscle contractions. It applies to all aspects of our behavior, good and bad, such as greed, compassion, and generosity. And it applies to our various mental capacities and abilities as well.

Doesn't it strike you as extremely unlikely, virtually inconceivable, that data dealing with every human characteristic are distributed according to the normal curve, but data dealing with body fat percentages are not? Yet, the public is led to believe there is a specific percentage of body fat that is ideal for all men and another percentage that is ideal for all women — and that people who are above these percentages are too fat. This "decree" is akin to saying there is an inherently ideal height for men and an ideal height for women, and that being above that figure means a person is too tall. The idea of a specific height, or a specific percentage of body fat, being ideal for *everyone* is hogwash.

Even if "ideal" were defined as average, the term should not be interpreted as implying value. A man who is 5 feet 1 inch tall, or 6 feet 9 inches, is not necessarily better or worse than a man of average height, which in the U.S. is roughly 5 feet 10 inches. By the same token, a woman who has a body fat percentage of 10% or 40% is not necessarily better or worse (or healthier or unhealthier) than a woman with the average body fat of about 25%. Keep in mind that this latter figure has not been engraved in stone by a thunderbolt. Each study comes up with a different number, and "average" is not synonymous with "best" anyway. What is *best* depends upon a variety of individual factors. In athletics, for instance, a woman would want very little body fat if she aspired to be a topflight mile runner. On the other hand, a long distance swimmer would want much more than average body fat for insulation, energy, and buoyancy.

It can be argued that "average" means "normal" and that variation from average is automatically abnormal. Abnormal is not necessarily undesirable, however. After all, Albert Einstein had abnormal intelligence, Meryl Streep is an abnormal actress, "Sugar" Ray Leonard and Greg Luganis are abnormal athletes, Luciano Pavarotti has an abnormal operatic voice, Itzak Perlman is an abnormally skilled violinist, and Marilyn Monroe had an abnormally voluptuous figure according to today's hard body devotees.

But was Monroe excessively fat? This brings us once again to the nagging question that is so difficult to answer: "At what point is any individual excessively fat?" *An aver*age percentage of body fat does indeed exist—relative to optimal health. For the sake of discussion let's assume that percentage is 25% for young women. But—and this is very important — when applying the concept of the normal curve, it is inconceivable to expect *every* woman to be at her healthiest at precisely the same percentage of body fat. While most women could be expected to be at their healthiest when fairly close to the hypothetical 25%, others would be healthiest at 30%, 35%, 40%, or even 45% or more. By the same token, some women would be healthiest at 20%, 15%, 10%, or even 5% or less.

The public is often given summarized information in the form of an average — and that is quite all right as long as they understand how "scores" are normally distributed about that average. The vast majority of people do not understand this normal curve, though. Even when they do, they do not automatically apply it when an average is stated. As a result, the single central score usually assumes far too much importance. People tend to slavishly accept the inflexible "magical" average when in reality all it does is provide a *starting point* for understanding summarized information.

The second major purpose of statistics is to allow generalizations to be made about an entire population from a small sample. This shortcut can save a researcher a tremendous amount of work, but it is vital that the sample be chosen to accurately reflect the population from which it is chosen. If this requirement is violated, the data collected from the sample is flawed and the research may be meaningless.

For instance, the forty-six person sample discussed previously does not necessarily reveal anything about the average height of people in general. If the *sample* group consisted of women from the U.S., no generalizations can be made about the height of men in the United States, pygmies in Africa, or women in Japan. If the data was obtained by measuring the heights of women on a U.S. high school basketball team, it can't even be used to make a statement about U.S. women in general. In fact, the data can not even be used to make absolute predictions about the height of women basketball players in the U.S. It could be that the measured team had, by chance, especially tall players or especially short players. To give any meaning at all to the data, every female player on every U.S. high school basketball team would have had to have an equal chance to be chosen for the sample — and even then there is still a chance of error.

In statistical jargon, height is called a *variable* because it is a measurement that can have different values. Height is a variable that can be very easily and accurately measured. As shown above, though, problems can still arise in the most basic of statistical procedures such as the collection of data. These problems are compounded when the results of the simple procedures are used in more complex statistical procedures — which, in turn, have their own built-in faults.

Even when data is fastidiously collected and all of the statistical procedures are followed perfectly and without bias, research conclusions can still be completely false. All that scientists can do is to try their best to increase the *probability* that their findings have truth. Again, research never proves anything. At most, it just gives indications or suggestions of truth. This fact must be kept in mind when a statement begins with "research shows." These two words inspire too many people to figuratively fall to their knees and clasp their hands reverently as if the information had a celestial origin.

As pointed out in the October, 1989, newsletter from the School of Public Health at the University of California, Berkeley, a tremendous number of research findings are published each year. For instance, about 240,000 biomedical articles in English alone are indexed each year by the National Library of Medicine. Obviously, if every study proved something, there would be very few questions left unanswered. Even when a study is done at a highly respected institution and appears in a prestigious journal, it should be viewed with skepticism.

The article also lists three practical points to keep in mind. One, a single research effort cannot prove anything; it must be duplicated. And that does not provide proof either. Two, even if a finding is acclaimed in the media, wait and see what follow-up studies show. A classic example are the cold fusion studies that originated at universities in Utah. And, three, be *especially* suspicious of research that is cited to help sell something.

If such an uncomplicated variable as height can be so complex statistically, it is easy to see how infinitely more complicated the subject of fatness can be. Along with hereditary differences, there are the well-known metabolic and dietary factors that can vary so much between individuals. Not so well known are the variations in the fatness "set-point," and the hunger and satiety control centers in the brain. There are also a variety of metabolic diseases, brain disorders, and hormonal disorders that affect fatness. The most mysterious of all the variables are the psychological ones.

Very little is known with certainty about fatness, particularly the ideal percentage for any individual as it relates to health and longevity. Scientists in general readily admit it. It's the middlemen "experts" who read the conclusions of a few studies, which may or may not be close to the truth, and then proclaim to know it all — and pass it along as fact.

The third function of statistics is to enable researchers to compare one variable with another variable. Many studies, for example, have been done to determine the relationship between the variables of body fat and longevity. Most studies, particularly those conducted in the United States, suggest that fat people die sooner than people of average body composition.

The basic assumption of this relationship research is that "all other things are equal." When relationships between variables are studied, it is of paramount importance that this assumption be true. Otherwise, an uncontrolled variable may be responsible for a study's findings. This point is supported by an excerpt from *How to Tell the Liars from the*

Statisticians by Robert Hooke.

> *Ceteris paribus* means "other things being equal," and I drag in this bit of Latin to suggest the antiquity of the phrase. Often we assume that other things are equal without saying so, and then we may forget the assumption was made. Data pushers like to profit from our habit of making this tacit assumption.
>
> During the 1970s a report was issued describing data for crude cancer mortality rates in two groups of ten American cities, one group that had added fluoride to the drinking water and one that had not. Between 1950 and 1970 the cancer mortality rate rose in both groups of cities, but it rose considerably faster in the fluoridated group. Some data pushers were more than willing to attribute the difference to the fluoride, without pointing out that they were assuming "other things being equal."
>
> The National Cancer Institute asserted that indeed other things were not equal and that the difference between the two groups of cities was explained by differences in the age, race, and sex distributions of the two groups of cities; these three demographic characteristics all have known effects on cancer mortality rates. In Great Britain the Royal College of Physicians asked for comment from the Royal Statistical Society. Two statisticians were chosen to analyze the data and here is what they found.
>
> The cities that were to be fluoridated already had, before fluoridation, an excess of cancer deaths over the "control" cities that went unfluoridated. Between 1950 and 1970 the demographic differences between the two groups became even greater. Taking onto account the known effects of age, race, and sex on cancer rates, they found that the remaining unaccounted-for part of the cancer mortality rate was actually somewhat smaller in the fluoridated cities than in the others.
>
> Which all goes to show that *ceteris* are not necessarily *paribus* and that the reason things are not what they seem is that we may be assuming things about them that are not true.

In fatness/longevity research, the longevity of fat people is usually compared with the longevity of average weight people. The assumption is that the subjects are equal in all other aspects such as heredity. Of course, the chances that a fat group and average group are identical, except in body fat, are so astronomically unlikely, they are inconceivable. Yet, when inequalities are not taken into account in research, conclusions can become meaningless.

Some of the inequalities between groups in fatness studies simply are not known and therefore cannot be taken into account. Many inequities *are* known and are simply ignored. Differences in emotional stress between fat people and those of average weight, for instance, have not been studied.

Stress, with its myriad physical and psychological ramifications, results from anything that threatens a person's sense of well-being. Being the unrelenting target of negativity is certain to result in unhealthy stress. Therefore, it is quite likely that a large majority of people who are considered to be fat by our society suffer illnesses and die prematurely, not due to being overweight, but due to the stress resulting from the constant harassment by the FATISTS in our thin-crazed society. The deprecation by others is bad enough, but the constant stress of self-hate has to be far more damaging.

Reduced longevity based upon stress is hardly a far-fetched idea. African Americans have a much higher level of high blood pressure than their white counterparts. In fact, blacks are three *times* as likely to have severe hypertension. A recent study indicates that genetics may well be a factor, but many researchers believe the difference is also closely related to the stress that African Americans face as a result of discrimination — real and imagined. It is also well-established that people who are perceived as being fat are also commonly discriminated against both socially and in the business world.

It is probably impossible for people of average weight to have a clear idea what it is like to be fat and to suffer persistently the scorn and contempt heaped upon them by society *and loved ones* — even when it is done subtly. For many fat people the torment and its stress must be awesome.

A much greater burden, though, is imposed when a fat person — no matter how lovely, inside and out — is finally brainwashed into believing the negative propaganda spread by FATISTS. A close look into the eyes of a fat person so indoctrinated will reveal the shame and guilt she feels. It is heartbreaking and so unfair. Many fat people, understandably, tend to become paranoid after awhile. They begin to think everyone who looks at them is thinking negative things about them and their fatness — and their level of stress continues its upward spiral.

The emotional stress of being fat, in the United States, is not unlike that experienced by soldiers who spend long periods in a combat zone. Battle fatigue, of course, is more intense but at least soldiers can be sent to rest and rehabilitation camps or sent home. Fat people, in the modern western society are generally victims of excessive emotional stress during their entire lives. There is no relief even in solitude. It is easy to tell them to just lose weight, but that is virtually impossible for some people. Further, losing weight may adversely affect the health of many people who are considered to be fat, but who in reality are not.

The harmful effects of chronic stress upon health and longevity is solidly established and alone could account for the statistical evidence that fat people die prematurely. Yet, stress has never been "factored" into fatness research.

There is also the likelihood that fat people who, after many reducing failures, just give up on practicing sound health measures in general. If a balanced diet and sound exercise program are not followed, health and longevity is bound to suffer, no matter how fat or thin, a person is. Once fat people give up on attaining good health, their sense of shame, guilt, and failure is bound to escalate — along with their weight. The result is a vicious, self-defeating cycle in terms of both physical and psychological health.

Even if there is an actual direct relationship between fatness and a reduced life span, it does not automatically mean fatness is the *cause* of reduced longevity. It could be that the two variables are related genetically. That is, the gene that determines fatness may be closely related to the one, or ones, that determines a person's longevity potential. Sickle cell anemia, for instance, is limited to black people, but skin color has nothing to do with causing the disease. If it did, bleaching cream would cure the anemia. The disease has a genetic origin and the causative gene is carried by a significant proportion of people of African descent.

There are countless numbers of genetic factors that affect a person's longevity, but in the interest of saving space just one will be discussed — heart beats. By relying on the normal curve it can be logically assumed that some people genetically are allotted a high number of heart beats while other people have been short changed in that regard — and research strongly supports this assumption. It may well be that the maximum number of heart beats each of us is "born to have" is genetically linked to the propensity for being fat.

In addition, some cases of obesity are caused by medical conditions such as metabolic abnormalities and damage to the hypothalamic area of the brain due to injury or disease. These victims do die relatively early in life. Still, it cannot be stated that excessive body fat is the cause of their deaths. Fatness is just one of the symptoms of an underlying disease and losing weight — even if it were possible — may have very little, or no effect at all, on the longevity of the afflicted people.

The relationship between excessive fatness and reduced longevity is not unique. People who are very short or very tall also tend to die sooner than people of average height, particularly when the extremes are caused by disorders of the hormonal system. Excessive levels of the human growth hormone, for instance, causes acromegaly (giantism) with its myriad health and longevity problems. Even though all of the intricacies of the disorder have yet to be uncovered, it is clear that abnormal height is not the problem but is only one of the symptoms of the disorder. Similarly, extreme fatness may not be a health problem as much as it is a symptom of an underlying disorder.

Another major problem with research is the common practice of studying extreme situations and applying the findings to moderate situations. For instance, extremely obese subjects typically are used in "fat research" and conclusions are then applied to people who are only slightly or moderately overweight. Such extrapolation is quite unsound since extreme fatness is far more likely to be the result of a biological or psychological disorder than is a moderately fat condition. The approach is akin to studying extremely premature babies, who are very likely to suffer a number of life-threatening health problems, and then applying that information to babies born only a little early. Similarly, many millions of women are only a little overweight — even by today's stringent standards — and they are made to believe the condition is unhealthy.

In summary, although the mathematical science of statistics has considerable value in the collection and organization of data, it also has many inherent deficiencies. These can cause confusion in research and result in gross inaccuracies in conclusions. The major weakness of studies dealing with the relationship between fatness and health is that (1) not all of the variables pertaining to fatness have been discovered and (2) those variables that *are* known have not been sufficiently controlled in fatness/mortality studies. But, and this is extremely significant, even if all of the variables were known and "factored in," it would still be impossible for statistical techniques to determine at what point any *individual* is excessively fat. Some common sense is required in this regard and subsequent chapters help to provide more insight into the matter.

7

FATNESS AND BODY TYPES

Some health professionals admit there is no precise ideal percentage of body fat, but say there is an ideal *range*. That range is typically expressed as being a specific amount below and above the average. As with the average, the range is always arbitrarily chosen. For the sake of discussion, however, let's assume the ideal body fat percentage (for women) is 25% with the range being from 20% to 30%. This range concept is certainly more realistic than a precise ideal figure, but it is still far from satisfactory as shall be shown in this chapter.

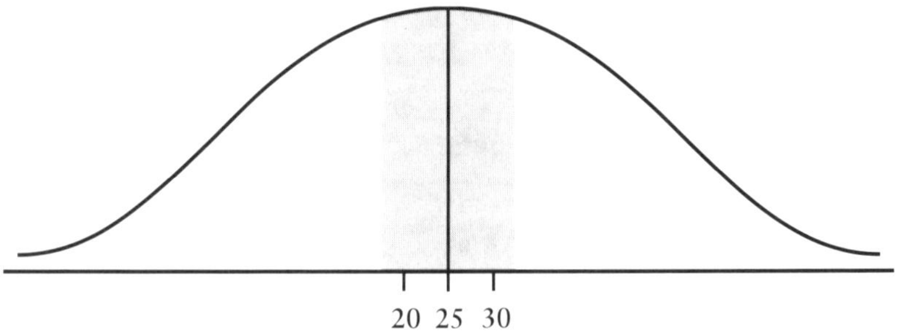

An Arbitrary Range of Ideal Body Fat Percentages.

From the normal curve, it may seem logical to assume that the further people are above the average percentage of body fat the more likely it is that they are excessively fat. And this would be true *if* everyone was born with exactly the same body type. Such is not the case, though. This additional variable makes the idea of a single "best" level of body fat completely unrealistic.

It has been known for a long time, probably even in prehistoric times, that not everyone has the same type of body. In historic times, it is believed that Hippocrates (around 450 B.C.) was the first to come up with a system of classifying body types. Since that date various other systems have been devised periodically. Except for terminology all are essentially the same, but the most well-known system today is the one devised in the 1930s by William Sheldon, a former Director of the Constitution clinic and Laboratory at Columbia University's College of Physicians and Surgeons. There have been improvements in his measuring techniques, but the basic concepts remain unchanged. Since the Greek word for body is "somato," Sheldon used the term "somatotyping" for his system.

According to Sheldon's system, every person's body type, male or female, consists of three basic components. The first component is called endomorphy, the second is mesomorphy, and the third is ectomorphy. The three components are named after the three primary layers of tissue in the human embryo — the endoderm, mesoderm, and ectoderm.

In Greek *endo* means "inner" and *derm* means "layer," so endoderm refers to the inner layer. This tissue gives rise to the lining of the abdominal organs. *Morph* is Greek for "form" so endomorphy refers to a body type wherein the digestive viscera are dominant and large. The chief external characteristic of an endomorph is a soft, rounded, fat-covered figure. This person seems to gain weight just by smelling food.

The mesoderm, or middle layer, of the embryo gives rise to muscles, bones, and connective tissue. A mesomorph, therefore, is characterized by having strong, thick bones, and large muscles. This physique is "squared" and hard.

From the outer embryonic layer, the ectoderm, is derived the skin and nervous system. An ectomorph, therefore, has relatively little body mass with a lot of surface (skin) area. In other words, the physique is linear and fragile. A person with this body type can seemingly eat constantly and never gain a pound.

It would be simplistic to believe that fatness, muscularity, or thinness are the only differences between the three basic somatotypes. They are merely the most obvious. A more complete picture of each component follows. *They apply to females as well as males.*

Because an endomorph's mass is concentrated in his large, round trunk region, particularly the abdomen, he has a high waist. Not surprisingly, his liver, stomach, intestines, and most other abdominal viscera are quite large. On the other hand, his heart and kidneys are usually of moderate size. His arteries vary from moderate to small size. This discrepancy in organ sizes may by itself account for the somewhat higher mortality rate in people with this body type.

An endomorph has relatively short, tapering limbs with the soft, "hammy" upper arms and legs being predominant over the shorter lower sections. His hands and feet are small and pudgy. Because he has a short neck, he appears to have "high" shoulders. His head is large and almost spherical; even his ears lie flat against his head and his nose does not protrude very far. Facial expressions tend to be bland.

As are his muscles, an endomorph's bones are small and weak. The lower part of his chest is wide and the front-to-back diameter tends to equal the side-to-side diameter. From the side view his vertebral column is relatively straight; it does not have the pronounced "S" curves seen in mesomorphs and ectomorphs. Males are rather feminine in appearance because of the fat deposits on their breasts, hips, and legs. This effect is enhanced by soft, smooth, velvety skin. It remains smooth and fresh looking even to old age but is very sensitive to the sun and is easily sunburned. An endomorph's hair is finely textured. The hair on his head lies flat and is easily combed, and there is a tendency for premature baldness. Generally, the loss of hair begins at the top of the head, toward the rear, and spreads to create a highly polished circular area. Genetic baldness is seldom seen in women of any body type.

The large bones and massive musculature of a mesomorph give him a stocky appearance, but the prominent muscular ridges are clear evidence of a hard, powerful body. Since his thorax is much larger than his abdomen, he has a low-waisted look. Unlike an endomorph's thorax, which is rounded like a barrel, a mesomorph's thorax is noticeably wider than it is deep. The upper part is also relatively wide. His limbs are generally longer than an endomorph's and his upper arms and forearms are about the same length, as are his upper and lower legs. A mesomorph's forearms, wrists, and hands are exceptionally powerful, as are his lower legs. His neck is fairly long and the sloping trapezius muscles at the sides make the shoulders seem low. His rectangularly "squared" head may be large or smallish, but its strong musculature, squared jaw, and thick bones (particularly around the eyes and cheekbones) may give him a bit of a brutish look. It is not necessarily unattractive, however — a point which I hasten to make should an offended mesomorph consider pounding on my door (with his forehead) late one night to discuss the issue.

In the *Canterbury Tales*, Chaucer introduces the miller as being, ". . . a very husky fellow, tremendous of bone and brawn . . . He was stocky, broad, and thickset. There was no door he could not pull off its hinges or break by ramming it with his head." This describes a mesomorph to a "T." The bony structure of his shoulder girdle is particularly heavy and broad and the width is increased by large muscles. His pelvis is also rather wide. The curve of the vertebral column in his lower back is prominent and further accentuated by muscular, protruding buttocks. His waist is relatively narrow and the front abdominal muscles show a distinct rippling.

Due to the considerable amount of underlying connective tissue, a mesomorph's skin is thick and coarse. It is also firm and elastic. When wrinkling occurs, it is heavy and coarse. The skin tans easily and maintains it for a long time. With consistent exposure it becomes permanently darkened and acquires a rich, leathery quality. A mesomorph's hair is generally also coarse. When a mesomorph become bald, the loss usually begins at the forehead and progresses rearward.

An ectomorph is the precise opposite of an endomorph. Chaucer's reeve (an overseer of an estate) is typical of such a person. "He was a slender, choleric man . . . His legs were as long and lean as sticks, completely lacking in calves." An ectomorph's small trunk has a front-to-back flattened look. His abdominal organs are small. Both the small and large intestines, for instance, are thinner and only about half as long as an endomorph's intestines — 10 to 15 feet versus 20 to 25 feet. As a result he does not absorb food nearly as readily into his body. Forced feeding to gain weight may merely result in a protruding abdomen.

An ectomorph's small central mass along with his long, "skinny" limbs result in a linear, fragile appearance. Not only are his bones thin and delicate, so are his muscles. The forearms and lower legs tend to be longer than the upper counterparts. His fingers and toes are long and fragile with small joints. Although his long, weak-chinned, triangular head seems large for his body, it too is rather small with sharp, fragile, sensitive features. The ears, particularly the upper part, are large and stick out conspicuously to the sides. His long, slender neck on the other hand projects forward and his "Adam's apple" is prominent. The curve in his lower back is flat but the curve in his upper back is quite pronounced. This gives him a characteristic stoop-shouldered look.

Because an ectomorph's skin has very little underlying connective tissue, it is thin and dry and acquires fine wrinkles at a fairly young age. Its color is pale and usually ashy in color. When exposed to the sun, the skin does not tan well; it burns easily and quickly peels. The amount of body hair is variable as it is in all three somatotypes, but it may seem more sparse on ectomorphs because their hair is usually much finer in texture. Because the hair on the head typically grows in several directions, it is rather unmanageable. Baldness is not common in ectomorphs.

Since somatotypes are a measure of shape, not height, any body type can be any height. Ectomorphs, however, due to their stretched-out-ness, tend to be the tallest of all the types. Endomorph's on the average are about a foot shorter while mesomorphs tend to fall midway between the extremes.

Sheldon and his associates initially used 4,000 eighteen-year-old college males of European ancestry to develop his somatotyping system. A later study using a wider range of ages involved 46,000 men. From front, side, and back photographs of nude men, the scientists measured seventeen diameters ranging from the width of the skull to the width of the ankle. Other research showed that somatotyping could be used just as effectively to classify the body types of Orientals, Semitics, and African Americans.

The attempts to classify women according to their somatotypes have not been nearly as extensive as those for men. A major reason seems to have been a difficulty in finding large numbers of women with a wide variety of body types who would agree to pose nude for the required photographs. Of the studies that have been done, though, the same body types identified among men have been found to exist among women. As would be expected, the endomorphic component is more prominent in women while that of mesomorphy is more common in men.

A major criticism of somatotyping is that its photographic and measuring procedures are laborious and subjective. This detraction may have been valid at one time, but it has been weakened tremendously with the vast improvements in technology. Computer use would greatly increase the ease and objectivity of the somatotyping method — as well as its accuracy. With modern technological advantages, long-term studies of individuals (ideally from infancy to old-age) would give even more information and insight into the subject of somatotyping.

Even with the weaknesses of Sheldon's technique, the fact that people have inherently different types of bodies cannot be, and never has been, challenged. And although this chapter stresses the relationship between somatotypes and ideal fat levels, there is much more to the subject of body types. For example, studies suggest that a person's body type may be linked to a wide variety of other characteristics such as juvenile delinquency, personality, moods, mental illnesses, academic success, and health. It would certainly behoove researchers to further investigate these relationships.

Assuming there are only three types of bodies — endomorphs, mesomorphs, and ectomorphs — and that everyone falls precisely within one or another of the groups, it is easy to see the untenability in establishing a *single* ideal range of body fatness that would apply to *all* people. It is totally inconceivable that every individual could attain and maintain such an arbitrary level. An endomorph would have to endure a lifetime of starvation and an ectomorph would have to continually gorge. If as a result these people lived a few years longer, which is very unlikely, would the daily torture be worth it? The extension would only prolong the agony of either starving or stuffing. As a long time dieter once explained to me, "With dieting you don't live to be a thousand years old, it just seems like it."

If everyone was either an endomorph, mesomorph, or ectomorph, common sense suggests there would be three normal curves for body fat percentages. More specifically, there would be three ideal body fat *ranges* instead of the single one that is generally promulgated. The drawing below shows the extreme variation in the range of ideal body fatness. The average for each of the body types was arbitrarily chosen but is probably not too distant from reality. Mainly, though, it helps to develop the concept of differentiation. The drawing also shows that an endomorph with body fat of, say, 25% would be greatly underweight for her body type, while an ectomorph with the same amount of body fat would be greatly overweight.

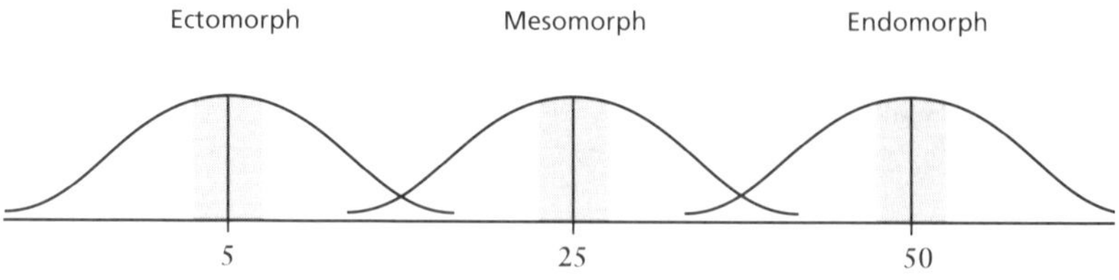

Variations in Ideal Body Fat Percentages (three body types).

With three distinctly different somatotypes the idea of a single ideal percentage of body fat becomes unacceptable. But there are not just three types of bodies. As stated previously, there are three primary *components*. The body type of each person on Earth is a combination of those components. In Sheldon's ingenious, yet simple, system, each of an individual's three components is ranked on a scale of from 1 to 7. Using endomorphy as an example, a score of 1 indicates a minimal manifestation of that body type; 7 indicates a maximum manifestation; and 4 is the mid-point. A person's somatotype is expressed in terms of a three digit number — one number for each of the three primary components. The score for endomorphy is always stated first, followed by the score for mesomorphy, and finally the score for ectomorphy.

In the illustrations below, subject "A" is obviously an extreme example of endomorphy. His somatotype score therefore would be 711 — 7 (for endomorphy), 1 (for mesomorphy), and 1 (for ectomorphy). There are no zeros in somatotyping because everyone has at least a minimal degree of every component. Even a 711 endomorph, for instance, does have some muscle tissue and some length to his neck (traits associated with mesomorphy and ectomorphy, respectively). Subject "B," an extreme mesomorph, would have a 171 somatotype—and "C," an extreme ectomorph, would be a 117. For all body types, females tend to be heavier in the buttocks and thighs than are males. An excellent example of a female endomorph is the Venus of Willendorf on page 16.

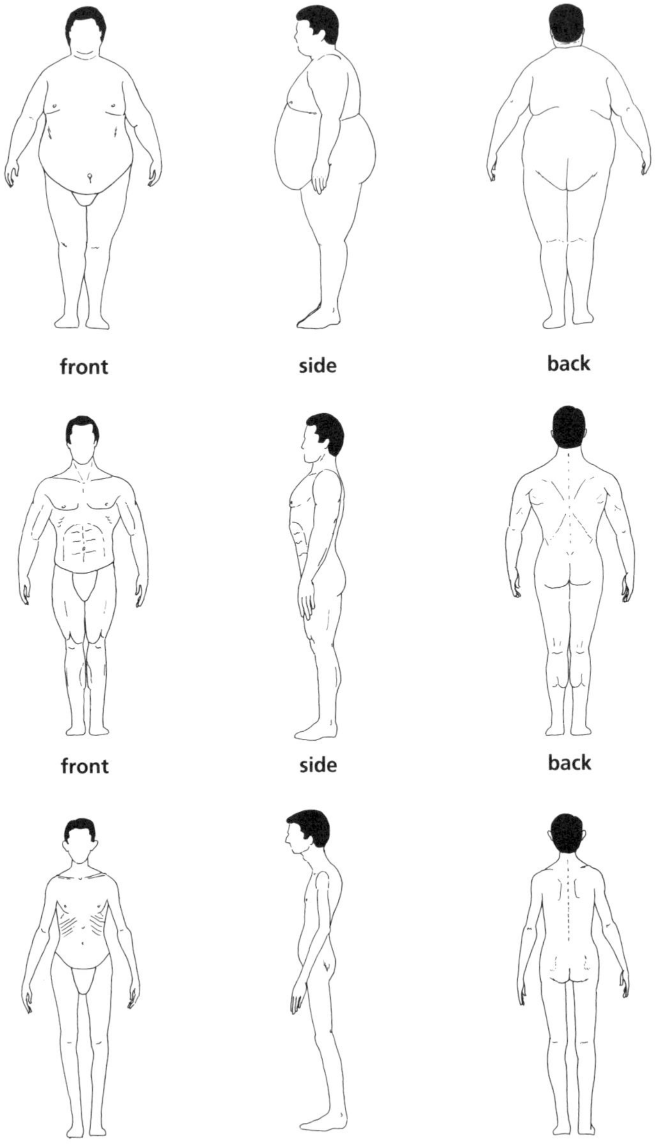

Drawn from Photographs in *The Varieties of Human Physique*,

with Permission of the Trustees of the William H. Sheldon Trust.

Perfect examples of extreme endomorphy, mesomorphy, and ectomorphy are rare. More common somatotypes have such descriptive names as "moderate endomorph," "mesomorphic endomorph," and "ecto-mesomorph." Although it is not within the scope of this book to include matching photographs for a wide range of somatotypes, such a volume already exists. Authored by William Sheldon and others, it is appropriately entitled, *Atlas of Men* and makes for fascinating reading. Many libraries have a copy. A perusal of the book will give you a clear understanding of the various somatotypes and will help you determine your own type. Such knowledge will give you some insight into estimating your ideal fat-percentage range. For the highest accuracy, though, precise measurements of various body dimensions should be evaluated by somatotype experts — if you can find one.

Generally the body types in the middle ranges, the three and fours, are called balanced somatotypes. They are the most common. For males a somatotype of 343 is considered to be the "average" male body. Females, genetically, tend to have a higher first component (endomorphy) so a somatotype of 433 would be more representative of a average women. That is similar to Albrecht Durer's ideal female figure (page 25). Sheldon referred to the very endomorphic 621 women as being "soft-round," "shapely," and "comely." Indeed, he named it the "Cupid" somatotype. Cupid was the Roman god of love. Previously to that, the

343

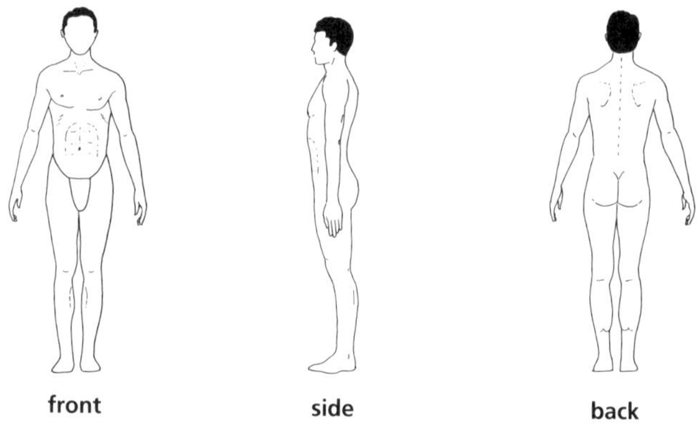

Drawn from Photographs in *The Varieties of Human Physique*,

with Permission of the Trustees of the William H. Sheldon Trust.

Greeks called him Eros. Interestingly, Freud chose the term "Eros" to refer to the instinct of sexual desire. As suggested in Chapter Three, perhaps men do have an inborn attraction to fat women.

Statistically, there are 343 possible body types when only the whole numbers, 1 through 7, are used in somatotyping. But Sheldon also advised the addition of half-numbers for more precise classifications; this results in a 13-point scale. When this scale is used, there are 2197 possible body types. In reality, then, there are many body types each of which has its own range of ideal percentages of body fat. The drawing below, using just seventeen ideal ranges, gives some idea of how the total range of ideal body fat percentages is extended by the overlapping ranges. It shows how the ideal body fat percentage, based upon one's genetics, may well range from less than 5% to more than 45% depending upon one's body type.

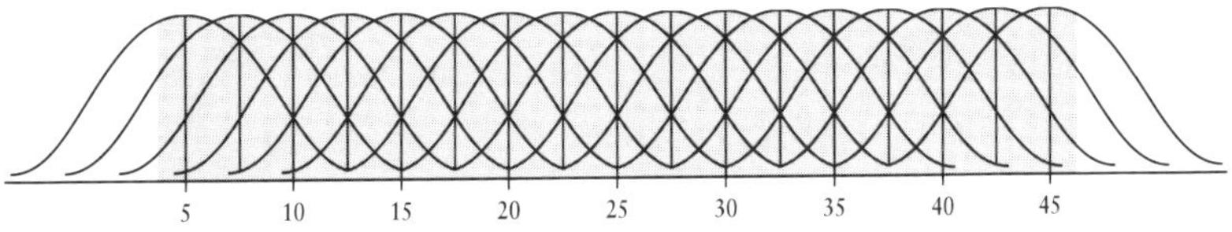

An Extended Range of Ideal Body Fat Percentages (assuming seventeen body types).

At this point the concept of an *single* "ideal" percentage of body fat that applies to everyone is ludicrously indefensible. In the 1930s Sheldon himself wrote:

> We do a great unkindness to those trusting people who still believe in the divinity of the printed word when we allow the usual publications of height-weight-age norms to go unexplained. It is sorrowful to hear the lament of a 632 (somatotype) who is already 30 pounds underweight, but who daily reads on the printed scales that she is 30 pounds overweight. And the poor 117 who weighs 99 pounds reads with horror that he should weigh 178. This kind of foolishness gives some of our best people inferiority complexes, and they have to be analyzed or sent to church.

Many so-called fat people who are trying to lose weight can be compared to the white person who devotes hours to lying in the sun to get a tan. Like being thin, a tan is fashionable and is thought to make a person look healthy. A suntan is not healthy, though; it ages the skin tremendously and greatly increases one's chances for getting skin cancer. Working against one's genetics for appearance's sake does not make a lot of sense as far as fatness is concerned either. Even when unnatural thinness is attained, it is usually an unpleasant experience and requires a lot of time, effort, and motivation — and excessive thinness is far from being healthy.

Expecting every person on Earth to conform to a fixed ideal percentage of body fat is an incredibly unrealistic situation. The feelings of inadequacy, shame, and guilt that have been instilled in people who, by nature, are unable to "toe the mark," are the most grievous legacy of such illusionary expectations. If this concept of a single ideal fatness level was a problem back in the 1930s, just imagine the degree of emotional suffering the idea causes today with the unrelenting emphasis on being thin.

Complicating matters even further, vastly so, is the fact that one part of a person's body can be one somatotype while another part can be a far different somatotype. Although there may be many subregions, to facilitate his study of this phenomenon Sheldon divided the body into five major regions:

the head, face, and neck
the upper trunk (thorax)
the shoulders, arms, and hands
the lower trunk (abdomen)
the legs and feet

Of the 4,000 young men Sheldon studied, he found that every single one showed some degree of somatotype variation between the regions. For instance, an individual's lower body can be somewhat endomorphic while the upper part can lean toward ectomorphism. Women for some reason tend to show much greater differentiation between regions of their bodies than men. This concept of regional variations not only vastly complicates somatotyping, it completely shatters the idea of a single ideal level of fatness that is bandied about in our society with such smug assurance.

Because each person is born with a particular body type, that does not mean the shape of one's body cannot be modified. It can be changed a lot. Diet, exercise, and drugs can reduce body fat, for instance, and produce increases in muscle mass. Wide variations in the color and texture of skin and hair can also be achieved through drugs, and cosmetics. Hair patterns and density can be altered through techniques ranging from plucking and electrolysis to implants. Ears that protrude laterally can be "tucked" back.

Although many physical characteristics can be modified, it is extremely important to remember that a person's somatotype will *always* remain the same. Skeletal dimensions, for example, cannot be altered, except through surgery, nor can the length and diameter of the intestines, the width of the pelvic structure, or height be changed. The number of muscle fibers cannot be increased. Nor can the number of fat cells be decreased, except through surgery. Yes, endomorphs can be starved to the point of emaciation, but they will always be endomorphs. Their bodies, for instance, will always have a strong inclination to revert to the body fat percentage that is associated with endomorphy.

To expect an endomorphic person to maintain the low level of fat that is arbitrarily fixed by society as being ideal is clearly delusive. Studies show that it is virtually impossible to do so on a permanent basis. Even if a person did manage to conform to society's thoughtless edict, doing so would be detrimental to his or her health.

To attack the character of an endomorph for lacking the will power to maintain a low percentage of body fat is not merely indefensible; it is grossly unfair. For a FATIST to know this and still accuse a fat person of having such negative traits as laziness, stupidity, gluttony, and immorality, is itself a sinful act. To compound the unfairness, in our thin-oriented society, women, who naturally tend to be fatter than men, suffer the greatest pressure to lose weight.

Since a woman's somatotype has a great bearing upon what her ideal degree of fatness should be, common sense suggests there has to be some way of relating her ideal percentage of body fat to her somatotype. One key to such a method would be the use of precise photographs and an expert somatotypist to analyze them. Because there are no more than a few of these specialists in the entire world, this is currently an impractical solution. Therefore, a simple, alternative method for determining a person's ideal fatness, based upon research and tempered with common sense, is developed in this book.

8

THE ANTIFAT INDUSTRY

Although fat people are currently the target of zealous condemnation in our culture, there is no record of this type of attack throughout all of previous history. On the contrary, fatness was generally considered to be a sign of prosperity in men and beauty in women. And when fatness was in vogue, thin people were never systematically reviled, scorned, and ridiculed — as fat people are today. What is the driving force behind this unique social phenomenon that finds a particular body type so firmly associated with such a wide variety of repugnant traits?

Not many questions have simple answers but this one does. Fat presently has an extremely negative image due to the intense and persistent efforts of a massively powerful antifat industry. It is an industry that in 1988 was fueled by thirty-three billion dollars a year in the U.S. Thirty-three *billion* dollars! That is more than *six times* the annual rip-off by the burglary industry! By the mid-1990s it is anticipated that the antifat harvest will increase to fifty billion dollars. Is it any wonder that so many enterprising entrepreneurs are jumping on the antifat bandwagon? Because people have become so paranoid about fat — any amount of fat — it is almost impossible not to make money with an antifat product. It's like having a license to steal.

Attitudes toward fatness fluctuated repeatedly in the twentieth century. It was as if America could not make up its mind. In the early 1900s, it was only gross obesity that was looked upon as a negative condition — and then only because it was harmful to health. Besides, people realized that most cases of excessive fatness were the result of medical problems. By the roaring twenties thin was "in," but people generally understood it was only a fashion just as fatness was the earlier fashion. A person's value as a person was not associated with his or her body weight.

By the early thirties fatness was making a comeback. In all likelihood, most people who were mired in the Great Depression thought a person was damned lucky to be overweight. Physicians, nutritionists, and other health professionals were denouncing the "boyish-build" look for women. Food manufacturers proudly announced the high number of calories in their products And fashion magazines contained articles like *Vogue's* "How Not to Be So Thin."

In the forties the trend to fleshiness continued. I recall (though, I was quite young at the time, mind you) that I and my equally odious cohorts would tease girls who were fat . . . but, heck, we teased every girl for one thing or another. Nobody's perfect; they all had some characteristic we could sink our teeth into, figuratively speaking. Now that I think about it, boys were also victims of our taunts — if they weren't too big! We were obnoxious little bastards, but we weren't suicidal.

As the fifties approached, I became a teenager and my perceptions changed dramatically. As if by magic, practically every girl suddenly looked really great to me. At the risk of incurring one of my gentle wife's rare flashes of testiness, I must admit they still do — fat, thin, or medium. The point is, my lack of objectivity in evaluating members of the opposite sex remained unchanged. My prejudice merely shifted from a negative to a positive frame of reference.

A more detached view of the concept of beauty in the middle 1940s requires turning to the pages of women's magazines of the period. That these publications had very few antifat articles or advertisements for weight reduction products was strong evidence that fatness was still no big deal — no pun intended. Indeed, according to the *Reader's Guide to Periodic Literatur*e, the number of articles dealing with fatness (corpulence) amounted to only a few per year. The number, however, shot to fifty-four between 1951 and 1953. Since then there has been a progressive increase; by the eighties it was almost impossible to find a popular women's magazine without an article on losing weight — and the trend has continued into the nineties.

Publications are awash with weight-loss ads. For some reason, the tackier the magazine, the more articles and ads there are dealing with weight-loss. I haven't given the circumstance a lot of thought, but it has to mean something.

The reasons for the increase in antifat interest are complex. The trend may have started because people felt guilty at suddenly having so much food compared to the deprivation of the war years. The advent of the television set, of course, would have showed women viewers across America how they were supposed to look — namely thin. Models, actresses, and beauty contest winners reflected, and thus reinforced, that belief.

The single most important peg for the antifat factions to hang their hats on popped up in 1951 with the phrase, "Obesity is America's No. 1 Health Problem." It would not have carried so much weight if it was not uttered by Louis I. Dublin, the chief statistician and "publicist" at the Metropolitan Life Insurance Company (MLIC) for almost sixty years. With fanatic zeal, he disseminated his beliefs through a prolific writing and speaking schedule.

By 1960 he had practically singlehandedly convinced the medical profession and the public that being fat was a dangerous threat to health. But there was still very little harassment of fat people regarding their appearance, intelligence, morality, etc. Significantly, there were very few advertisements for weight-loss products.

But some entrepreneurial eggs were scattered about, ready to metamorphose into a kind of larvae that feeds rapaciously upon the vulnerability of fat people. These creatures figured that in a thin-oriented society they could make a lot of money from people who did not conform to the modern view of the "ideal" body shape. History shows that the aspiring tycoons had hit the nail right on the head. Other entrepreneurs picked up the scent of opportunity and a modern version of the gold rush, based on fat, got under way.

The "larvae," nourished by antifat forces, quickly grew and combined to form an enormous industry that stops at nothing to convince people to lose weight. Magazines currently abound with ads for weight-loss products. Why are antifat companies developing such products? Because they are concerned with people's health? Or with the more than thirty-three billion reasons mentioned earlier? With that much lucre swirling about, there are bound to be scams aplenty, particularly since there is such ineffectual policing of the industry, internally or externally. Indeed, the antifat industry is infested with Money Acquisitive, Grotesquely Greedy, Obesity Tyrants — or to use the singularly appropriate acronym — MAGGOTS.

Most advertising people understand that good health is not a top priority for many people. If it were, people would not indulge in the exceedingly distasteful, pathogenic habit of smoking cigarettes. People want to be beautiful. Advertisements, therefore, stress the message that beautiful people smoke and, if others want to be beautiful, they too will also smoke. Unbelievably, millions of people "fall" for the ridiculous message.

Due to the flood of ads that stress "Get rid of ugly fat and flab" or "Lose weight and be beautiful," the public is similarly convinced that fat is not beautiful. Convince people that losing weight will make them beautiful and they will beat down doors to buy weight-reducing products. Realizing this, the antifat companies constantly pound into the public mind the idea that fat is ugly; that it is a four-letter word.

MAGGOTS are masters of innuendo. As an illustration, the statement in one ad, "You'll be gracefully thin," implies that fat people cannot be graceful. Yet, anyone who has seen a fat person gliding across a dance floor knows they can, in reality, be exceedingly graceful. In 1388, Chaucer, in *Somnours's Tale* described a character as being, "Fat as a whale and walkinge as a swan." It is true, though, that people who are self-conscious about their weight, or anything else about their appearance, will tend to move in an inhibited, awkward fashion.

People, naturally, want to be loved. They also want to be successful in life and they want loved ones to be proud of them. The quotation below, including the bold lettered words, is typical of antifat ads that capitalize on these normal desires.

> Enjoy the pride of a **slender, more beautiful and younger-looking you.** You will become that trim, exciting and attractive man or woman, who is envied by all of your friends and co-workers. Your husband or wife will be proud of the new you. You will **enjoy greater self-confidence** and lead a greater social life and might even be promoted at your job.

Does a person's fatness have any bearing on the characteristics that have to do with one's *real* value? Of course not. Anyone with a fat mother, grandmother, or daughter can attest to this, as can anyone who is happily married to a woman who is perceived to be fat by society.

Still, the antifat industry has relentlessly attempted to brainwash the public into believing fat people are not nice to be around. As ridiculous as this message is, many people fall for it. I will never forget a lean, muscular woman in one of my exercise classes who told her friends, with a shudder, "I simply refuse to associate with fat people." That woman probably does not realize it but it is *she* who has a serious problem. The overwhelming sorrow, though, is that a lot of fat people have, themselves, been convinced they are not fit to be loved.

Of course, the antifat companies are counting on the creation of such negative feelings to goad overweight people (and many who are not overweight at all) into buying their products. Now, making money is one thing, but doing so at the expense of making vast numbers of people feel miserable is quite another. But that is exactly what the MAGGOTS are doing.

Fat people are not miserable by nature. In fact, psychological studies of endomorphs indicate their natural temperament is just the opposite. They tend to be the most social of all the somatotypes. They participate easily with other people and enjoy making them feel at home. Endomorphs have, and are able to express, a warm interest in others and to show a sincere tolerance for different personalities. This observation did not originate in the 1900s. Nearly two thousand years previously, Plutarch, in his biographical work, *Lives*, had Julius Caesar say, "I am not much in fear of those fat, sleek fellows, but rather of those pale, thin ones."

Later, Shakespeare, in *Julius Caesar*, would have the Roman leader express the sentiments more poetically:

> Let me have men about me that are fat,
> Sleek headed men, and such as sleep at nights
> Yond Cassius has a lean and hungry look;
> He thinks too much. Such men are dangerous
> . . . he loves no plays . . . he hears no music.

As the last line indicates, it is not solely a modern idea that endomorphs also have a keen sensual appreciation. This contributes to their being creatures of comfort. They radiate it and they typically want such things as soft furniture and luxurious surroundings. Good food and ceremonious dining are very seductive to them.

In spite of the natural propensity of fat people to enjoy life, the antifat forces have nonchalantly made a large percentage of fat people feel wretched and worthless. Happy lives are thereby destroyed. The MAGGOTS have committed these atrocities for one reason — so they could sell their antifat merchandise. Compounding the sin is the fact that their products are rarely successful in helping people achieve a permanent weight loss anyway.

Wha . . . what? That's right; they are not successful. Common sense reveals that. Some of the world's wealthiest women, Elizabeth Taylor and the late Christina Onassis to name but two of the best known, with all of their money and fame were unable to find the answer to a permanent weight loss. Both women spent fortunes going to "fat farms" and "fat doctors," and taking a wide assortment of "fat pills." All of those programs resulted in, at most, only temporary successes and merely led to the nearly inevitable phenomenon of weight "yo-yoing" — and escalating weight gains. If these wealthy women, who had access to the best informed, best trained, highest priced physicians and experts, could not find the answer to a permanent weight loss, how can an average person expect to get the answer by sending in twenty or thirty dollars to a mail order firm?

If common sense does not convince you, perhaps a few words from America's grandmother, Ann Landers will. If you cannot believe her, whom can you believe? The following is from her December 20, 1988 column.

> DEAR ANN: I keep reading about an amazing new pill developed by two prominent doctors at a world-famous hospital in Los Angeles.
>
> With this pill, you can continue to eat anything you want and you will lose weight without exercise. The pill is called a fat magnet because it breaks into thousands of particles, and each particle acts like a tiny

magnet, attracting and trapping fat particles. This is 100 percent safe and not a drug. The price for this miraculous weight loss pill is only $38 for 180 pills.

Tell me, Ann, do these pills work? — Too Much Me (Tulsa)

DEAR TULSA: Yes, they will work wonders — for the people who sell them. They will get rich. The so-called magic diet pills are a total rip-off. What you read was not a news story. It's an ad. Papers that accept such ads do their readers an injustice if they fail to clearly identify them as such.

When such an ad *is* identified as being an advertisement, the word is typically in very small print, compared to the printing in the ad, and is not very close to the text. This makes the identifying word easy to overlook.

The question that is apt to pop into most minds is, "But how about the ads that promise a 100% full money back guarantee?" Ah yes, that ranks right up there with the ever-popular, "The check's in the mail," "Trust me," and other more colorful pledges.

MAGGOTS are despicable creatures, but they are also cunning. They realize most fat people have a mind-set for failure when it comes to losing weight. They have failed at so many reducing attempts, with or without "reducing aids," they automatically blame themselves when yet another product fails. Even if people want to write for a refund, they tend to be embarrassed at having to admit to another failure. They just want to try to forget about it.

There are, of course, the rare individuals who do write for a refund. How do they fare? I'll let Ann handle this one, too. The letter from her April 23, 1989 column, was written by a typical victim of yo-yoing.

DEAR ANN: I have dieted all my life, lost at least 1,000 pounds over the last 20 years and gained it all back. Now I am heavier than ever.

I am looking at two newspaper advertisements, and they both sound convincing. I don't know which one to choose. One is a pill. It breaks into tiny particles and acts like a magnet. It attracts the undigested fat, which is flushed out of the body because it cannot be absorbed. This is guaranteed to work or you get your money back. The price is $35 for 180 pills plus $3 for handling.

The other is called "the lazy way" to lose weight — as much as 10 pounds a week while eating six meals a day. And you can eat anything you want. This is based on the ketosis theory that makes your body go into a fat-burning frenzy. The cost is $17.95 plus $2 for handling. Money-back guarantee if not satisfied. What do you think, Ann? — Desperate in Denver.

DEAR DENVER: I think they are both ripoffs and the real miracle is how they stay in business. Many people have written to say they have asked for their money back and their letters have been ignored.

Do you think an antifat business expects anyone to sue them to get a refund? Of course not. Who's going to hire an expensive lawyer (now, that *is* a redundancy) to try and recover twenty or thirty dollars — especially if the deceptive firm is located in another city or state? Since the companies often do not intend to refund the money, you may wonder why they don't offer a "*double* your money back" guarantee. Actually, some do — and don't be surprised if before long you see a promise of "triple your money back."

Why is the antifat industry so successful? One reason is that some marketing and advertising geniuses have chosen to use their talents in corrupt ways. They are masters of misleading insinuation and at using fancy charts and information from obscure scientific studies — that are often irrelevant to their products anyway. Most of the entrepreneurs, however, are just people of average intelligence who have a lot of gall coupled with an aptitude for lying. Moreover, the public tends to believe any ad they see in print or on television. Fat people are particularly vulnerable because they want so much to believe. Even when lay persons have the expertise and financial wherewithal to research all of these products, they do not have the time. They are too busy earning a living.

Besides, they probably think the various governmental agencies — federal, state, and local — are vigilantly protecting the public from phony reducing schemes. Logic, however, suggests that if the agencies were effective, there would not be so much false advertising or so many "worthless" products flooding the marketplace. This is not a condemnation of governmental agencies. Oh, there are plenty of things for which those institutions *can* be blamed, but they do not deserve sole blame for their ineffectiveness. They sometimes try, but it is just too expensive for prosecutors to bring all of the unscrupulous companies into a court system whose dockets are drastically overcrowded as it is.

Not only are legal actions against weight-reduction scams rarely undertaken, successful prosecutions are often meaningless anyway. A manufacturer who is making a million dollars per year from a bogus product can retain a lawyer and for a surprisingly small fee keep the case from being heard for years. When the manufacturer is finally ordered to "cease and desist," and perhaps pay a relatively small fine, he will have lost an inconsequential sum compared to the huge profits he had been raking in all along. Even as swindlers are laughing their way out of the courthouse, they can already have a slightly different product ready to foist onto the public under a different name or company — perhaps in another state.

While specific individuals are initially cheated by a manufacturer, the public ultimately has to pay the substantial court costs through their taxes. In other words, even when the government wins, the people still lose. Governmental "watch dog" agencies through experience have learned they are attempting to stem the flood of dishonest companies with a teacup. The antifat industry is gleefully aware of the government's nearly futile position. The best protective advice to the consumer is *caveat emptor*. If you learn only one Latin phrase in your entire life, let it be this one. Essentially it means, "Buy at your own risk." It's the most important advice anyone will ever get when it comes to purchasing anything.

If you feel a local company is committing fraud by selling a product or service, you can voice a complaint with the Better Business Bureau. For national firms, contact the local office of consumer affairs or state attorney general's office. They can direct you to the appropriate federal agency such as the Federal Trade Commission, Consumer Product

Safety Commission, or Food and Drug Administration. You might want to contact the National Council Against Health Fraud — Task Force on Victim Redress. This non-governmental agency helps consumers find legal and medical assistance. The ultimate move may be to catch the attention and aid of Ralph Nader, a defender of consumer rights and one of the few current American heroes. The FDA, incidentally, has identified a number of categories in which medical fraud is most frequent; figure enhancers are at the top of the list.

The antifat crowd is successful in convincing people that fat is awful stuff because the industry has learned the effectiveness of the "Big Lie." That is, the bigger the falsehood, the more likely the public is to believe it, particularly if the lie is told often enough and loud enough. The Big Lie technique worked for Hitler's Minister of Propaganda, Joseph Goebbels, and it works just as well for MAGGOTS.

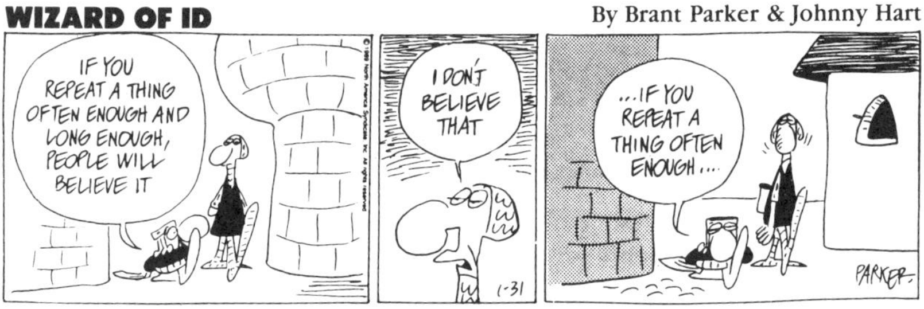

By permission of Johnny Hart and NAS, Inc.

The efficacy of the Big Lie soars when the public does not have the opportunity to hear the truth — the whole truth. This is why a dictator always suppresses freedom of speech immediately upon gaining power. The public only hears one side — his side. Even when a society *does* have freedom of speech, though, the truth can be withheld effectively from the population by slick marketing experts. A prime example of this deception is seen in the antifat industry. It spends vast sums of money each year to denigrate fatness — not just excessive fatness, but fat in general. A favorite ploy is to publicize information from research which lends credence to their claims, and to withhold information which debunks their claims. The results are half-truths which tend to be more deceptive, and even more effective, than outright lies.

The rationale behind freedom of speech is clear. It gives every faction in an argument the opportunity to present its case to the public, which presumably is then able to make an intelligent decision. Unfortunately, our founding fathers did not envision the run-away capitalism that exists today. In such situations ethics takes the backseat to the almighty buck. The dollar is the "bottom line." A motion picture, *Crazy People*, released in 1990, gives a satiric view of the sad state of ethics in the advertising industry. In real life, lies and deceptions are not nearly as funny.

Not surprisingly, the people with the most money have the loudest voices. They are in the driver's seat as far as the Big Lie is concerned. Antifat companies are in an especially advantageous position. "Suckers" are constantly pouring huge sums of money into their coffers, a large portion of which the companies can devote to advertising. This process helps them sell more of their products and put even more dollars into advertising. In addition, the smell of "easy" money — like garbage to flies — constantly attracts other sleazy entrepreneurs. The result is a vicious cycle that spirals ever upward in terms of both antifat business and antifat propaganda. With this cycle in mind, it is easy to understand the persuasive power of the antifat companies.

Who is going to dispute their misleading claims? Few individuals have the time or financial resources to present an opposing viewpoint. Other businesses are not going to lead the way because there is little or no money to be made in such an endeavor. There *is* an organization called the National Association to Advance Fat Acceptance (NAAFA). Basically, it is dedicated to fighting prejudice against fat people and working to end discrimination in employment, education, access to public accomodations, and adequate medical care. These goals are undeniably commendable. The efforts of the NAAFA to reduce antifat attitudes would be much more effective, however, if they would attack the roots of fatism by exposing the purely mercenary aims and fraudulent methods of the antifat industry.

Even if the NAAFA broadened its objectives, however, it would still be largely incapable of achieving them. Because the organization lacks the money to effectively disseminate information, it has very little chance in getting across *any* message. An indication of the group's inability to inform the public is revealed in the fact that very few people have even heard of the NAAFA, and it has been in existence since 1969. With a monthly *NAAFA Newsletter* circulation of about 3,500, the odds that they are going to significantly increase their financial base in the near future and improve their capacity to speak effectively on behalf of fat people are negligible.

Due to the lack of informational balance, the public only hears one side of the fat story — the unfavorable side. Can you imagine a judge hearing only one side of a case and attempting to arrive at a fair decision? It is impossible. It's difficult enough after hearing both sides, which is why there are appellate courts to review decisions made by lower courts — and supreme courts for further appeals. Even they sometimes reverse their decisions.

While it is true that *excessive* fatness is, by definition, unhealthy, that's all it is. Excessive fatness does not necessarily mean a person eats intemperately or is slothful, or is mentally or emotionally deficient, or immoral. Unfortunately, when brainwashed into believing such things are true, people will generally be willing to do or take anything to lose fat — even if they are manifestly underweight. At this stage of indoctrination, they become easy prey for MAGGOTS.

It is not difficult to see how people can be victimized by the antifat industry into developing a fat paranoia. That includes well-meaning health professionals in such fields as medicine, public health, and education who preach an antifat doctrine. It would not be fair to call these people MAGGOTS, of course; they have just been deluded, along with the rest of society, by the Big Lie.

That should come as no surprise. Having grown up in an antifat culture, these respected professionals have acquired the same negatively biased attitudes toward fatness as everyone else. It is well-known that attitudes instilled in childhood tend to be remain fixed when one becomes an adult. Mark Twain, who was as much a philosopher as a humorist, observed in, *Is Shakespeare Dead*?

> I am aware that when even the brightest mind in our world has been trained up from childhood in a superstition of any kind, it will never be possible for that mind in its maturity to examine sincerely, dispassionately, and conscientiously any evidence which shall seem to cast a doubt upon the validity of the superstition.

This persistent narrow-mindedness leads to "tunnel vision" in health professionals. That is, their brains absorb only that information which confirms their profoundly entrenched beliefs.

A reluctance to change is no modern phenomenon. It is the reason many of Aristotle's false conclusions held sway for more than 2,000 years — and Ptolemy's "Earth is the center of the universe" idea was dogma for nearly 1,500 years. Today, intolerance for new ideas and truth is not limited to the health-related professions. It is rampant in all academic disciplines. Indeed, such intolerance is the logical outcome of our educational system wherein students, above all, must demonstrate the ability to be parrots.

This parrot mentality is most deeply ingrained in university faculties. Teachers, who aspire to become respected professors and leaders in their fields, quickly learn that any deviation from academic orthodoxy leads to denunciation — and has a stifling affect on their careers. As columnist Joseph Alsop wrote about the halls of academia, people who see their position being blown apart by new evidence also see their prestige, careers, and everything else being "blown to hell." Of course, this servile adherence to ideas that are politically correct is the opposite of what a university should be. An exchange of ideas should be encouraged; that process is *essential* in seeking truth.

Certainly no group is more aware of the current resistance to change than the professors themselves. Father Andrew M. Greeley, a sociologist with the National Opinion Research Center at the University of Chicago, observed that fashionable beliefs leave "little room for dissent." He proceeds to observe that the typical academic "is serenely confident of his own judgment and thus assumes that those who dare to disagree with him are not only wrong but are either stupid or in bad faith or, quite conceivably both . . ."

George Orwell, in a rejected preface to *Animal Farm*, also observed that anyone who challenges prevailing beliefs is silenced with surprising effectiveness. He states that this oppression would be bad enough, but the people who *do* think and are able to arrive at new perspectives are held up to ridicule as if they were crackpots by their more conservative colleagues.

It is from such inflexible, unenlightened clouds that pour the flood of antifat dictums. And information, like water and other far less savory material, flows downhill. Public health departments unquestioningly suck up the effluence and pump it on. The Fourth Estate, print and broadcast, which depends chiefly upon experts for information, picks up the information (unaware of its biased source) and disseminates it to an even more naive constituency. From thence the news spreads by word of mouth. This brings to mind the old dictum, "A lie makes two trips around the Earth while the truth is just getting to its feet." No, most health professionals do not purposefully mislead the public, but they certainly give a lot of "rotting meat" to MAGGOTS who know how to best use it for their avaricious purposes.

Taking into account their societal and professional environment, it is not difficult to see how well-meaning health professionals can unwittingly contribute to the perpetuation of antifat propaganda. It is understandable and can be forgiven. When highly trained professionals purposefully metamorphose into MAGGOTS, that is quite another story. Few character flaws are as contemptible as the selling of one's ethics for material gain.

It is even more reprehensible when physicians "fall from grace." They have taken the Hippocratic oath to serve their fellow man. Lay people expect them to be saints and the American Medical Association over the years has done its best to foster that image. Well, there are very few saints around—even though I suspect that physicians as a rule come a lot closer to that ideal than any other professional group. Unfortunately, a certain percentage of people in any group will take unethical shortcuts to financial gain. When physicians abuse the public trust in their revered position, they become the slimiest of MAGGOTS.

That some medical doctors do succumb to financial temptation is reflected in the strong trend for unsavory antifat companies to have them on their payrolls. Indeed, more and more antifat organizations are adopting medical-sounding names that are designed to lend credence to their operations. Apparently they hope such catchwords as "doctors," "physicians," "nurses," and "medical" will lull their prey into a false sense of trust. Unfortunately, the technique is a very effective one.

I recall an obese student asking me about a hospital-associated weight-loss program she had joined. Upon learning that its main feature was an expensive liquid protein supplement and that the program cost more than $3,000, I told her it smacked of skullduggery. "But, it's with a hospital!" was her astonished, incredulous reply. Since she was obviously "hooked," I merely changed the subject. The woman did go on to lose a lot of weight. About a year later she stopped by my office and gloatingly rubbed her much reduced body in my face — figuratively, of course. I was fond of the woman and was pleased that she was happy. Not surprisingly, however, when I spotted her in a mall a few years later, she was larger than ever. Puddings and milkshakes apparently lose their appeal after awhile.

Hospitals are businesses in what has become a very competitive field. According to the National Association for Hospital Development, most private (non-tax supported) hospitals in this country are suffering from a malady called "red ink" syndrome and their financial situation is desperate. Requiring weight-loss patients to undergo tests, and have periodic examinations and counseling can bring in a lot of money — from $2,000 to $6,000 per patient. It is impossible to fault the concept of medical supervision in weight reduction, but the programs would be much more credible if the hospitals would simply sever their associations with the liquid protein companies and concentrate on life-style changes based entirely upon a sensible, and effective, program of exercise and a balanced diet.

Sometimes a hospital's antifat advertising seductively cries, "Come to our *free* seminar to learn about our program. Hurry, space is going fast!" It's a nice marketing touch. The seminar, of course, is a hard-sell promotion for their program. Can you imagine a used car dealer using this sales approach? "Come to a *free* seminar to learn about our cars.

Hurry, space is going fast!" You would break out laughing. The main difference between used car salespeople and the hospital's liquid diet salespeople is that the latter wear starched, white coats. By joining forces with a "nutrition" company whose only concern is to sell their products, these health professionals are walking a very thin ethical line. There is truth to the adage, "You are known by the company you keep."

Some medical doctors have dashed across that thin line by selling their souls and becoming MAGGOTS themselves. Apparently, there are enough of these Hippocratic defectors (and impostors) to have their own mailing list. As a result, falling for one of the doctor's ads means a person will soon be getting information from a bunch of other "fallen" doctors who smell fresh meat. My wife got on the mailing list after I had asked her to respond to one ad that had a distinctly MAGGOTY stench about it.

The ad in question was an unobtrusive little three or four liner from a "Board of Medical Advisors" in North Miami Beach, Florida. By deviating from the typical large, flamboyant ad, it was an effective — and very inexpensive ploy. The ad indicated the board was involved in fat research and needed participants. Those who qualified for the "once in a lifetime" program were promised a $1,000 U.S. treasury bond.

When the brochure arrived (from Dayton, Ohio) it claimed the board consisted of a Ph.D. and four M.D.s — one of whom was a psychiatrist. The latter could conceivably be of some use since a person would have to be crazy to fall for the scheme. The board was merely a front for an organization that sold the "Ultimate Solution Diet Program." Their offerings included puddings, shakes, and wafers, along with little goodies called "Super Energy Plus Diet Pills" and appetite suppressors. Included, too, was the latest wrinkle — *nighttime* diet tablets. All of the containers were wrapped with blue labels emblazoned with a flag-like pattern of red and white stripes. It seemed as if buying the stuff would be a patriotic act.

Oh yes, to qualify as a subject for the "research" a person had to pass a test to meet the qualifications. It was not difficult. Mainly, a person had to buy at least a two-months supply of the product. The cost was a minimum of $229.90 — and the company "graciously" allowed a person to buy the stuff even if test participation was declined.

Still, getting a $1,000 bond for signing up does not sound like a bad deal until one learns, *after* signing up, that the bond is not worth $1,000 when it is received. It is worth a small fraction of that amount. The exact amount depends upon a variety of factors including the number of decades required for the bond to mature and the market cost at the time of purchase. I checked with an economics professor at the time of the offerings and she estimated the bond's cost, considering twenty-five years for maturity, to be $115.00 or less. Not a bad business to be in! Not only did the Board of Medical Advisors make a substantial profit on the bonds they were "giving" customers, they also sucked the people into laying out at least $115.00 a month for their outrageously over-priced product.

Shortly after receiving the so-called research material, other "medically" related antifat ads began littering our mailbox. One arrived in a plain white envelope with a hand applied stamp. Both the return address and destination address appeared to have been hand-typed on a machine with a worn ribbon — a very folksy touch. We did not recognize the name, which made the letter very intriguing. We thought it must have been sent by an acquaintance we had not seen in a long time. There was no hint of "junk mail" about it, although later I did notice the telltale "bulk rate" printed in small letters on the postage stamp. Overcome with curiosity, we tore open the bulging envelop to reveal a very slick, large, full color brochure for an HGH (human growth hormone) stimulant. Strangely, although the return address of the doctor (he claimed to be a Doctor of Osteopathy) was in Norcross, Georgia, in his brochure he claimed to be practicing in California. You may appreciate the opening sentence of his letter.

> Dear Dieter: It's very unusual for a doctor to ever endorse any kind of diet product, but a diet aid has finally been perfected with such astounding weight loss potential that I feel I must speak out and tell everyone about it.

Gosh, what a public spirited fellow! We laughed so hard at the ploy, and our gullibility, tears came to our eyes — which proves that junk mail can have some amusement value. At one time it may have been unusual for a doctor to be involved in such a scam, but this is no longer the case. Still, one has to admire the ingenuity of the man's approach. I doubt if anyone would have thrown the letter away without reading it, and that clearly was the intent of the plain, but enticing, envelope.

In my case the doctor's subterfuge was unnecessary since I collect such antifat junk. Maybe I'll open a MAGGOT MUSEUM some day. Logically, it should be in Bridgeport, Connecticut, next to the newly renovated Phineas T. Barnum Museum. P.T. has gone down in history as the man who observed, "There's a sucker born every minute." He would really appreciate an antifat museum.

Shortly after the appearance of the D.O.'s letter, another antifat epistle arrived using the same persuasive approach and a similar product. It was even from the identical address in Norcross, Georgia (it must get a tad crowded in that office). The only thing different was the doctor's name. In his letter he said:

> Dear Friend: It's about time you were told the truth about dieting . . . the American public has become addicted to dieting . . . and dieting failure.
>
> This is why a group of physicians and researchers formed the Medical Council for Weight Loss. We decided that in order to expose the truth about dieting we would have to form a professional association to stand up against the multi-billion dollar business of selling diets.

Large letters in their brochure proclaimed, "YOUR BODY WAS MADE TO BE SLIM." The proclamation, which conflicts completely with somatotype studies, immediately casts some shadow on the credibility of the self-esteemed Medical Council. This group also resorted to the use of a well-worn gimmick — a "free gift." The offering was a facial cream that, ". . . is so powerful, it has been proven to help restore and heal severely damaged skin. In fact, it showed 'excellent' results and improvement *within just 16 hours.*" Of course, if their antifat product was so effective, they wouldn't need a gimmick. And if the skin gunk was so marvelous, they would not be giving it away. People with fistfuls of dollars would be beating down the company's doors. Still, a more devastating one-two sales punch is hard to imagine.

The most ingenious, most underhanded, sneakiest "letter" my wife ever received came from California. It consisted simply of a newspaper clipping about a dietary plan — with a handwritten message that read, "Judy, I thought you might be interested in this." There was no hint of the sender's identity. It was, of course, most intriguing. The mystery was solved about a year later when I was discussing antifat schemes at a women's club. I did not bring up the "California clipping" because it had never crossed my mind that it was a ruse. One of the women, however, mentioned offhandedly that she had received such a clipping. At least one-third of the women joined me in laughingly shouting, "I got one, too!" Until that moment they had been mystified also.

The classic example of a MAGGOTY association between an antifat company and health professionals was revealed in the "superpill" scandal of 1987. Dietary supplements manufactured by United Sciences of America, Inc. (USA, Inc.) claimed in their ads to help those who were "Overworked. Stressed. Always tired. Overweight. Underweight." The firm's primary attraction was its advisory board of "internationally acclaimed scientists and medical professionals." Their photos and quotes were liberally displayed in the firm's promotional literature. The M.D.s and Ph.D.s got between $10,000 to $15,000 each for lending their names. As Frederick Stare, Harvard professor emeritus of nutrition, suggested — if the money had not been so generous, his colleagues would have exercised more critical judgment before allowing "their names and the institutions where they work to be used for such shoddy commercial purposes." Indeed, after the dangers and dubious values of the company's products were exposed, most of the experts practically fell over themselves in dissociating themselves from the company. The fact that they had usually been misquoted, or their words taken out of context, accelerated their retreat.

It must be granted that most health professionals are as ethical as could be reasonably expected. No doubt most of them also know that the vast preponderance of weight reducing products are worthless. Why then do they not speak out and expose the MAGGOTS? The health pros just do not have the time or financial means to do so. They also realize that by speaking out they can be dragged into court by the powerful companies — and justice, unfortunately, does not always prevail. It has long been said, and for good reason, that justice is primarily for rich people — and in these types of cases the allegation is even more likely to be true. Even if justice were to prevail, and a health professional exonerated for revealing the truth, the cost of legal protection would still be financially destructive. Understandably, many concerned professionals just stick their heads in the sand. If it appears as if the antifat industry has all the cards stacked in its favor, that is very close to the truth. Again, the *caveat emptor* advice cannot be overemphasized!

Why am *I* being so "courageous" in exposing the antifat crowd? Simply because I have very little to fear. First, after more than thirty years in the health and fitness field, primarily as a university professor, I can retire anytime I want. This gives me the luxury of being able to speak the truth even if it does go against the grain of my profession and lead to ostracism. Second, it would be a waste of time for the MAGGOTS to sue me; I frankly do not have enough money to make it worth their while (and, fortunately, I don't need very much). True, they may be able to legally force me to recant my position because I do not have the financial resources required to defend myself against a massively funded industry, but the truth is already out.

Maybe I'm not courageous at all. Maybe I'm just tired, and angry, at seeing fat people suffer at the hands of insensitive people. That refers to strangers as well as friends. It's heartbreaking when you see a fat person, almost always a woman, and by her demeanor you know she feels worthless and undeserving of love — just because she is fat by today's standards. For a long time I've been standing with my hands in my pockets saying, "Tsk, tsk, isn't it awful the way the antifat bullies are hurting a large, innocent segment of our society?" Well, I took my hands out of my pocket to write *Fat is NOT a Four-Letter Word*.

I jokingly tell people this book is my ticket to Heaven. Maybe it is more than a joke, though; maybe it's wishful thinking. I have known for many years that fat is not a four-letter word, but did not start writing the book until I had an extremely close brush with death. Such an experience can give a person a new outlook on life, ethics, and priorities. If anything I have done in my somewhat checkered life is a ticket to Heaven, I firmly believe this comes the closest. And while the antifat crowd is admittedly very powerful on Earth, I have a hunch it's a whole new ball game on the Other Side — and justice a lot less complicated.

Deceptive marketing, of course, is certainly not unique to the antifat industry. The public is particularly gullible when it comes to "beauty" products. For instance, women have been beguiled into believing they have to remove hair from their legs, that underarm hair is gross, that walking into a room without first using a feminine deodorant spray will cause people to gasp and pass out, and that perspiring is an abomination against God. When you come right down to it, most so-called beauty aids actually have an adverse effect on the user's health. The current obsession with cleanliness, for instance, destroys the beneficial bacteria and dries the skin; hair colorizers damage, sometimes severely, the very thing they are supposed to enhance; and the FDA says there are nearly five hundred toxic agents found in cosmetics. Feminine douches are not only unnecessary for the overwhelming majority of women, they interfere with the natural healthy environment of the vagina and lead to problems.

The preoccupation with every aspect of physical appearance has gotten out of hand, but has reached its greatest obsession in the antifat miasma that pervades our culture. An obsession is an psychiatric term meaning a fixed idea or feeling, usually irrational, over which a person has little conscious control — it can also mean domination by an evil spirit. It is easy to think of MAGGOTS in this latter sense. Their constant gnawing has profoundly damaged the physical and psychological well-being of multitudes of undeserving people. If that is not evil, what is?

At this point the reader can be excused for believing this to be a pro-fat book. However, it most assuredly is not. Its aim is not to persuade people to become fat. In fact, people who are truly excessively fat and who want to lose weight should be encouraged to do so. But they should do it for reasons of their own, not to conform to a society's narrow-minded dictates.

No, this is not a pro-fat book. It can most accurately be called an *anti*-antifat book. As such, it is staunchly against the denigration of fat people — ranging from those who are morbidly obese to those who are not fat at all but who have been bullied by an antifat social environment into believing they are fat. Major goals of this book are to shed light on the concept of excessive fatness and health, and show that a person's percentage of body fat has nothing to do with her or his value as a person. To accomplish these aims it is essential to expose the intentions and deceptions of a massive antifat industry that is infested with MAGGOTS. Vastly compounding their sins is their cultivation of legions of lackeys, called FATISTS. These small creatures arise from beings who in general lack sensitivity, compassion, and strength of character. No, fat is *not* a four-letter word. The same cannot be said, however, of MAGGOTS and FATISTS.

9

ANTIFAT PILLS AND POTIONS

The medical profession has not always routinely treated fatness as a disease. That makes sense since, generally, it is not a disease — although, in a small percentage of the cases obesity is a *symptom* of a disorder. Before 1950, physicians sensed that the vast majority of those who are today called fat people were within the normal range of fatness for their body types.

Then in the 1960s, due to some studies that showed extreme obesity to be related to various illnesses, many doctors began treating all "fat" people as being diseased. The medics' chief approach was to prescribe such remedies as appetite suppressants, diuretics, thyroid hormones, and even digitalis (a highly toxic heart stimulant). The weight losses were, disappointingly, only temporary. Also, judging from the drugs' effects on millions of human "guinea pigs," the potions were far more of a threat to a person's health and well-being than was fatness — particularly in people who were not excessively fat to begin with.

Amphetamine, a nervous system stimulant, was the main prescription appetite suppressant. The problem is that it also has serious adverse side effects. Often sold under the name of benzedrine, and commonly called "bennies" or "speed," regular use of amphetamines can cause, among other problems, ulcers, strokes, cardiovascular collapse, and death. Behavioral modifications include insomnia, increased irritability, aggression, delusions, and symptoms of paranoid schizophrenia.

Coming down from an amphetamine high can lead to acute depression — and suicide. To top it off, users can get "hooked" on the drug. After facing all of this in order to suppress the appetite, people experience a rebound effect when they stop taking speed. With the dramatic increase in appetite that occurs, the percentage of body fat usually rebounds to new levels. Although there has been a crackdown on the dispensing of amphetamines, there are still many "diet doctors" who prescribe them.

Common over-the-counter (OTC) appetite suppressants include

Acutrim II, Appedrine, Control, Super Odrinix, Prolamine, Permathene-12, Hunger-Plus, Dexatrim, and Grapefruit-Plus. All of these, including the latter, have precisely the same active ingredient, phenylpropanolomine (PPA), and the same daily dose (75 mg). The words "safe and effective" are typically prominent in large, colorful letters on the containers. Warnings, however, are listed on the backside of the package in tiny print. One has to wonder how many customers read this information or take it seriously. After all, in bold letters the products are proclaimed to be safe. Below is the small print from a typical OTC appetite suppressant. You can judge for yourself if such a product sounds harmless.

> If you have or are being treated for high blood pressure, diabetes, or heart, thyroid, kidney, or other diseases, or depression, or are pregnant or nursing, do not take this product except under the supervision of a physician. If you become nervous, sleepless, or dizzy, stop taking the medication.

The warning does not indicate the *severity* of the risks for some people, particularly those with the disorders mentioned. Further, millions of people are unaware that they have "high blood pressure, diabetes, or heart, thyroid, kidney, or other diseases." Risks increase with prolonged use but there are cases of convulsions and strokes occurring after taking only a single dose. Virtually all of the risks can be attributed to PPA.

Unfortunately, there is a very small margin of safety with PPA. That makes it particularly easy to overdose on the pills for users who believe an increase in the dosage will increase their rate of weight loss.

Even without this misguided belief it is easy to overdose on PPA because other OTC drugs also contain PPA. The most common are the cold remedies, such as Contac, Dimetapp, Comptrex, Walgreens' Cold Capsules, and Alka-Seltzer Plus. In addition, the risk of PPA is increased with the consumption of caffeine which Americans ingest in vast quantities in coffee, soft drinks, and chocolate. And caffeine is not all that innocuous by itself, especially for consumers who also smoke cigarettes.

In addition to the common beverages, caffeine is also found in such products as No Doz, Vivarin, and Pep-Back. In fact, that drug is the only active ingredient contained in these sleep retarding tablets. The caffeine may be called a different name, such as Stimucin (in Vivarin) or Eleveine (in Pep-Back) — which, of course, misleads consumers. At least No Doz is not deceptive; its package clearly states, "caffeine tablets."

These caffeine pills are advertised as being for students, drivers, and *dieters*. The back of their packages list warnings such as: too much caffeine may cause nervousness, irritability, sleeplessness, and rapid heart beat . . . for occasional use only . . . do not give to children under 12 . . . if you are pregnant or nursing a baby, consult a doctor before using . . . in case of overdose see a doctor or contact a poison control center immediately. One warning is rather amusing: "If sleep or drowsiness persists, consult a doctor." See a doctor! What's wrong with foregoing the caffeine product, and lying down and sleeping when you are sleepy? Jay Leno, the comedian, observed on NBC's Tonight Show that, "Colombia is responsible for 75% of our nation's addicts — and that's just the people who drink coffee." In a more serious vein, the containers of products with caffeine never warn the consumer that the drug is addictive or that it increases the risk of PPA reactions.

In spite of their "safe" claims, OTC appetite suppressants are not as harmless as their advertising would lead a user to believe. To those who may believe the risk is worth taking in order to lose weight, it must be added that none of the products are effective anyway except in the short term — at best.

One popular weight-loss product, Ayds, is a lozenge whose active ingredient is a local anesthetic called benzocaine. The rationale behind the product's alleged effectiveness is that by numbing the tongue and reducing the sense of taste, eating will be less attractive — and the user will eat less. A stick of Slim-Mint gum, which advertises itself as an appetite control product, has the same amount of benzocaine. When results are achieved with this drug, they are also of a short term nature.

It is not unusual for a product to combine active ingredients. Thinz: Back-to-Nature pills and Stay Trim gum, for instance, both contain PPA *and* benzocaine. The combination does not make them any more effective than the other "aids."

Some people smoke cigarettes believing it helps them to lose weight. Indeed, the tobacco industry fosters the belief by using always thin models in their ads. Or do you think that is just a coincidence? Smoking does have an appetite suppressing effect, and because it makes the heart work harder, it does increase a smoker's metabolic rate. As such, it generally results in a weight loss of about five to ten pounds. But smoking killed more than 400,000 people in the U.S. alone in 1991. The "cigarette diet" is far-and-away the most deadly of all weight-reducing schemes.

Diuretics, including many OTC products such as Aqua-ban and Diurex, are often used by people who want to lose weight. The products do not contribute, however, one iota to helping a user lose *fat.* Since diuretics cause a person to urinate more often than normal, any reduction of body weight is merely due to a loss of water. When the water is replaced, people gain the weight right back. To keep the weight off, the water intake must be continually restricted. This results in dehydration, which can be very detrimental to health.

Some physicians do prescribe diuretics to weight reducers. Apparently those doctors feel a weight loss is more important than the depletion of such substances as potassium from the body that is caused by the pills. This depletion can cause lightheadedness, weakness, and muscle cramps. Diuretics do have legitimate medical benefit in disorders such as high blood pressure, but a few extra pounds of body weight due to natural water levels is hardly a medical problem. Besides, since every drug has risks, it does not make sense to take needless risks just to lose a few pounds of water weight. Unfortunately, when physicians will not prescribe diuretics, people can waste their money and build up false hopes by purchasing over-the-counter diuretics.

Nearly all bodybuilding contestants take diuretics so they will look more muscular. The procedure is particularly effective since steroid use results in water retention and a bloated appearance. As a result of the diuretic abuse, however, severe dehydration is common. The contestants are flirting with death. Some, including professional champions, have needed emergency treatment backstage to save their lives. Indeed, a world champion named Hans Sallmeyer died as a result of taking diuretics before a contest.

Paradoxically, the best natural diuretic is water itself. Drinking large quantities of water depresses the body's level of antidiuretic hormone (vasopressin). That causes the kidneys to secrete more water and sodium, thereby *reducing* fluid retention. In addition to being safe, drinking a lot of water is beneficial to health in a number of ways.

A popular antifat prescription, especially among women, is the thyroid hormone, thyroxine. It increases the rate at which the body burns calories. That sounds fine except that people who are considered to be fat seldom have a true thyroid deficiency or a low energy expenditure to begin with. Giving them enough of the hormone to significantly increase their metabolic rate requires levels that are generally toxic. In addition, thyroxine usage can upset the balance of the entire endocrine system. That is really treading on dangerous ground. One specific hazard is the alteration of the contractile properties of the heart.

This is not to say that all doctors who prescribe thyroid hormones (and other weight-loss preparations) are irresponsible pill pushers. Some are compassionate people who feel sorry for patients who are trying desperately to lose weight. The shame is that society puts such pressure on these people — many of whom are not overweight at all for their genetic make-up and may even be too thin.

For some reason "weight-reducing" hormones are very popular. Perhaps the medical ring to "hormones" impresses people. In addition to the thyroxine already discussed, there is human chorionic gonadotropin (HCG) which is obtained from the urine of pregnant women. Its purveyors claim its use produces weight losses, but recent studies show that its injections have no more effect than ordinary salt water.

Anabolic steroids were the rage of the 1980s and are still used by large numbers of people, particularly males, to lose body fat and build muscle. There is substantial evidence, however, that the drugs are quite hazardous. For instance, after about three months of use a man's testicles start shriveling. That alone should give a male user some pause for thought. There are many other potential problems associated with the hormone, though, including headaches, rectal bleeding, cancer of the liver, kidney disorders, cardiovascular diseases — and really distressing problems like acne and premature baldness. Anabolic steroids can also upset the body's enzyme systems and breakdown genetic patterns in the nuclei of cells. Behavioral changes, called "'roid rages" include extreme aggressiveness, violent outbursts, and suicide.

Paradoxically, a male user of steroids can develop gynecomastia or as it is known in gyms, "bitch tits." They are the result of the body producing excess estrogen to counteract the tremendous increase of injected testosterone. These bulbous swellings, under one or both of the nipples, are especially likely to develop when a man stops taking the drug. Ben Johnson, whose steroid use was exposed during the 1988 Olympics, experienced these symptoms. He also had the moon-faced appearance and puffy looking physique that are indications of steroid use — due to its water retention effect.

As discussed in Chapter Four, anabolic steroids are undoubtedly even more harmful when women use them. One has to wonder if all of the hard work, time, dieting, and chemical abuse needed to acquire a fashionable body is really worth it. Are the hard bodies of today's female bodybuilding champions more attractive than those of traditional "full-figured" women? Is the epitome of the male body, as displayed by today's physique contest winners, more pleasing to the eye than, say, Michelangelo's *David* which was sculpted nearly 500 years ago.

A recent "body-shaping" pharmaceutical is the human growth hormone (HGH). Some antifat enterprises obviously felt they had to turn to a new gimmick when anabolic steroids began receiving a lot of bad press, including being banned by most athletic regulatory organizations. Sadly, all the publicity surrounding steroids has probably increased their use. Legions of aspiring young athletes apparently are thinking, "Hey, if Olympic and professional athletes are risking their health and serious punishment by taking steroids, it must really help to improve their athletic performances."

Many antifat moguls are pushing HGH just in case steroid sales do plummet. The growth hormone, in synthetic, injectable form, is being sold on the black market in much the same fashion as steroids. HGH is also banned by most athletic regulatory agencies including the U.S. Olympic Committee, The National Collegiate Athletic Association, and the National Football League. The sales pitch is that HGH helps increase a person's muscle mass while at the same time reducing body fat. There is some truth to the claims — but only if users are deficient in HGH to begin with or if they use huge, dangerous injections of the very expensive hormone.

A prospective buyer should be aware that HGH, which is extracted from the pituitary glands of cadavers, effects the growth of every organ in the body except the eyeballs and the brain. Unfortunately, the internal organs may grow even faster than the musculo-skeletal system and space can get a bit crowded inside the thorax. The heart may enlarge so much that congestive heart failure occurs. As pointed out by Robert Voy, M.D. (chief medical officer for the U.S. Olympic Committee) in an April, 1987 congressional hearing, other problems include diabetes, thyroid disorders, decreased sexual desire, and a shortened life span.

The most visible result of elevated HGH levels is acromegaly. Although it may be a cute word, acromegaly refers to a condition that is characterized by a Frankensteinian look — which is not cute at all. The bones of the feet, hands, forehead, nose and jaw enlarge, along with the cartilage and soft tissue of the nose, lips, naso-labial folds, and tongue. In addition to the wide range of disfiguration, the joint distortions lead to pain and a decrease in ranges of motion. Acromegaly occurs naturally when a person has a disorder of the pituitary gland that leads to an excess production of HGH. The condition, however, can also result from HGH abuse.

When HGH is not kept refrigerated, even during shipping, it loses its potency. Although its users are being "ripped off," in reality they are lucky when it's weakened; it is less harmful. In addition, as with most illegitimate drugs, HGH is often mislabeled. Many buyers are actually only getting saltwater — extremely expensive saltwater. These users, in terms of health, are the most fortunate of HGH consumers.

HGH must be purchased on the black market; commercial channels are too chancy even for MAGGOTS. Some have found a way to circumvent the law, however. The latest scam from the antifat industry involves amino acids that purportedly stimulate a person's body to produce its own HGH. The potential adverse side effects are never listed in the sales literature. On the contrary, they proclaim, "It's safe, natural, and works with your body instead of against it."

This identical proclamation was once the safety rationale behind birth control pills and anabolic steroids, which also achieve their objective by tampering with the body's endocrine system. Today, however, there is a long list of *known* contraindications, precautions, and adverse reactions associated with both types of these hormone products.

One reason the list is not as long for the HGH "releasers" is that they have not been around very long. The "guinea pigs" who take them are really taking a chance with their health. One sobering fact is that HGH is produced by the pituitary gland, the gland that is commonly called the "master gland." This gland, located at the base of the brain, controls the activity of all the other endocrine glands. If there is one gland a person should not tamper with, it is the pituitary. Legitimate doctors do prescribe HGH for pituitary dysfunctions, but not for people with normal pituitaries — the reasoning being, "If it ain't broke, don't try to fix it." That's a sound policy for anyone contemplating the use of *any* drug.

The dangers of taking various amino acids to release HGH may be, admittedly, a tempest in a teacup. There are no published accounts of research showing that the use of amino acids supplements can in fact increase HGH. Of course, this would mean there are no muscle building or fat burning benefits. There are still disadvantages, however. Studies show that the ingestion of individual amino acids results in amino acid imbalances which can actually cause a *decrease* in muscle building processes. Further, side effects include an increase in uric acid which can lead to such disorders as gout and kidney disease. With this information in mind the taking of amino acids to lose weight simply does not make sense. If people want to increase the HGH level in their blood, there is a safe, natural way to do so — moderate exercise.

By the end of the 1970s many reputable physicians had stopped prescribing any drugs for weight reduction or even attempting to treat it. Run-of-the-mill fatness was still commonly considered, erroneously, to be an illness but many physicians shied away from dealing with it because they realized they did not have enough understanding of the condition or the proper training.

Their new approach was, and still is to a large extent, to counsel fat patients to eat less and exercise more. Since the two ways a person can reduce body fat is to 1) take in fewer calories and 2) burn more calories, the advice seems logical. It is not that easy to follow, however, as any person who has tried to lose fat well knows. When the advice does not bring lasting results, which is almost always the case, a doctor will usually in frustration castigate patients for their lack of will power and send them on their bewildered, disappointed ways. The truth is, unless people have a medical condition that is responsible for their fatness, this procedure is about all a physician's training qualifies him to do. At least he, or she, is not charging patients for treatments that are not going to produce results — or may harm them.

With the withdrawal of reputable physicians from the field, people who desperately wanted to lose weight had no one to turn to. But "a vacuum is abhorred" in the medical world as well as in the natural world. If science cannot help a group of patients, disreputable characters will quickly slither into the breach with any number of worthless products and treatments. Quack promises are made for practically every disease from arthritis to cancer, as well as for a number of non-medical problems such as baldness — and, in most cases, fatness.

As mentioned in the previous chapter, the latest trend is for doctors to once again become involved in the very lucrative field of weight control. Dr. Robert D. Gillette of the St. Elizabeth Family Health Center in Youngstown, Ohio, expressed the opinion in the Letters Column of the *Journal of the American Medical Association* (April, 1989), that the increase in health care costs in the U.S. can be attributed in part to the tendency of doctors to treat variants of normal as diseases. This variation of normality is precisely the situation that exists for most people who are considered to be fat.

Many people who want to lose weight do not feel the need to seek expensive medical advice since non-medical MAGGOTS are offering a surfeit of potions and elixirs. Typically, the products are advertised as containing "miracle" ingredients such as royal jelly, ginseng, tryptophan, cider vinegar, garlic, and seaweed. A few catchy words such as organic, natural, and herbal will often be included in the ads as additional bait to ensnare desperate and naive customers.

That these "weight-loss" products are merely worthless is bad enough. Far worse are the ones that are also harmful to a user's health. Most of these products fall into the drug category. A drug is any substance taken into the body, other than food, that causes a change in the body.

The certification of all legal drugs to be safe is the responsibility of the Food and Drug Administration. It attempts to accomplish this with information based upon research. Usually the research for a drug is conducted by the manufacturer itself which is akin to installing Warren Beatty as housemother in a sorority house. Ideally, the FDA itself should do the testing, but they are grossly underfunded. And there is, of course, the corruption that nearly always exists whenever large sums of money are involved. An example of falsified test results, bribery, and fraud in the FDA, occurred in 1989 and involved the five billion dollar a year generic drug industry. Happily, there is now new leadership at the FDA and strong evidence of improved ethics and consumer protection. The new commissioner, David Kessler, is a physician and a lawyer. He says, "This agency means business" and the increased activity of the FDA shows he is serious.

There are so many antifat pills and potions on the market, with new ones proliferating like flies (What would you expect from MAGGOTS?), it is impossible to discuss all of them in this book. A general approach to the subject is the only practical course. Basic to this approach is the fact that every human being is unique. This individuality is widely known as far as finger-prints are concerned, but it also applies to practically every aspect of the body and mind.

The biochemical uniqueness explains why every drug, including medicines, affects each of us differently. Remember, even the finest, most unbiased research only reveals probabilities. The odds that aspirin, for instance, will relieve a headache is quite high. Yet, millions of people have such adverse side effects to aspirin that they cannot tolerate the drug. In addition to an individual's biochemical make-up, the severity of a drug's side effects depends one's age, sex, and weight. This situation applies to *every* drug, legal and illegal, and is a major reason why 125,000

Americans die each year from prescription drugs alone while millions upon millions suffer *known* adverse effects.

A person cannot know how any drug is going to affect him or her until it is taken. Further, a drug may affect a person one way one time and another way another time depending upon such things as the quality, dosage, and age of the drug. Other factors include a user's health, mental attitude, expectations, environment, time and method of administration, and frequency of dosages. Much also depends upon other drugs that have been taken, recently or concurrently. A drug may cancel, or heighten, the effects of other drugs — or a combination may even give rise to an entirely new set of physiological or psychological responses.

Moreover, drugs can break down and recombine with others to form new mixtures. This is true for practically all elements and compounds. Table salt which consists of sodium (Na) and chlorine (Cl) is a classic example. Sodium by itself is a soft, white-silver metal that is so light it will float in water. And it is so volatile it bursts into flame when it comes into contact with water. Chlorine is a greenish-yellow, foul-smelling, poisonous gas. Neither element would be a big hit at a smorgasbord. But, when Na and Cl combine, chemically, they produce "table salt" (NaCl) which adds considerable zest to our food. It is also vital for our bodies to function properly.

If two such simple elements as Na and Cl can combine to produce such a remarkably different compound, can you imagine the recombinant possibilities of two drugs with complex formulae? A famous example of drug interaction was seen in the Claus von Bulöw trial — *the* trial of the 80's. In the first trial he was found guilty of twice trying to kill his wife Martha ("Sunny") with insulin injections. He denied the accusations. During the second trial, it was found that Sunny had been injecting amobarbital and valium in a saline solution — and that this combination often shows the presence of insulin when, in reality, there is none. Apparently, Sunny's self-administered injections produced the "insulin" overdose that resulted in her falling into a profound coma. Von Bulöw was acquitted.

The number a possible drug interactions is mind boggling. Vastly complicating matters are the scores, perhaps hundreds, of "hidden" drugs we are ingesting each day. These hidden drugs come in such forms as food preservatives, taste enhancers, colorizers, residue from pesticides and insecticides, and chemicals (some of which are known to be carcinogenic) that are fed to animals to make them grow faster with less feed.

How do these drugs, *individually*, affect us in the long run? No one knows. We are all guinea pigs. Occasionally we learn that long term use of one these products or another is a severe health hazard. After a brief commotion, the offending drug is taken out of use and is replaced by another one — whose long-term effects we may learn about, if fortune smiles upon us, after another few decades or more. Infinitely exacerbating the problem is the *interaction* that takes place between these hidden drugs and the ones we knowingly take. How the interactions affect any specific individual are rarely known — until after the drugs are administered.

Drugs that are used to treat illnesses are called medicines. People take them because they figure they must in order to get well. In most cases the medicines seem to work; all you can really do is cross your fingers and hope. Still, it usually makes sense to take them because the alternative, not taking them, may be worse.

To take a drug, however, when there is no medical reason to do so is — how best to say it? — dumb? Yes, that's the best way to say it. It is DUMB! Why heighten an already largely unavoidable, potentially disastrous drug problem? Due to all of the hidden drugs and the medicines that we often cannot avoid taking, we are all playing Russian roulette. Why knowingly slide some *antifat* "bullets" into the chambers? The main reason people do so is because the antifat industry has such tremendous persuasive power. Over the years they have so frightened the masses with their propaganda that fatness, any amount, is now not only detested but is feared by vast numbers of people.

The antifat ads promise everything fat people want to hear, such as "Eat all you want, no exercise, safe, and 100% guaranteed." "Kiss your fat goodbye forever." More sophisticated approaches include wrapping the claims in a package of slick-sounding, pseudo-scientific jargon, and tossing in a free string of real faux pearls. "Faux," the French word for "false," is a particularly appropriate word considering the products with which the adjective is associated. Of the hundreds of weight-loss pills and potions I have ever seen advertised, I have *never* seen one that did not have a MAGGOTY stench about it. The simplest of common sense suggests that if a safe, bona fide product existed, it would not need advertising. It would be emblazoned across the front page of every newspaper and blare from every T.V. news program in America — and three seconds later the American Medical Association would probably see to it that you needed an expensive prescription to get it.

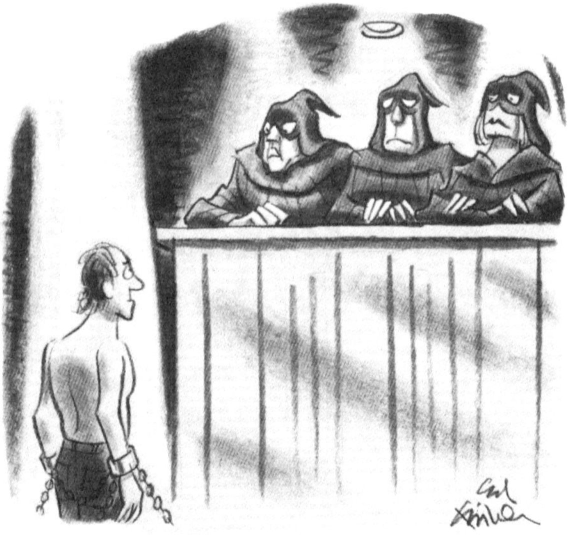

"You are charged with preaching wrongful, deviant and pernicious doctrine about weight loss."

The antifat industry is particularly adept at using a deception technique called "doublespeak." This term originated with an informative and amusing book entitled *Doublespeak*. Its author, William Lutz, shows how doublespeak is a:

". . . language that pretends to communicate but really doesn't. It is language that makes the bad seem good, the negative appear positive . . . language used to mislead, distort, deceive, inflate, circumvent, and obfuscate..."

Of Lutz's many military examples, my favorite was the way the Pentagon referred to their airborne invasion of Grenada. They called it "a predawn vertical insertion." It sounds as if the generals were confusing combat with sex. Indeed, upon reflection, that confusion may be the reason there are so many wars in the first place. At any rate, it makes one wonder about the general who came up with the ever popular "thrust from the rear" tactic.

Lutz is especially informative when it comes to the the world of advertising. He says their most popular words are "new," "improved," "virtually," "better," "extra," "fresh," "clean," "beautiful," "free," "great," "light," "helps," "acts," "works," and "fast." He calls these "weasel words" because they are as "hollow as any egg sucked by a weasel." In addition to the above mentioned words, some favorite weasel words employed by anti-fat companies are "safe," "doctor," "like magic," and "guaranteed."

A typical example of doublespeak was promulgated by Herbalite International in 1986. Authorities had charged them with making false claims in promoting its nutritional and weight-loss products. The company settled by agreeing to pay $850,000 and changing some of its claims. Afterwards, Herbalite's president issued the following press release:

> Today represents a milestone for Herbalite — a solid foundation that is built on the confidence given to us today by statements issued by state and federal regulatory agencies. I am pleased to announce that, after more than a year and a half of negotiations with the Food and Drug Administration, the California State Attorney General, and the California Department of Health, all three agencies have independently determined that Herbalite products have been and still are safe for the American public. Furthermore, all of our claims, labeling and marketing material are now in conformance with the spirit and the letter of both federal and state law.

Talk about making chicken salad out of chicken manure! The release almost makes it sound as if the government gave the company a good citizenship award. And you can bet that plenty of readers were duped.

More recently, Joe Weider, whose company grosses 250 million dollars a year, had to pay a $400,000 an out-of-court settlement to the Federal Trade Commission. It seems his "Anabolic Mega-Pak" and "Dynamic Life Essence" pills did not deliver the muscle growth promises as advertised. Don't feel sorry for Joe, though, he has plenty of other "nutritional" products for sale.

Almost humorous is the antifat industry's penchant for using in its print ads that most convincing phrase, "As seen on TV!" To the millions of viewers who worship that technological icon, that phrase is unassailable confirmation of the veracity of an ad. That Americans tend to believe everything they see on television is understandable since commercials can indeed be quite convincing. Especially effective are the slickly produced 30- and 60-minute programs that frequently appear on cable stations and sometimes on the networks. Often these shows are hosted by a movie star or a famous personality. Such programs, replete with MAGGOTY experts spewing deception, can be easily mistaken for documentaries or news shows — which is no coincidence. Adding to the deception is the fact that the programs are not listed as "advertising," but as "paid programming" — a classic example of doublespeak.

The marketing scheme for practically every antifat product relies on selective truths and half-truths to sell its product. Any person who has ever sold a house or automobile knows how that goes. The antifat people, however, have scraped the bottom of the pit when it comes to bald-faced lies. An entire book could be devoted solely to exposing the deceptions that appear in weight-reducing ads. But that is not the primary aim of this book. The fictitious **ObesiVac-10^6** ad that follows, however, includes many of the "red flags" to watch for when evaluating the veracity of such advertisements. As a rule of thumb, if a product sounds too good to be true — it is!

Assume that one week after a person takes **ObesiVac-10^6** his I.Q. drops by 90%, all of his hair falls out, and his anal sphincter goes into a permanent spasm. Should these side effects be mentioned? Nah! None of the other antifat companies mention their potions' adverse side effects.

MEDICAL BREAKTHROUGH! THE SECRET IS OUT! MEDICAL BREAKTHROUGH!

ANCIENT FORMULA PROMISES A **PERMANENT CURE** FOR ALL **OVERWEIGHT** PROBLEMS!!!
Medical and Pharmaceutical EXPERTS are astounded!

ObesiVac - 10⁶

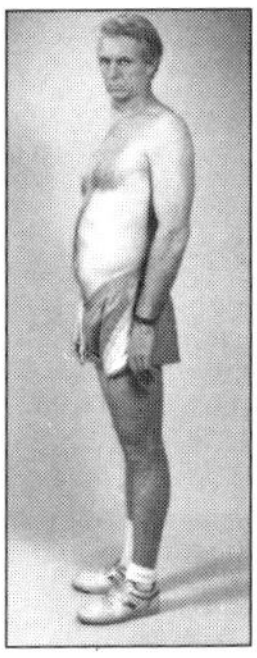

5:07

As seen on **TV**

(Unsolicited testimonial)
Dr. CRS - Memphis TN
Age 53 - May 4, 1989

"I lost 9" of fat from my waist!"
("...and gained 9" around his head! Editor)

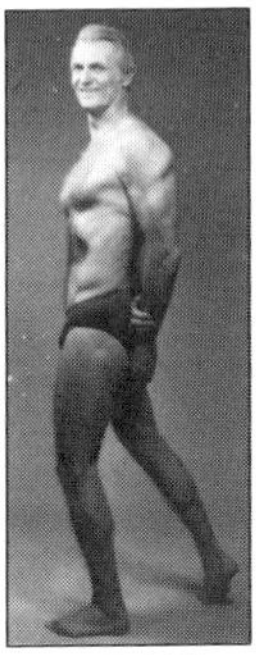

5:08!!

"...a disgusting slob - - then I took **ObesiVac - 10⁶** - - now I'm magnificent!"
"Girls hurl themselves at me!"
"Mom doesn't even recognize me - but who cares?"

It's a Miracle!

Breathe off UGLY Fat!!

(Not in months - not in weeks - not in hours)

IN MINUTES!

No Self-Control Needed!

EAT CONSTANTLY - Fatty bacon, cheese, pastries, butter, heavy cream, chitlins, etc... the more you eat the more you lose! Best of all - **NO** sweaty, tortuous **EXERCISE!**
All other weight reduction claims are now completely obsolete!

Your body has 60,000 miles of blood vessels. They pass by every cell of your body, including your fat cells. **ObesiVac - 10⁶** magically converts your red blood corpuscles into tiny **vacuum cleaners.** These powerful little suckers draw the fat (and cellulite) from your fat cells and carry it to the alveoli in your lungs. There, due to the adiposity pressure gradient, the fat from your red corpuscles diffuses into your lungs. Therefore, every time you exhale, you discharge hundreds of molecules of fat into the air! When you reach your desired weight, merely stop taking **ObesiVac - 10⁶**. Fat stays off **forever!** (Clinically tested and certified by the Federal Association of Reduction Therapists.)

Made from organically grown Oriental plants, this ancient **Tibetan formula** is jealously guarded by nasty-tempered, fanatical monks and cannot be duplicated by modern scientists. Only a very limited supply was smuggled out of the hidden monastery by an internationally known **Professor** from a prestigious **Caribbean Medical University.**

Don't wait! You must **order**
Once in a lifetime offer!
Absolutely **safe!**

NOW!

Lifetime supply!
(or one week-whichever comes first)
~~$29.95~~ SALE PRICE **$19.95**

300% guaranteed!!!

Buy one vial — get TEN free! SEND CASH and get a valuable string of Genuine Arkansas faux pearls.

Send to: LOTSA LUCK PHARMACEUTICALS, Box 0003, Trianketchus, Alaska

Except for the photographs in the **ObesiVac-10^6** ad, which actually were taken about a minute apart, and the fact that the average man really does have about 60,000 miles of blood vessels, the rest of the ad is sheer hogwash. This proportion is consistent with most weight-loss ads. The **ObesiVac-10^6** ad was intended to be a humorous imitation of the actual ads, but the latter are typically so ludicrous it was impossible to top them. For this reason, several obviously ridiculous statements were included in the **ObesiVac-10^6** ad so readers would realize it was a parody. I did not want the postal service to be inundated with money-stuffed letters sent to a fictitious Trianketchus, Alaska.

Before leaving the topic of weight-loss concoctions, I have to mention my favorite — not that it is any more effective than the others, but because of its name — "Granny's Fat-Off Formula." What an ingenious approach. The probable rationale, or hope, is that nobody's going to distrust a product with a name like that. Granny's other unique gimmick is to offer a different formula for different blood types. Some suckers are bound to fall for it. Before long I fully expect a company to come out with a weight-loss product that has different formulae for different ethnic groups.

For purely mercenary reasons, the antifat industry has propagandized society into believing that fat people are less than desirable in a wide range of ways. Promising to make fat people more attractive, worthwhile, and healthy, the industry has callously flooded the market with "weight-loss" drugs, pills, and potions. Not only do these products result merely in short-term results — *at best*; they are themselves health hazards. And the insatiable MAGGOTS know it!

10

ANTIFAT GADGETS AND LOTIONS

It must be conceded that some antifat products have a kind of twisted merit — none of the drugs, of course, but some of the mechanical gizmos and lotions that multiply in the commercial environment like fungi in a rain forest. This does not mean the gadgets and lotions help users lose weight. But some are so bizarre as to be laughable, and anything that inspires amusement cannot be totally lacking in value. Of course, the products lose a considerable portion of their charm when dupes realize the junk is a waste of money. To help keep people from being cheated, this chapter is devoted to unmasking some of the gimmicks. Most of the information can be applied to other products. When specific products are mentioned they are merely examples. The singling out does not mean they are any worse than others of the same ilk.

There are hundreds of silly devices that are advertised as aids to people who want to lose weight. The "squealing pig" figurine is typical. It is placed in the refrigerator and "oinks" every time the door is opened. On the pig's shirt are the words, "U-Pig Diet Plan." This little jewel, which does little more than humiliate fat people, is advertised in a novelty catalog. You can tell it is from a really classy company; next to the pig advertisement are ads for the Condom Repair Kit, the "urinal" snack bowl, and the baseball cap with a coil of feces (presumably fake) on the bill.

Of the serious "fat reducing" gadgets, one of the most comical ever devised was based upon a rolling pin design. It had several longitudinal rows of suction cups attached to the roller. Although the device appeared in the 1970s at some prominent department stores, the idea was hardly original. An almost identical device was advertised nearly a hundred years previously in a 1884 edition of a ladies' fashion magazine.

The rolling pins, while amusing, are merely a kind of massaging device. Massages in general can be delightfully enjoyable and relaxing, and are highly recommended for those reasons. It is fanciful, however, for a massagee to expect one speck of fat loss from any kind of stroking or passive manipulation.

This calorie burning relationship also pertains to the application of any of the numerous "body firming" creams on the market. When an ad says its product "dramatically improves the biomechanical properties of the skin" it is merely another example of doublespeak. These creams create a firming illusion with ingredients that shrink the skin. Since the skin shrinking effect is only transitory, the small print will usually advise consumers to use the product daily "for maximum benefit." Of course, daily use will result in the selling of more of the expensive gunk.

A favorite ploy is to advertise such creams as being "the cellulite solution." That is a catchy little phrase, all right. The use of the term "cellulite" does provide a service to potential customers because it is often the first clue to other deceptions in an ad. Cellulite, by the way, is pronounced "cell-u-*leet*" by its proselytizers. According to them only the gauche call it "cell-u-*lite*." No matter how it is pronounced, cellulite is just ordinary fat and all of the fancy pseudo-scientific arguments cannot change this fact. The substance is not a quagmire of "toxic wastes" as some MAGGOTS would have consumers believe. It has been fourteen years since the *Journal of the American Medical Association* stated unequivocally, "There is no medical condition known or described as cellulite in this country." Yet, so-called cures continue to flourish on the market.

The dimpling appearance of "cellulite" is caused by fat deposits pushing up between "walls" of fibrous tissue that extend from the skin to underlying muscle tissue. Since the outer layers of skin are thinner in women than men, the dimpling is far more obvious in women. And women have a greater tendency to store fat in their hips, thighs, and buttocks, therefore the cellulite is most prevalent in those areas. In addition, some women are more prone to show the condition than others due to genetics. People who have tight skin, for instance, are much less likely to have the dimpled appearance than those born with looser skin. Because connective tissue loses its elasticity as people get older, their skin gets more slack and cellulite becomes more obvious.

Some purveyors of cellulite products do admit that cellulite is just ordinary fat, but say it refers to fat that is located just under the skin. If they want to give this fat a special name, that's okay, but to imply that cellulite has special properties and requires special techniques for elimination is a blatant hoax. No cream on the market can reduce this fat. The overlying skin can be shrunk to reduce the dimpling for a few hours but the fat will not have gone anywhere. Not even liposuction works; the fat mass can be reduced but the connective tissue that creates the dimpling will remain.

"Heavy duty" kneading massage can reduce the cellulite considerably in some people but it requires an ongoing program. Stop the program and the dimpling soon returns. The most effective method of reducing the cellulite is to exercise, avoid the sun, eat a balanced diet, and drink a lot of water.

The French word for cream, incidentally, is *crème*. When the term is used on the label of one of these "body firmers," it merely means a customer can expect to pay more for it. Scientific sounding names are also popular. The makers of *Biotherm's Serum Contour* claim its Lipo-Active Body Contouring Treatment helps, "to keep orange-peely skin at bay. . . and that means away from your legs!" It's price? $32.50 for 4.2 oz. That's $123.81 per pound, plus tax! That's a tad expensive even if it actually got rid of the dreaded cellulite — which it absolutely does not.

Similar concoctions are also touted to firm and lift the breasts. One company claims its products contains, "Natural vegetable and biological extracts — like sage, hops, aloe, and geranium — make up our bust beauty treatments. They firm, tone, and tighten the breast's skin envelope and keep skin healthy by nourishing and strengthening its cells." Another company offers "plant milk for breast beauty." There are also "breast contouring cremes" and "translucent firming throat and breast masks." These products sound like miracle substances, all right. But Dr. John E. Sherman, a plastic surgeon at New York's Beth Israel Medical Center, has stated that short of surgery there is nothing a woman can do to help sagging, except to try to prevent sagging in the first place. That translates to, "Wear a brassiere." By counteracting gravity the practice keeps the ligaments in the breasts from stretching.

As could be expected, soap manufactures were not long in picking up the cellulite scent and producing their own products. The ads for one ingeniously named brand, Cellusoap, instructed its users to,"Simply massage its pearly lather into your skin . . . refreshes, cleanses, and moisturizes cellulite afflicted areas." The doublespeak implication is that the soap is beneficial in reducing cellulite. In reality, the ad merely says the soap "refreshes, cleanses, and moistures," none of which has anything to do with cellulite reduction. The dictionary, by the way, defines *affliction* as, "a state of pain, trouble or distress; misery. SYN: wretchedness, tribulation." Cellulite sounds like really bad stuff, all right — worse than the "heartbreak of psoriasis." Actually, cellulite is really an infinitesimal "affliction" unless a woman becomes obsessed with the condition. Let that same woman get cancer and see how insignificant her cellulite becomes.

As might be expected, the "reducing" lotions are not without their antecedents. In 1920 an ad in *Eve Pictorial* promised:

> A hot bath to which a packet of Clark's Reducing Salts has been added is delightfully fragrant and refreshing, and those who follow this treatment can grow slim without rigorous dieting.

To most Americans anything foreign is automatically imbued with mystical qualities of indisputable value. Associating a product with Europe is a common marketing stratagem. The terms "French" and "Swiss" seem to be particularly effective. Nothing, however, causes American eyes to glaze over and start American arms reaching for plastic faster than the words "Oriental" or "Chinese."

Acupressure is the latest of a long line of Eastern imports that purport to reduce body fat. If it is more appealing than its western counterpart, massage, it is probably because acupressure is less strenuous and can be self-administered. Supposedly, all a person has to do is squeeze an ear lobe, or whatever, and the desire to eat will disappear.

Since even ear lobe squeezing to diminish one's appetite requires some effort, some enterprising soul came up with the idea of stapling an ear. That's right, a U-shaped piece of metal with pointed ends is actually stapled into the ear cartilage. To eliminate hunger pangs all a staplee has to do is massage the metal device. A friend of mine, who succumbed to having the procedure done, complained that it was painful and made her nauseated. Not surprisingly, the staple idea never "caught on." It is no doubt true that getting sick at one's stomach would detract from the desire for food, but Americans are not, as a rule, particularly fond of a steady diet of pain and nausea.

This is where some MAGGOTY genius came up with weight-reducing earrings. They were not effective, either, but at least there was no discomfort. One positive note is that they did not sell well. It's a welcome sign that there may be a limit, after all, to the gullibility of Americans.

Then again, maybe not. Not long ago doctors were putting balloon-like devices in patients' stomachs to help them lose weight. When inflated, the device took up a lot of space in the stomach and only a small amount of food was necessary to make a "balloonist" feel full. While the idea seemed logical, it did not produce any better results than conventional weight-loss programs which are likewise ineffective. Besides, the stomach balloon had its dangers. Nearly one wearer in ten, for instance, developed serious complications such as ulcers and intestinal blockage. The contrivances are no longer on the market in the U.S. although Europeans are still swallowing the claims — and the balloons.

Having a gastric balloon implant may seem a tad drastic until you consider such procedures as jaw-wiring, stomach stapling, and intestine stapling. Stapling the ear is merely silly, but stapling organs inside the abdomen is something else. For instance, Dr. Paul Ernsberger (in *Radiance*, Summer, 1988) reported there were thirty-seven complications associated with the intestinal stapling. They include severe malnutrition, nerve and brain damage, immune deficiency, liver damage and failure, stomach cancer, irregular heart beat, and pernicious anemia. Within six months of the operation ten percent of the patients develop ulcers. Two to four percent die within days from other causes. If it sounds as if a person might be better off just staying fat, that is certainly true in all but the most extreme cases of fatness. The mortality rate of women who have the operation is nine times higher than those who do not!

The latest "miracle" for getting rid of body fat is liposuction. In this operation a pencil-sized steel tube (cannula) is slipped through a small incision and repeatedly and vigorously rammed through the fatty layer under the skin to suck out fat cells. In seven years the procedure has rocketed from being an obscure operation to becoming the most popular cosmetic surgery in America in 1990. Ninety-four percent of the patients are women. Dimensions may be trimmed off "problem" areas, but the surgery is not a solution to obesity. No more than four pounds of fat can be safely taken off at a clinic; removing six or seven pounds requires a blood transfusion and a night in the hospital; more than seven pounds would result in such large shifts in internal fluids that a patient could go into shock.

Doctors are flocking to get a piece of the action. All they have to do is attend a weekend training course. Yes, virtually all of the surgeons are "board certified," but there are more than a hundred "boards" with professional- sounding names that are *unregulated.* And ninety percent of the cosmetic surgery in health conscious U.S. of A. are being committed by surgeons who are unregulated! The profits of liposuction are enormous. A two- to three- hour "thigh job" (the most common procedure) costs from $2,000 to $3,000.

The extraction from the pocketbook is only a part of the pain and suffering associated with liposuction. A patient can expect about ten days of bruising and discomfort along with such risks such as infection, shock, and fat embolism (which can clog the arteries in the lungs or brain). There is evidence that a liposuctioned body still wants to maintain its original percentage of fat. When the fat is regained, though, it does not go back on the suctioned areas but on other areas — which can result in, as one doctor said, "bizarre looking bodies." In addition, many women are dissatisfied with such results as baggy skin, the fact that the dimpled cellulite appearance remains, and the occasional gross disfigurement.

Its promotional material makes liposuction sound like the answer to a fat woman's prayer and the risks are naturally pooh-poohed by the people who are making a living with the procedure. Amazingly, according to a spokesperson for the American Society of Plastic and Reconstructive Surgeons, no one is even keeping track of the ultimate adverse side effect — death. In 1987, however, a survey of 100,000 liposuctions did reveal 11 documented deaths. Other sources claim that at least 67 American women have died up to 1988. These are not large numbers, unless you are one of the victims or a member of their families. Reprehensibly, this surgery is often perpetrated upon lovely, healthy women who very often are not overly fat to begin with. They just have the misfortune to live in a culture that has coerced them into thinking they are so fat and ugly—and hating their bodies enough to subject them to such drastic treatment.

After a close look at the work of the French doctor who developed the technique, the American Society of Plastic and Reconstructive Surgeons told its members that liposuction is effective in trained and experienced hands. But they also concluded that:

1. the surgery does not cure general obesity since it only effects localized fat deposits.

2. the final results are not visible for weeks or months.

3. clumsy or excessive fat removal can lead to serious complications or permanent irregularities of shape.

4. the possibilities for misuse of the procedure are vast.

Caveat Emptor!

Currently taking the place of the "reducing" balloons in American are fiber products such as FiberTrim and Slim With Fiber. These substances are supposed to curb a user's appetite by expanding when they reach the stomach. They have not been found, however, to be effective for long term losses. Adding PPA to the product, as done in Fiber-Rich, does not help.

The Phoenix Natural Fiber Cookie was marketed primarily as a high-fiber product that can be an aid in losing weight. In 1990, however, the FDA charged the maker with using false and misleading labeling. More specifically, the cookie's labeling falsely indicated there was scientific evidence that it helped prevent or treat diseases, including diabetes, diverticulitis, colon cancer, and cardiovascular disease. The FDA classified the cookie as a *drug* because of the therapeutic claims — and therefore the company was ordered to present scientific evidence that it was safe and effective. It was unable to do so. But even if the cookie was marketed as a food, the FDA said the product would still be misbranded due to the extensive nutritional claims without the required labeling. The company's brochures indicated that each cookie had 126 calories, 5 grams of protein, 22 grams of carbohydrate, 2 grams of fat, 10 grams of fiber, and no cholesterol. When the cookie was ana*lyzed* by the Mississippi State Chemical Laboratory, though, it was found to have twice the calories, half the fiber and fives *times* the fat that was stated in its brochure!

Although the rolling pins and earrings share the prize for being most ridiculous antifat products, runners-up are the various types of "reducing" belts and pants. The simplest kinds are nothing more than wide constriction bands. Most are designed to be wrapped around the waist. They do result in a *temporary* decrease in girth, but there is no loss of fat. Besides being ineffective, these bands are dangerous because they restrict the flow of blood from the legs to the heart. That makes the heart work harder and encourages the development of varicose veins.

More sophisticated reducing belts and pants are made of rubbery plastic and fit snugly around the body. One, called the Astro-Trimmer, was hailed by its manufacturer as, "THE MOST ASTOUNDING ***WAIST AND TUMMY REDUCER*** OF ALL TIME!" It was guaranteed "to reduce your waist and abdomen 4 to 8 inches in just three days or your money back." The ad also promised results, " . . . without dieting and in only 5 to 10 minutes a day."

As impressive as those claims were, they were rather modest compared to the Sauna Belt whose makers proclaimed, "There are those who have lost as much as 3 inches from their waistlines from jus*t o*ne session with the 'magic' belt." All a person had to do was, "Slip the belt around your waist — inflate — and you are ready to do your two 'magic' waist reducing exercises: 5 to 10 minutes." Incredibly large numbers of people fell for this drivel.

The advertising for another product, Trim-Jeans, was refreshing for its relative honesty. Its manufacturer admitted that, "Not everybody may lose 7 inches in just one session and 14 1/2 inches in 3 days . . ." You can *bet* not everybody did. In fact, I would like to meet *anybody* who did — legitimately.

The most ridiculous "reducing" pants were the ones that attached to a vacuum cleaner, "to create a super new inch reducer so far ahead of its time that it reduces excess inches 7 times faster than 'crash diets." The ad goes on to claim losses of, "Over 8" from abdomen — 7" from waist: these are just some of the fantastic inch losses achieved by Slim-Skins users in just one to three days on a special slimming test conducted by a prominent American physician." Do you ever wonder why the names of the "prominent" doctors in these kinds of ads are rarely given? In keeping with the Big Lie, it seems the more incredible the advertising claim the more likely people are to believe it

As far as I could determine, the "Slim-Skins" hold the record for preposterous claims. A woman from San Francisco was quoted as saying she, " . . . took off 19 inches in just one day — more than I could ever lose with dieting!" Of course, her statement ended with the exclamation mark that is liberally sprinkled throughout MAGGOTY ads in general. What was the theory behind the vacuum pants? Its ads did not elaborate, but it is easy to envision the fat being sucked right out of her body. A more perceptive person would envision dollar bills being sucked out of the woman's purse.

Judging from the *before* and *after* photos of the models in the antifat ads, the products must also improve the posture of users. For some reason the poses are also far more attractive in the *after* pictures, and the models' clothes are more fashionable and their hair always neatly arranged. The apparent improvements never impress me, though, because I showed more improvement in my Obesivac - 10^6 ad in just *one minute* — and all I did was sip some water, suck in the "stomach," and flex some muscles!

One sneaky and very common ploy employed by the antifat industry is to use the entire photograph of a person in the BEFORE picture, while using a cutout of the person in the AFTER picture. Naturally, there is usually some "scissor reduction." Usually the scissoring is accomplished with admirable skill and the trimming of the body is nearly undetectable. Some ads, however, show outrageous arrogance in their grossly inept scissoring. They must think consumers are completely daft. Unfortunately, many are. The reader will understand why companies would not be inclined to grant permission for such ads to be reproduced in this book, but it is regrettable since some are quite amusing. The ads are unmistakable evidence that their products should be accepted for what they really are — con jobs.

It can be argued that these advertisements are ripoffs only if people fall for them. And there is some truth to that. Consumers have to accept some responsibility; they have to use some common sense. *CAVEAT EMPTOR*!

Just when I detected a shred of honesty in the aforementioned Slim-Skin ad, it went and burst my bubble. Near the bottom, the ad described a user as having a trimmer, tighter, *leane*r figure after the very first session. "Leaner" means a person will have less fat. The statement must have been a slip because the ads for reducing belts and pants rarely claim to reduce fat—just measurements. A claim of fat loss is usually too much of a misrepresentation even for a MAGGOT. Their *modus operandi* is, through deception, to merely imply a loss of fat.

Apparently, if a bogus claim is not challenged by the massively overburdened consumer "watchdogs," the industry considers the claim to be legitimatized. The claim can then blatantly be used by other producers of weight-loss trash. Of course, each subsequent claim tends to be further inflated. As a result, the falsehoods escalate ever upward. This is why the makers of one of the latest of the tight fitting reducing "belts," called Better Sweaters, felt free to blithely and erroneously announce that its product works to "reduce excess flab and water." If "flab" refers to "fat," the claim is absolutely false.

Advertisers, naturally, prefer half-truths to outright lies. The half-truths make it a little easier to put their hands on a Bible and swear to the veracity of their claims. And it *is* true that the belts, pants, or type of girdles, especially when used with movement, will help to reduce a person's measurements. The reduction occurs because the contrivances squeeze fat out of the compressed regions and into adjacent regions. If only the waist is squeezed, it will lose fat cells — but the areas above and below the waist will gain the fat. This latter point is, of course, never mentioned.

Moreover, if the girth of the waist is reduced by half an inch, a women can measure her waist at six different levels and claim that a total of 3 inches has been lost from her waist in a period of, say, 15 minutes. For a greater reduction she can merely measure her waist at more levels for the *after* measurement. But, she must measure quickly because as soon as a compression device is removed, the displaced fat starts oozing "back home." After a few hours her measurements will be the same as they were originally. If a person measures herself before and after each session, a three-inch loss can be detected each time. When added together after three sessions, the total loss will amount to an "amazing" nine inches in three days. Of course, the measurement will always be the same at the beginning of each session. This ploy is a classic example of the use of a half-truth.

The measurement reduction by compression is the same type that is achieved when a person uses a vibrating belt. These machines consist, basically of a wide belt that is attached to an electric motor. The user puts the belt around his or her waist and expects the fat to be shaken off. In reality, the device would have to be used for fifteen minutes every day for an entire year for a pound of fat to be lost. The intense itching sensation that follows each session use is a symptom of the irritation and harmful breakdown of connective tissue that lies under the skin of the "treated" area. These machines can lead to serious skin problems.

Roller machines are commonly seen in exercise studios. Typically, one consists of a rotating drum with about a dozen knobby, wooden dowels around the edge. A user leans a body part against it and is lead to believe the underlying fat is liquefied so it can be removed faster during exercise. The machines are completely worthless. They are also dangerous for people with varicose veins or other circulatory problems.

Most "reducing" belts and pants can more accurately be called heat garments. They fit snugly against the skin and make the wearer sweat. Because of this effect, manufacturers of these products claim the devices result in spot reducing. The implication is that fat is the substance being reduced. When the heat garments are removed, the liquid one sees is water, along with important electrolytes (mainly sodium, chloride, and potassium), but there is not one iota of fat. Dehydrated cells quickly refill after a few glasses of water are ingested. In reality, the only results of heat garments are a temporary water loss and a reduction of a buyer's bank account.

An adventurous friend of mine once spread a liniment, called Atomic Balm, on the inward side of a reducing belt to augment its heating effect. As he quickly realized, the fiery gel was aptly named. He never repeated the experiment. As it turned out, however, his inventiveness was a forerunner of a product with the oxymoronic name of Sweet Sweat. It is a concoction whose promotional material claims, "Sweating burns calories and Sweet Sweat lets you break a good sweat on your problem areas." It's amazing how one short sentence can sound so impressive and be so misleading. Although sweat glands do burn calories to create sweat, the amount is so slight it is negligible. Even *if* the amount were significant, breaking a "good sweat" on a "problem area" would not burn any more calories (or fat) from that area than any other part of the body. The remaining fat would be redistributed according to the pattern determined by one's genetics. There is no such phenomenon as "spot reducing" as far as fat is concerned.

The heat belts and pants are just miniature variations of the plastic sweatsuit. Some women may prefer to call them "perspiration ensembles" or "glow garments." Whatever they are called, the outfits can be very dangerous because they severely restrict the evaporation of sweat. Since the cooling effect of vaporization is eliminated, a wearer sweats profusely in a futile attempt to cool the body. Sitting in a steam room has exactly the same effect.

Sweat *can* evaporate in a sauna room due to the low humidity of that environment. Therefore, practitioners may be fairly dry. In actuality, though, they also will be sweating a lot. Because the sweat evaporates in a sauna, the skin (and body) is cooled; much higher air temperatures therefore can be safely endured.

Several pounds of weight can be lost per hour by sitting in a "heat room" or encasing a body in a heat suit. Again, though, it is not fat that is being lost, but sweat — or more precisely, water and many vital salts. Since so much water can be lost, if it is not carefully replaced, one can quickly become dehydrated. A water loss equivalent to 1% of body weight is no problem; a person will just salivate less and be thirsty. When more than 2% of body weight is lost through dehydration, however, it begins to adversely effect the heart rate, body temperature, and central nervous system. As the deficit increases it will result in irritability, lethargy, fatigue, loss of appetite, and an even faster heart rate. At levels above 5%, dehydration starts becoming dangerous due to heart irregularities and changes in kidney function. More severe dehydration leads to delirium and eventually to death.

Ingesting water alone to prevent and treat dehydration is not enough. The salts that are lost in sweat must also be replaced. A sodium deficiency, for instance, can result in fatigue and cramps. People who are not acclimatized to the heat must be especially aware of replacement since they can lose as much as ten times as much sodium per quart of sweat as those who *are* acclimatized. Acclimatization is achieved by exercising, sensibly, in the heat.

People, particularly those with kidney impairment (which is not uncommon), may experience water intoxication when only water is replaced. The symptoms include headache, "heat" cramps, dizziness, vomiting, diarrhea, and convulsions. Replacing the electrolytes lost in sweat is best accomplished by eating a balanced diet — with an emphasis on citrus products, potatoes, nuts, and bananas to replenish potassium. Sprinkling a bit more salt than usual on food may be desirable to replace sodium and chloride. Salt tablets are not necessary.

Exercising while wearing a plastic sweatsuit is dangerous even if a person drinks enough salt-laced water. Sweat must evaporate if it is to cool the body — and the suits *prevent* evaporation. Since the garments prevent the loss of heat from the body, a person's temperature can quickly rise to result in heat exhaustion or, worse yet, heat stroke. Exercising on a hot, humid day is almost as foolhardy as exercising while wearing a plastic sweatsuit.

Sweating apparel is actually counterproductive when it comes to losing fat. Since much of the output from the heart is diverted to the skin in a doomed attempt to keep the body cool, not as much blood can be sent to active muscles. As a result a person cannot exercise as strenuously, and burn as many calories, as is possible in a cooler environment.

"Body wrapping" has added an interesting new twist to "reduction" garments. A spa or salon employee may wrap a client in long strips of material so she that resembles a mummy and then the client is dunked in a solution that contains an astringent. An occasional dousing with a bucket of the mixture helps to intensify the "Magic." Another method is to wrap a client with hot, soaked strips of cloth and then encase her in a rubberized suit that is tied at the wrists, ankles, and neck to retain the heat.

Since the solution causes skin to shrink, a person's measurements do decrease. One ad promises, "Lose 4 to 15 inches in one hour with our European body wraps." The number of measurement sites, of course, are not stated. The ad also neglects to mention that the effects of the astringent begin to wear off in several hours and the original measurements return. Nor is it revealed that the technique is potentially hazardous due to dehydration and heat illnesses. Some establishments emblazon across their ads, "Lose 10 pounds, 10 inches in 10 visits . . . !" In the tiny print of the fancy-bordered guarantee, however, they usually admit, "For the loss to be lasting, our patrons must lose weight. This can be accomplished by spa treatments and a sound nutritional program."

For the money these joints charge you would think they could at least show some creativity and refer to their process with some fancy name such as the *Pharaoh's Phantasy*. Not only it is suitably exotic, it contains some truth since phantasy means "unrestrained imagination." They could also add a little class to their ads by saying something like, "Soak in the Pharaoh's eleven secret herbs and spices!"

Some of the more commonplace MAGGOTY devices that promise to help people lose weight have been discussed here. Regrettably, not all such ripoffs have been exposed; due to a lack of space, a line had to be drawn somewhere. Besides, even if all of the fallacies of the bogus weight loss products were exposed, and people stopped buying them, new products would pop up overnight like mushrooms, anyway. And hopeful, but unenlightened, dupes would line-up to buy them.

This chapter should help potential victims recognize some of the more common deceptive advertising techniques employed by the antifat industry to sell worthless gadgets and lotions. It has been said that, "To be forewarned is to be forearmed." Hopefully, that is true. Let the buyer beware!

The antifat industry is not the only one engaging in deceptive marketing. Such techniques are common throughout the business world. But the antifat industry is unique in that its chi*ef modus opera*ndi is to publicly degrade its victims to set them up for plucking — a mean and despicable technique. Even worse has been the creation of hordes of FATISTS who delight in ridiculing people who are fat or who have been led to believe they are fat. The antifat industry's greatest sin, however, has been the convincing of fat people that they have little value as human beings and are not deserving of respect — which is utterly ridiculous. This crime, which has caused immeasurable pain and suffering in millions upon millions of people, is inexcusable — and the cavalier manner in which the industry's propaganda is spewed forth only compounds its moral transgressions.

11

FATNESS AND HEALTH

The public is constantly being deluged with dire warnings that body fat is a health hazard. Excessive fatness, of course, *is* unhealthy. But at what point can fat be considered excessive? There is no clear-cut answer — in spite of self-serving proclamations by the antifat industry.

Ultimately, each person's desirable level of fatness is an individual matter that depends upon your body type, way of life, and personal priorities. Considerable thought should be given to these factors before people make a commitment regarding their own fatness.

The Height-Weight-Mortality Ratio Table, devised by Louis I. Dublin of the Metropolitan Life Insurance Company, is the standard most often used to determine if a person is excessively fat. The information contained in this table has long been considered gospel in the health related fields because millions of subjects have been used in compiling the data. Because the table is highly regarded, its data are often quoted as unassailable proof that fatness is a health hazard. Metropolitan's mortality ratio is defined as "the ratio of the actual deaths for a particular height and weight group to the expected deaths among policy holders . . ." A score above 100 indicates a greater than expected chance of dying while a score below 100 indicates a less than expected chance — for a particular height. In other words, the lower the score the better.

Unfortunately, there were many flaws in the compilation of the mortality table. For starters, the conclusions were *arbitrarily* based upon data pertaining only to Americans of Northern European ancestry. Would conclusions apply equally as well to Americans of African, Mexican, and Japanese descent? No one knows.

The insured people also tended to have higher incomes than average which suggests they probably had better than average medical care. They were relatively free of serious medical diseases and generally were engaged in safer occupations than the uninsured people. These circumstances would certainly affect the application of conclusions to the public in general.

The mortality table is reproduced below. It was published by the Metropolitan Life Insurance company's *Statistical Bulletin* (Jan-Mar 1984) and is based upon their latest collection of data. It is suggested that you study it for a few minutes and see what conclusions you make.

MORTALITY RATIOS ACCORDING TO RANGE OF WEIGHTS (1983)

Height (In Shoes) *	Range of Weights † (In Indoor Clothing) ‡	MORTALITY RATE		
		Weight Below Range	Weight Within Range	Weight Above Range
		MEN		
5'2"	128 – 150	114%	106%	125%
5'3" - 5'6"	130 – 164	115	100	108
5'7" - 5'10"	138 – 180	114	97	111
5'11" - 6'2"	146 – 197	115	96	114
6'3" - 6'4"	158 – 207	98	94	119
		WOMEN		
4'10"	102 – 131	197%	104%	116%
4'11" - 5'2"	103 – 143	144	95	101
5'3" - 5'6"	111 – 159	127	99	104
5'7" - 5'10"	123 – 173	145	102	109
5'11" - 6'0"	135 – 179	¶	134	365

SOURCE: Metropolitan Life insurance Company. "Measurement of Weight," Statistical Bulletin 65 (January - March 1984): 23.

* Shoes with 1-inch (2.50 centimeters) heels for both men and women.

† From 1983 Metropolitan Height and Weight Tables

‡ Indoor clothing 5 pounds (2.3 kilograms) for men and 3 pounds (1.4 kilograms) for women.

¶ Ratio not computed; fewer than 10 deaths.

Compare your conclusions, if you will, with the one below. It appears in *Health*, a college health textbook published in 1986 by the Charles E. Merrill Company.

HEALTH CONSEQUENCES OF OBESITY

Men and women who weigh more than the standards on the height-weight tables can be expected to have a higher mortality ratio than

> individuals whose weights fall within average limits (see Metropolitan table above). An overweight 6'3" male, for example, has a 25 percent higher mortality ratio than his average-weight peer. For many people, excessive weight gain is accompanied by a higher incidence of diseases . . .

Health is one of the fairest health textbooks on the market in attempting to show both sides of the fatness issue. Still, the bias of the authors clearly shines through. They pick out a single set of data from the Metropolitan table — namely, that of an overweight 6 feet 3 inch male, and point out that he has a higher mortality rate than his average-weight peers. They might have pointed out that the *underweight* males in this height group also have a higher mortality rate. They might also have stressed that between the heights of 5 feet 3 inches and 6 feet 2 inches, which includes the huge majority of men, the mortality ratio is actually a bit higher for underweight men than the overweight ones.

If the emotional stress so unfairly imposed upon fat people were taken into consideration, it might even show the overweight group to have the lowest mortality ratio. It must be mentioned that in this latest Metropolitan table the weight range for the average-weight group has been sharply revised upward. In other words, with a stroke of the pen millions of people were no longer considered to be dangerously fat. Because their "paper" health had improved, it was likely that their actual health also improved due to reduced anxiety and worry.

By far the the most dramatic data in the table has to do with women. From just a cursory look at all of the categories from 4 feet 10 inches to 5 feet 10 inches, which includes the vast majority of women, it is evident that being underweight is *far* more detrimental to longevity than being overweight. Simple computations reveal that the increase in the mortality ratio for underweight women is about seven times greater than the increase for overweight women. Seven times! Now that statistic practically reaches off the page and grabs a perceptive reader by the ears; yet, health professionals never mention it. All they say is that the Metropolitan table shows it is hazardous to be overweight.

It is not being suggested that health professionals are purposefully trying to deceive the public. Not at all. Their comments merely reflect their deep-seated antifat bias due to their having been raised in a society that is persistently being bombarded with MAGGOTY propaganda.

Incidentally, the mortality ratio for very tall women has little practical meaning since there were so few subjects in this category; it would not take many accidental deaths to affect the findings. People who are extremely tall or extremely short tend to have a higher than average mortality ratio anyway.

One of the most misleading aspects of the mortality table is that it is based upon Louis I. Dublin's 1942-1943 publication of "Ideal Weights" for men and women. His "ideal weights" were not "average weights," they were weights *he* felt everyone should strive for. Since his ideal weights were considerably less than the average weights, many people of average weight were placed in the overweight category, thus considerably increasing the number of people in the overweight group. A cynical person might find this a tad suspicious since overweight people had to pay higher premiums to the company Dublin worked for—a neat little twist to the "fox in the hen house" scenario. Besides, the ideal weight is not the same for every individual; in fact, the average ideal weight for an entire population is not even known. Durbin's "ideal" body weights were strictly *arbitrary*.

Yet, because these "ideal weight" tables were widely disseminated through popular magazines, doctors' offices, and public scales, they became universally accepted as being the correct standards for body weight. The tables failed to point out that there was a range of about 30 to 40 pounds, for each "ideal" weight, where life expectancy would be average or above. Dublin apparently felt the broad range gave too much leeway so he divided people into three categories of frame size. The glaring problem was that the frame sizes were *arbitrarily* assigned; that is, none of the policyholders' frames was actually measured!

When the 1983 tables were updated, policyholders were told to compute their frame size by measuring the elbow joint with the thumb and finger and then measuring the digital gap with a ruler. This is a laughably imprecise method of measurement, and evidence that it reveals anything about an individual's frame or healthiest weight is scarce at best.

Even the accuracy of the policyholders' heights and weight are suspect. These measurements were obtained with subjects in street clothes and shoes—and estimates were then made of the effect of clothes and shoes upon measurements. More astounding is that at least twenty percent of the insurance applicants merely reported their measurements to the examiner! Self-estimates are fraught with errors even when people attempt to be honest. Studies show that women, for instance, tend to under-estimate their weight while men tend to over-estimate their weight.

But how do you think applicants would state their weight if they knew overweight people had to pay a higher premium? Smart, if not ethical, overweight people would logically tend to put themselves in the normal weight group. In 1959 the Society of Actuaries found this was indeed happening. Overweight people, on the average, reported themselves as being ten or more pounds lighter than they actually were—thus discrediting the theory that "fat people are stupid." This cheating meant that many of the average weight insurers in the mortality table were actually overweight — and many of those in the overweight group weighed more than was reported. And mortality statistics were based upon these inaccuracies.

Logically, since overweight people had to pay higher premiums for Metropolitan's life insurance, a healthy overweight person was not as likely to buy insurance as an unhealthy overweight person. This circumstance would certainly increase the mortality ratios for fat people.

A major failing of the Metropolitan table is that it does not take age into account. Dublin's tables were based upon the belief that everyone should weigh what was ideal for a twenty-five-year-old. Since then, however, Dr. Reubin Andres, clinical director of the Gerontology Research Center at the National Institute on Aging, has found that it is healthier for adults to gain weight as they get older. Using the latest Metropolitan data (1983), he found the tables to be satisfactory for people around forty but that twenty-year olds should weigh considerably less and sixty-years olds considerably more to increase their chances of good health. Dr. Andres' findings themselves are based upon averages and therefore have little meaning when applied to any particular *individual* because differences in body type, and a lot of other significant factors, were not considered.

Perhaps the most glaring flaw in the MLIC Mortality Ratio Table has to do with the frequency of weighing policy holders. Incredibly, they were only weighed when they initially purchased their policies unless they bought a new policy or reapplied to change their risk category — presumably a lower risk category, for lower premiums. But studies clearly show that people nearly always gain weight as they get older. How many fifty-year-old people do you know who have not gained weight since they were twenty-five?

Using this weighing policy, Dublin's data *did* show that heavier people had a higher mortality ratio. But because age, and weight gains and losses, were not factored into the long-revered table, all the statistician actually discovered was that older people die more frequently than younger people. Not a particularly shocking revelation.

In sum, the MLIC mortality ratios are just too simplistic to have much meaning, except for people who are extremely underweight and overweight. Yet, for more than forty years the table has provided a fertile breeding ground for MAGGOTS. And now that the U.S. is completely infested, the vermin are swarming into other nations.

Although the amount of fat on a person's body generally has very little influence on his health, *where* the fat is deposited most abundantly is very important as it relates to increased health problems, particularly cardiovascular heart disease. Fat that is stored on the buttocks, hips, and thighs poses little threat to health because it is located directly under the skin — and tends to stay there. Due to this inactivity, however, it is difficult to lose.

Fat that is stored on the mid-section, on the other hand, tends to be quite harmful. First, much of the fat is stored inside the abdominal cavity. Second, that fat breaks downs readily. Third, the blood supply in the abdomen drains directly into the liver. When the fat cells in the abdominal region get full they dump the fat back into the bloodstream where it is carried to the liver. This "active" fat interferes with the liver's control of insulin levels and it stimulates the liver's production of artery clogging cholesterol.

Since women tend to store large percentages of their body fat on their buttocks, hips, and thighs, they are said to be pear-shaped. Men generally carry more of their fat on their mid-sections and are said to be apple-shaped. Even though the fat of pear-shaped people offers a tiny fraction of the health risk compared to that found in apple-shaped people, women are the focus of far more pressure to lose weight. Once again the expectations of society is totally out-of-line with the dictates of nature.

To determine if you are an "apple" or a "pear" requires just two measurements. Measure the circumference of your waist about a half-inch above your navel and then measure the circumference of your hips where the buttocks protrude the most. Then divide the waist measurement by the hip measurement. If the number is more than 0.85, you are an apple, if it is less than 0.75, you are a pear. Values between these numbers are neutral. If the waist/hip ratio is higher than 1.0 for men and above 0.80 for women, the risk for various health disorders increases.

One advantage of the fat in apple-shaped people is that, being active, the fat is much easier to lose. Along with having a higher metabolic rate, this is why men tend to lose weight much more easily than women—and have a big advantage in "weight loss" bets with women. For women who are trying to lose weight, the waist-to-hip ratio is especially difficult to change. It can be achieved with a very large loss of weight, but losing ten to twenty pounds will not have much effect.

In spite of the variable and complex relationship between fatness and health, there is absolutely no mention of fat in the Metropolitan Table. The table is merely a comparison of *weight* and mortality ratios, and to use the company's own words from their *Statistical Bulletin* (Jan-Mar 1984):

> The concepts of obesity and overweight are often confused. Though sometimes used interchangeably, the term obesity usually indicates excess body fat while overweight denotes excess weight. Obesity can be determined by several types of skinfold measurements, or by tests in laboratories with special equipment designed to make complicated body density determinations. However, when skinfold measurements

> are not available, obesity is most often defined in terms of overweight because of the simplicity of the method.

"Ay, there's the rub," to borrow from Hamlet. The Metropolitan people say the concepts of "obesity" and "overweight" are different, but for simplicity's sake the company placed people of both types in the same group when the mortality table was compiled. What the researchers gained in simplicity they lost in accuracy. And which should have been more important? Accuracy, of course. The mortality ratios in the table would have given far more insight into the relationship between fatness and mortality rates, if the body fat of its subjects had actually been measured — instead of merely assuming that all the people in the overweight category were fat. The process would have been more expensive, but if worthwhile research is to be done, a high degree of meaning and accuracy should be aimed for. Even then, there is plenty of room for error. For instance, body-shape alone, apple or pear, is a major variable.

The weakness of standard height-weight tables in estimating fatness is dramatically revealed in studies using athletes as subjects. According to the tables, many powerfully built athletes are considered to be overweight, sometimes grossly so. Often, however, these same athletes have a lower percentage of body fat than do nonathletic men of similar height and who weigh much less. Not until 1942 was the first serious effort made to reveal the inadequacy of determining "ideal" weight from height-weight tables. The study used twenty-five professional football players, most of whom had been college All-Americans. It found that seventeen of the men were unqualified for military service or first class insurance because they were more than 15% above the average weight figures for their heights. Yet, eleven of the seventeen actually had exceptionally low levels of body fat! Such findings have often been duplicated.

None of this is meant to be a condemnation of the intentions of the Metropolitan Life Insurance Company. Its table is undoubtedly an honest attempt to shine some light into a very large, dark, and important corner. The main problem is that its data, along with countless others, has been grossly overemphasized, misused and misrepresented by the antifat industry for its mercenary purposes.

Some FATISTS are quick to say, "There are very few, very fat, very old people alive." The implication is that fat people die before they reach an advanced age. The truth is, many fat people do reach old age — they just begin losing weight as they approach "senior citizen" status. In fact, the results of a ten year study of 10,000 adults by the Department of Health and Human Services (1990) showed that men and women generally begin losing weight at about age fifty-five. It is not that they try; they just do.

Why does this weight loss occur? There are a variety of possible reasons. Many old people find themselves on reduced budgets and simply cannot afford as much food as they were previously able to buy — and they may not find canine cuisine all that tasty. The appetite declines with advanced age, anyway, because taste buds lose their acuity and food loses much of its appeal. If an old person lives alone, the motivation to prepare meals is diminished along with the social aspects which enhance the eating experience. Similarly, the death of a spouse can result in an altered life style and a diminished zest for life that is reflected in a loss of appetite. Old people also tend to have more wasting illnesses, such as cancer, that lead to a reduced body weight. Even if an illness does not have this effect, certain medicines can cause a loss of taste and appetite. In addition, simple things such as poorly fitting or misplaced dentures, can make eating a difficult and painful affair — and "gumming" a steak or an apple can take a lot of joy out of eating those and other favorite foods.

The public has been led to believe that *any* amount of body fat, above a mythical ideal, causes a number of very serious health problems. A close scrutiny of the research, however, refutes this. As far as health is concerned, the most that can be said is that there appears to be a positive relationship between obesity and some diseases. The operative word here is obesity, which means extremely fat. As explained in Chapter Six, when researchers investigate a relationship between fatness and a particular illness they typically use very obese subjects. By selecting these people, the researchers know they greatly increase their chances for finding a relationship. Even if they discover a relationship, though, it does not mean one exists for moderately fat people. But when a study does show an *apparent* relationship between extreme obesity and an illness, the antifat brigade broadcasts the "proof" as applying to fatness in general — and everyone has his or her own idea of what constitutes fatness. Some people who are in reality morbidly thin (say, 5% body fat or even less), think they are excessively fat.

As explained earlier, even if a positive relationship between fatness and various diseases were proven beyond a doubt, that would not mean fatness *causes* the diseases. A third factor, such as genetics may be the linking agent.

Since the antifat brigades are constantly bombarding the public with frightening pronouncements implying that heart disease, high blood pressure (hypertension), diabetes mellitis, and arthritis are caused by obesity, these relationships are discussed here. While this is not intended to be a textbook, footnotes are used in this section due to the controversial nature of the subject. Sources for information are listed under Footnotes in the back of the book. Instead of just using significant individual studies, *reviews* of research were also chosen because their conclusions are based upon a much wider range of information.

A study reported in the *International Journal of Obesity*[1] concluded that obesity, by itself, has often been found *not* to be a risk factor for heart disease, especially in population studies of limited size and duration. Of course, long term studies are far more meaningful. The often quoted Framingham (Massachusetts) project,[2] which has collected data on 5,000 subjects for about forty years, found that a risk did exist but only for severe obesity of long duration.

Even this moderate conclusion, however, has its detractors. Prominent among them is Dr. Dale Ahrens, a psychobiologist at the University of Sydney (Australia) where he heads an active interdisciplinary research group studying the psychobiology of energy balance. Ahrens found that although the results of the research were significant *statistically*, a more sophisticated analysis of the data showed the heralded findings to be practically devoid of any predictive power. In other words, the relationship between weight and cardiovascular disease was actually *medically* insignificant. Therefore, it could be concluded from the Framingham study that being overweight is only a minor cardiovascular risk factor.

This conclusion never reached the public because they were fed what the antifat forces wanted them to swallow. In addition, it is rarely reported that the thinnest men in the study had the highest mortality rate. Again, the MAGGOTS used half-truths to their greedy advantage.

The Framingham findings were not unique. A thirteen-year study involving hundreds of Swedish men indicated there was no relationship between fatness, by itself, and heart disease and stroke. It did, however, show that where fat is distributed on the body is significant. Specifically, fat is a health hazard only when it accumulates in the abdominal area — the typical male pattern.

The passage below is from Dr. Ahrens book, *Don't Diet.*

> In the classic Seven Countries Study, fat men were *less* likely to die from cardiovascular disease. The same finding has also been reported in men from southern Europe. In Finland, where cardiovascular disease is extremely prevalent, the men in the top 10 percent of the weight distribution were shown to have the lowest incidence of cardiovascular disease. Further, even in the United States, it is well-known that mortality from cardiovascular disease has been decreasing steadily, whereas fatness has been increasing. Another study compared 866 American soldiers who died of coronary causes with a similar group who died of various accidental causes. The two groups showed no differences in fatness either at the time of admission to the army or at the time of death.

One study of over twelve thousand white middle-aged American men showed that fatness was a cardiovascular risk only in those who were at least 30% overweight. However, even among the six subgroups that made up the study, there were major differences. Several groups showed an increased risk while several others did not. Clearly, the risk of cardiovascular disease is determined by a great many factors. The degree of body fatness appears to be one of them, but is probably not a major one — except at extreme levels. Body fat, however, has received the most attention and blame. Because other variables are not so obvious, or are much more difficult to measure, they are to easier to ignore. Mainly, though, the other variables do not have high-powered, well-financed groups, analogous to the antifat industry, continually propagandizing the public.

Even if going on a low-fat diet to lose weight would lower the chances for people dying of heart disease, it does not necessarily mean they will live longer. One reason is that losing weight appears to affect one's behavior in a negative way. That is revealed in a study by Jay Kaplan and associates.[3] Using several groups of monkeys, they found that a low-fat, "prudent" diet resulted in lower blood cholesterol. As the levels decreased, however, the animals started shoving, hitting, and biting 50% more than the fatter, more easy-going, monkeys on the high-fat, "luxury" diet.

These findings are consistent with research using human subjects. In a series of studies [4, 5, 6,7] M. Virkkumen and associates found that relatively low blood cholesterol levels (the result of a low-fat diet) were prevalent in people who typically engage in violent behavior. That included criminals diagnosed as having antisocial personalities, adolescent boys with both aggressive conduct disorder and attention deficit disorder, and impulsive fire setters. It would seem that the phrase "lean and mean" has some truth to it. And a glance at Picasso's Seated Nude (page 33) does nothing to refute that.

Data suggests that the level of cholesterol in the blood may not be as important, though, as a decline of 10% or more. It is believed by such experts as Matthew Muldoon,[8] internal medicine specialist at the University of Pittsburgh, that cholesterol is required for the body's cells to release a natural tranquilizer called serotonin. Therefore when the cholesterol level drops, the tranquilizing effect of serotonin is also reduced.

Such a reduction, of course, is likely to result in aggressive, antisocial, behavior — which could be decidedly unhealthy if one acts belligerently toward the wrong person. Indeed, studies do show that people on a low-fat regimen are more prone to accidents, suicide, and to being murdered than those on a high-fat diet.[9] It is well-documented that people on a high-fat *diet* have a relatively high rate of heart attacks. *All things considered*, though, there appears to be very little difference between the longevity of the high-fat and low-fat diet groups.

Logically, it seems that an increase in body fat should be achieved with low-fat foods. And to lower blood cholesterol, a very desirable goal, one should do it gradually — in ways that are discussed in Chapters 13 and 14.

It is obvious that obesity does not automatically cause high blood pressure since many extremely fat people do not have high blood pressure, and many extremely thin people do. It may be true, however, that fat people have a greater likelihood for high blood pressure. A lot of research does indicate that this is the case. On the other hand, reports in the prestigious *Circulation*[10] and *American Journal of Medicine*[11] suggest that body type is a far more important factor than obesity. Specifically, men with a large chest circumference, relative to their height and weight, are ten times more likely to have hypertension than slender men. In fact, body build had a nearly proportional effect on both systolic and diastolic blood pressure. Further, when blood pressure was compared with groups with the same body build, there was no significant correlation between obesity and high blood pressure!

Research has revealed that a fall in blood pressure follows weight loss in 50% to 70% of the time. But why not all the time? Is a loss of body fat actually the determining factor? No one knows. A report in the *New England Journal of Medicine*[12] suggested that a lower caloric intake would result in a reduction of sympathetic nerve impulses to the heart and thereby reduce one's blood pressure. This suggests that diet, not obesity, may be the significant factor.

Yes, studies have shown that hypertension is twice as common in overweight people as in those of normal weight.[13] Interestingly, though, this relationship is most striking in white women and blacks of both sexes. As discussed earlier, these findings could very well be a reflection of the stress associated with racism and the pressure imposed upon fat women to be thin.

In 1982 a very important "fat" study was published in *Lancet*[14] the British medical journal. The results of the research cast serious doubt on the findings of every study that had found a positive relationship between obesity and hypertension. The scientists discovered that when the blood pressure of obese people was measured with a *normal*-sized arm cuff, the readings would be much higher than their actual blood pressure — as measured by the extremely accurate, but invasive, intraarterial method. The researchers estimated that nearly 37% of the subjects with arm circumferences between thirteen and sixteen inches (large arms), who were found to be hypertensive when normal-sized cuffs were used, actually had normal blood pressure!

For accurate blood pressure measurements with arm cuffs, which is the standard method used, the inflatable part of the cuff should completely surround the arm. Yet this important factor had not been considered in previous obesity/blood pressure research. The discrepancy would obviously cause gross inaccuracies in the data of these studies and the conclusions made from such data would be greatly suspect.

As with hypertension, the public has been convinced by the antifat industry that fatness causes diabetes. The conclusions of two reviews of the literature by medical researchers, however, paint a far more moderate picture. In *Diabetes, Obesity, and Vascular Diseases* Berger and his associates[15] concluded:

> Although textbooks of medicine often refer to 'ample epidemiological evidence' linking the incidence rates of diabetes and obesity, critical evaluation reveals that adequately controlled quantitative data are available to a limited extent only.

A review, in *Diabetes and Obesity*, by Keen and his colleagues[16] described the situation in even stronger terms. They wrote:

> . . . despite strong and frequent assertions of the importance of obesity in the pathogenesis of diabetes, sound evidence of the frequency of obesity in established diabetes is scanty and contradictory.

These conclusions are from analytical *reviews* of the research . They are not from one or two obscure studies.

The simple fact that many obese people are not diabetic and that many thin people do suffer from the condition is solid evidence that *extreme* fatness (not to mention mild or moderate fatness) does not necessarily cause diabetes. It is also known that people inherit the propensity for becoming diabetic which means there may be little or no causal relationship at all between fatness and diabetes.

Yes, more obese people are diabetic than are thin people, but this does not mean obesity causes the disease. Indeed, it may be the other way around; diabetes may cause fatness. An understanding of the metabolic disorder strongly supports this supposition. Diabetes is basically an insulin problem. This hormone is necessary for the body's cells to take glucose from the bloodstream. Some people do not secrete enough of the hormone; others secrete plenty but an inhibiting factor keeps the insulin from accomplishing its function. In either case, the body's cells do not admit glucose so diabetics have chronically elevated levels of glucose in their blood. Although the use of glucose is impaired in diabetes, insulin's role in the promotion of fat remains unaffected. In trying to lower blood glucose the pancreas produces more insulin, and unfortunately, most of this increase is used to create more fat. With the increased fat, however, the body becomes even more insulin resistant. This vicious cycle causes the percentage of body fat to spiral upward. In some people the process eventually reaches a plateau; others have to take insulin shots. Losing weight helps to reduce the need for medication, but diabetics have an even harder time reducing fat than do nondiabetics. Exercise is usually quite therapeutic, even if the diabetic does not lose any weight.

There are studies which suggest that the manner in which people become fat has a much greater effect on their health than the degree of fatness. For instance, a repetitious cycle of weight decreases and increases, commonly called "yo-yoing," tends to redistribute body fat from the thighs and hips to the abdomen — a distinctly unhealthy shift. Further, in the middle 1980s Dr. Paul Ernsberger, a highly respected "yo-yo syndrome" researcher, discovered that yo-yoing greatly increases the risks of dangerously high blood pressure and congestive heart failure. In a simplification of his findings, the stress of overeating stimulates the production of a stress hormone (norepinephrine) that drives up blood pressure. The condition becomes permanent, though, only after repeated feast-famine cycles. Diabetes also appears to be linked to the weight gains associated with yo-yoing — not to fatness, per se.

Although fatness may not cause high blood pressure or diabetes, it must be emphasized that losing weight does help to ameliorate these diseases. Obese, hypertensive patients, therefore, are advised to lose weight — not by drastic calorie reductions — but by adhering to a sensible balanced diet and exercise program.

Fatness is also commonly linked with arthritis. This generic term refers to many joint diseases. Some of the one hundred known causes include tuberculosis, rheumatic fever, gonorrhea, and syphilis. A noninflammatory type of arthritis, called osteoarthritis, is age-related and leads to degeneration and deformation of joints. This is the type of arthritis that many health professionals feel is caused by obesity. Once again, though, the literature on this problem is contradictory. Fat women, for example, do have a higher than normal incidence of arthritis but fat men do not.

It does seem logical that a heavy body could be expected to cause more than normal trauma to weight bearing joints. One study reported in *Arthritis and Rheumatism*,[17] however, revealed that for older people who were 100% overweight, the incidence of osteoarthritis in the hip joint was only 12%. In addition, fat women are just as likely to suffer arthritis in the joints of their *hands* as in their weight-bearing joints! Can it therefore be concluded that the women do a lot of walking on their hands?

Instead of fatness causing arthritis, it may be that arthritis leads to fatness. The pain of movement assuredly restricts physical activity — and research strongly indicates that inactivity does lead to fatness.

Many respected studies may be interpreted as showing that being overweight, according to current standards, is actually beneficial to health. In an article by Joel Gurin in *American Health* (May, 1984) research is cited showing that a gain of about ten pounds per decade can in reality help keep a person healthy. Longtime survivors were found to be thin at age twenty and plump at age sixty. Gurin suggested, for instance, that a man of moderate weight might best weigh 150 pounds at age twenty and 180 pounds at age fifty. The conclusion was that good health does not require that a single, "ideal," body weight be maintained throughout life.

Again, it must be emphasized that many of the diseases associated with fatness may in reality be due to stress. There is a powerful biological rationale for this belief. Stress results in the secretion of hormones which reduces the effectiveness of the immune system. The body is therefore more susceptible to virtually every disease from asthma to ulcers — including heart disease, high blood pressure, diabetes, and arthritis.

At this point I have to admit to having selected studies that substantiate one particular viewpoint — namely that fatness, per se, is not necessarily the unhealthy condition it is often painted as being. This is not to say the research I have selected is more valid than those that put fat in an unfavorable light. Chapter Six (Fatness and Statistics) showed the difficulty in making such a statement. Since there is evidence for both points of view, it is clear that much more investigation needs to be done before sweeping generalizations can be made concerning the effect of body fat on health and mortality. Until that time, perhaps the most logical course would be to assume the truth lies somewhere between the extremes. That is, for any weight within a range of about 30 or 40 pounds of an individual's ideal weight, health and life expectancy should be average or better.

Even though there are widely conflicting positions regarding the relationship between fatness and health, the public is getting a totally unbalanced view. Whenever research can be interpreted as showing that obesity is harmful, health professionals smile smugly and the antifat industry gleefully increases the volume on its persistent bray that any amount of body fat is hazardous. The cry is a convincing one since each year the MAGGOTS spend massive sums of money to persistently pound their mercenarily inspired message into the public mind. As a result, a large majority of our population has developed a phobia toward fatness that has caused an immeasurable amount of physical, emotional, and social suffering — particularly among women. Unnecessary suffering! Unfortunately there is no organization to consistently and effectively counteract the massive antifat propaganda. And it is due to this unbalanced avalanche of biased information that fat has undeservedly become a four-letter word.

12

THINNESS AND HEALTH

Because of the ubiquitous, and iniquitous, efforts of the antifat industry, it is easy to see why losing weight has become a passionate quest for many people. Women are most vulnerable to the cruel antifat victimization. Not only do they have a greater genetic propensity for fat storage, cultures have historically placed greater pressure on them to have a pleasing appearance. And today the message is to be lean.

With such intense antifat propaganda it is no wonder that so many women become obsessed with their weight. This involves many millions of women who are not excessively fat at all — including many who are actually too thin, even morbidly thin. This point cannot be stressed too much.

Worst of all, the haunting drive to be thin encompasses large numbers of girls and young women. Boys and young men are not plagued nearly as much by this problem because society is not as demanding of them in this regard. Besides, they tend to be naturally leaner. And since they experience a prolonged rapid growth spurt at the beginning of adolescence, much of the food they eat is used by their bodies to support their vertical growth. Girls, on the other hand, have a much shorter period of rapid vertical growth. After that, they tend to quickly fill out into womanly contours which, sadly, they are currently led to believe is unattractive by a society that suffers from a fear of fat. Some people call this malady "fatophobia." Those who wish to impress others may prefer to call it "lipophobia."

Adolescence is a period during which conforming to group ideas and behavior is very important. Physical appearance has a special significance since it is visually more obvious than far more consequential attributes such as personality, intelligence, talent, and character. A girl's body image often reaches a low ebb during this period — and for many it remains there throughout their entire lives. Most girls believe to be attractive they must conform to the unnatural slenderness of women who adorn the popular glamour and fashion magazines.

Most girls and young women do not realize that the photos of these models are air brushed and often computer-enhanced. The latter technique allows body parts to be adjusted so that legs may be lengthened, hips reduced, busts enlarged, etc. A thoughtful observer might well see an analogy between the electronically produced images and Dr. Frankenstein's infamous creation. And just as that unfortunate surgeon was initially unaware of the suffering and death that could result from his work so, probably, are the modern "surgical" artists. This danger is no exaggeration as will be shown in this chapter.

A more charitable observer, however, would perceive the models as modern day Galateas; like Pygmalion's mythical creation they are artistic creations. The following list of credits for the April, 1989 *Cosmopolitan* cover girl is stark evidence of that.

> Photograph of Julie Anderson by Francesco Scavullo.
> Hair by Howard Fugler for Roger Thompson
> at Barney's, New York.
> Make up by Fran Cooper for Prescriptions:
> "Burnished Gold" Exact Color Makeup 1;
> "Neutral 3" Prescriptives A Better Powder;
> "Universal Eyes" Eyeshadow Powder Quintet;
> "Sable" Eyecoloring Pencil;
> "Basic Brown" Mascara;
> "Universal Blush" Powder Cheekcolor;
> "Henna" Lipcoloring Pencil;
> "Dramatic Warm" Classic Lipstick.
> Nails by Elizabeth Drabinsky.
> Clothing by Bob Mackie Sportswear.
> Jewelry by Kazuko Mitsushima at Artwear.
> Styled by Sean M. Byres.

If such credits were all-inclusive and candid, in many instances they would have to add something like:

Body Styling directed by Dr. Frank N. Stein for
Tackum and Tuckum of New York.
Ears; "Nautilus Sunrise" by Dr. Lobes.
Teeth; "Burnished Pearls" by Dr. Capps.
Breasts; "Vavoom Bozoom" by Dr. M. Planter.
Nipples; "Titillating Calibers" by Dr. Addum.
Hips; "Vacu-form" by Dr. Slerp.

Girls and women should realize the models in the glamour and fashion world do not necessarily have the body type females should strive to attain. It is not carved in stone anywhere that "Twiggy" models represent the ultimate in body shapes. Beauty is a matter of individual taste. In fact, the fashion industry, logically, does not particularly want to use models with attractive bodies. The women must be accepted for what they are, manikins for displaying beautiful products. Voluptuous bodies distract a buyer's attention from the clothes. The industry simply wants mobile clothes hangers. Unfortunately, the female public has come to believe that the skinny models have the ideal body type. This is one instance where the typical man knows better.

In attempting to emulate the models, many girls and women go so far as to engage in dangerous weight loss practices that lead to bizarre eating disorders — and severe health problems. One of the most widespread eating disorder is anorexia nervosa. This medical condition has been recognized at least as far back as 400 A.D., but only as a rare occurrence. Significantly, the first "outbreak" of anorexia occurred in the 1920s when extreme thinness became stylish for the first time in history. After that decade, the popularity of that severe body fashion subsided considerably. Then, shortly after 1960 the MAGGOTS started breeding in earnest. It is hardly a coincidence that since then anorexia has ballooned in direct proportion to the proliferation of that insatiable species. In the last decade, anorexia has reached epidemic proportions — almost exclusively in the middle and upper socioeconomic classes. The lower classes apparently do not feel it is a luxury to spurn food.

There has not been much research using subjects of *average* weight to study the effects of prolonged caloric restriction. A classic in the field, however, was conducted at the University of Minnesota by Keys (and colleagues) in 1950. Thirty young adults were placed on a prolonged semistarvation diet and their physical, psychological, and behavioral effects were recorded. After three months of normal eating and activity, the subjects' food intake was reduced by half, which is typical of women who are dieting. After six months of the restricted regimen, there was a three months normalization period.

Not surprisingly, after a few weeks of semistarvation the subjects became ravenous and felt strong desires to break the dietary rules. By the time they had lost about 25% of their original body weight they had become obsessed with eating and thoughts of food. Some resorted to eating binges and vomiting — followed by feelings of guilt.

Before the restricted period ended there were a number of physical changes including headaches, hair loss, sleepiness, gastrointestinal distress, and a lowered metabolic rate with its associated symptoms. Most of the subjects suffered psychological problems ranging from depression, hysteria, angry outbursts, anxiety, hypochondriasis, and even psychotic levels of disorganization. Common social disturbances included the loss of ability to operate effectively in the workplace and with friends. This was attributed to a lack of energy, apathy, social isolation, and a decrease in sexual interest. During the renormalization period, some of the subjects could not keep from eating continually. Others indulged in uncontrollable cycles of eating and vomiting.

The subjects were healthy, intelligent young *men* who had been measured as having high ego strength and emotional stability! It is not hard to imagine the severe effect chronic semistarvation would have on the physical, emotional, and social health of girls in the throes of early adolescence.

Actually, females have a greater minimum requirement for bodyfat than do males. This *essential fa*t is found in organs, muscles, bone marrow, intestines, and the central nervous system. In men the essential fat is about 3% of total body weight; in women it is 10% to 12%. These percentages refer to the amount of fat people need to support life processes — to stay alive.

Some experts believe there are two forms of nervosa — anorexia nervosa and bulimia nervosa. Both kinds of victims have an overwhelming terror of being fat. Anorexics, however, respond with prolonged periods of stringent food restriction while bulimics engage in frequent eating binges followed by self-induced purging (mainly vomiting, but also defecating).

Although the causes of anorexia are extremely complex and far from being completely understood, research suggests that a number of predisposing elements are involved, ranging from cultural attitudes, family interactions, and a victim's personality structure. One major element seems to be associated with the advances in women's rights. Young girls no longer are expected, or perhaps even permitted, to grow up and "merely" be housewives and mothers. They are under tremendous pressure to take advantage of the new opportunities to achieve in all areas—otherwise all the battles fought and won by their mothers and aunts would have been for naught. Some girls are reluctant to accept this awesome responsibility. One way to avoid it is simply to not grow up. Being very thin seems to be an effective way to become a female Peter Pan. After all, girls are bombarded with advertising that equates thinness with youth. Besides, stringent dieting delays the onset of the menstrual period, which is the most powerful evidence that womanhood and its obligations can be avoided. Significantly, 90% to 95% of the people who suffer from this eating disorder are females.

Many girls who develop anorexia come from calm, loving, but emotionally inexpressive families who are overprotective and have rigid expectations for their children. The girls feel that not living up to family expectations will lead to a feeling of not being loved. Such an environment stifles their social and personal growth. They know they do not have enough control of their lives but typically do not argue with their parents about it. Not realizing that "testing limits" and "acting out" (two terms which parents will immediately recognize as being blatant euphemisms) are signs of healthy maturation, the girls try to be model daughters. That explains why they tend to make good grades in school. Inspired by all of the antifat furor, however, they feel they can at least gain control of one aspect of their lives, namely, their weight.

Young women who develop anorexia tend to be introverted,

emotionally reserved, perfectionistic, self-abasing, socially insecure, have a drive for approval by others, are prone to be submissive, and are compulsive in general. Mainly, though, they have a strong desire to be thin and attractive. It is easy to see how such women would be especially vulnerable to the antifat propaganda that prods, "All alone? Embarrassed to face people? No friends? Listen to us! Get rid of repulsive fat! Be popular and happy! We have the answer!"

Yes, girls are especially fertile ground for the implantation of MAGGOTY larvae. Being inexperienced, they have a naive tendency to believe what they are told in advertisements and "paid programming" on television. Even if these girls do not purchase the antifat products due to insufficient funds, they still get the message loud and clear — "Fat is detestable!" Of course, the message is confirmed, and thereby strengthened, by a society that has already been thoroughly brainwashed into believing the same thing.

For some unknown reason, obese people practically never develop anorexia. It is also interesting that the thinner an anorexic becomes the more obsessed she gets about losing weight.

Typically, an anorexic starts her descent into the disorder during *early* adolescence. Initially, she is only slightly overweight according to current standards—which means she may not be overweight at all. After she loses, say, ten pounds through dieting and exercise, people start complimenting her on her more svelte shape. Encouraged by the control she has exerted over her body, she continues to lose. Before long she loses her healthy glow. Her continuing desire to lose weight, however, becomes irrational and starts dominating her life. Because of the obsession, she drops to about 15% below what is considered to be her ideal weight. At that point she is on the threshold of a full-blown case of anorexia. The resulting change in her body chemistry makes a reversal of the anorexic condition greatly resistant to change, and leads to low body temperature, low blood pressure, infertility, and heart damage. Since the phrase "ideal weight" is so ambiguous, a more objective indication of the eating disorder is the absence of at least three consecutive menstrual periods. An aversion to food and a fear of fat are the most characteristic behavioral symptoms.

At about this point, the danger of anorexia quickly intensifies since self-inflicted starvation distorts a person's perception. Even though she is approaching emaciation, she sees fat in the mirror — "ugly" fat. It is amazing how little food these starving people, males as well as females, can eat and how much much exercise they can perform in their drive to lose fat. Incidentally, the term anorexia, meaning "without appetite," is a misnomer since the victims are always extremely hungry until the last stage of the disorder — at which point death is imminent.

Treating an anorexic patient is maddeningly difficult because she strenuously denies having a problem — often even at the subconscious level. She is proud of her weight loss. Society idolizes thinness and she has undeniably achieved the ultimate in thinness. Besides, she finally has firm control of her body — and of her parents. The more her parents beg or threaten her to convince her to gain weight, the more resistant she becomes to their entreaties. And, of course, a looming MAGGOTY specter is constantly goading her to lose weight.

The eating disorder of bulimia has been recognized for almost as long as anorexia. Although the disorders may be related, they are quite different in terms of symptoms, the victims' personalities, and family environments. Victims usually begin their slide into bulimia during their later adolescent years. At the beginning, many of them are quite overweight. They may even view themselves as failed anorexics since they persistently give in to their hunger. To atone for each transgression they are driven to "cleanse" themselves by purging. As with anorexics, 90% to 95% of bulimics are females.

Far from being quiet, model daughters, bulimics tend to be lively, defiant, and headstrong. Due to overt parental conflict and a lack of emotional closeness in their family relationships, often fueled by physical or sexual abuse, they feel isolated. While their family problems are more chaotic and overt than those experienced by anorexics, their eating disorder is not obvious at all. The victims usually binge in secret and the purging helps them maintain a normal weight. Since the problem is hidden from view, bulimics are able to avoid treatment for a long time. As a result, the prognosis for curing these patients is considerably worse than it is for anorexics. The "hidden nature" of the disorder may also be one of the reasons bulimia is so widespread. And the number of victims is growing, especially among women in the last year of high school and the first year of college.

Purging involves spontaneous as well as self-induced vomiting, and the ingestion of massive doses of laxatives which lead to violent episodes of diarrhea. Virtually all of us have experienced vomiting and diarrhea as symptoms of various diseases so we know they are not acts in which people would normally engage if they had their "druthers." These unpleasant practices give some idea of the bulimics' intense motivation to lose weight.

Bulimia usually begins with weekly or monthly purgings, but for a young woman to be diagnosed as having *clinical* bulimia, she has to have at least two binge and purge episodes a week. Binges of 4,000 to 5,000 calories are not uncommon, and for patients who binge and purge 10 or more times a day the total caloric intake may be as much as 20,000 calories in a single day!

Observable physical signs of a person afflicted with bulimia are puffiness around the eyes, general edema, bruises and lacerations over the knuckles, broken blood vessels on the cheeks, and noticeably swollen parotid glands. These are the large salivary glands just in front of and below the ears. A long term sufferer will often have terrible looking, rotting teeth. And dental disorders such as caries, root canals, hypersensitive teeth, and chipping teeth persist for years after a bulimic kicks her habit. Other oral problems include jaw deterioration and dry mouth (from taking multiple doses of laxatives, stimulants, and vitamins — all of which reduce the flow of saliva). Also, after months of voluntary vomiting the stomach starts "thinking" it's supposed to vomit every time food is eaten. Women have told me that years after they have stopped purging, they "*still* feel like throwing up after every meal."

Although bulimics may try to atone for their gluttony by fasting, using diet pills, or by exhaustive exercising, purging is the most common step. Methods include vomiting and the use of diuretics or laxatives. All of these steps can cause health problems. When the harshly acidic contents of the stomach are regurgitated, the entire esophagus, along with the gums and teeth, are eroded.

Frequent vomiting can cause hiatal hernias or rupture the stomach! Even if that does not occur, the loss of acid in the stomach makes the blood more alkaline. This condition and the loss of electrolytes leads to a loss of circulating calcium, bone degeneration, tingling in the fingers, severe muscle cramps, epileptic seizures, and damage to the liver, lungs, and heart. Vomiting, along with diarrhea and the use of "water pills," results in dehydration that causes kidney damage and a loss of nutrients. Sodium and potassium deficiencies, among other problems, lead to further vomiting and dehydration, and eventually rectal bleeding and heart irregularities. As with anorexia, bulimia results in deficiencies in the immune system. In addition, the over-the-counter drugs that bulimics use to induce vomiting lead to irreversible neurological damage. This is usually manifested in an inability to concentrate and do well academically.

If females (and males) are trying to become sexier by starving themselves or by purging, they are headed the wrong direction. Due to hormonal imbalances, anorexics (males and females) lose their sex drives. The enjoyment of sex by bulimics, on the other hand, is thwarted by a powerful self-hatred of their bodies. Not only is the pleasure of sex largely diminished in anorexics and bulimics, it must surely result in reduced enjoyment for their partners.

A variety of methods are used to treat the eating disorders of anorexia and bulimia. Unfortunately, success is elusive. About one-third of anorexics get better, one-third stay the same, and one-third get worse. Bulimia has an even more bleak prognosis. Unfortunately, there are about six times as many bulimics as anorexics. Some experts estimate that as many as twenty percent of the anorexia and bulimia patients die. That is an extremely high fatality rate! It amounts to about 150,000 deaths each year among American women alone — according to the American Anorexia and Bulimia Association. That is 17,000 more fatalities than the total number of deaths caused by AIDS since it was recognized as a disease in 1980, to 1989 — in all the 177 countries surveyed by the World Health Organization. Up to half of the survivors of anorexia and bulimia *never* recover completely.

The illnesses and deaths associated with these eating disorders are particularly heart-rending because 1) the victims are nearly always young and 2) there is absolutely no reason for the disorders to occur. They are caused solely by society's distorted values — fueled largely by an grossly mercenary antifat industry. It may be melodramatic to say that innocent youths are being sacrificed on the alter of conscienceless profit, but that statement would also be accurate.

In both eating disorders, early detection and treatment, before the abnormal eating habits become firmly entrenched, greatly increase the chances for recovery. As with most illnesses, though, the best route is prevention. For young people with a personality predisposition to eating disorders, the best preventative measure would be for parents to instill in their children the feeling that they do not have to be perfect to be valued and loved — that no one *is* perfect — and that no one *can* be perfect. And a perfect child would not be very interesting, anyway. An obsessive drive to be perfect only leads to frustration and misery. Nowhere is this more evident than in the futile attempts to achieve "ideal" body shapes and weight levels.

Generally a small loss of weight within reason, through conservative methods of diet and exercise, is not harmful — and for people who are truly excessively fat, a loss is indeed beneficial. However, in susceptible females (and males) the fat reduction can get dangerously out of hand. Exact figures are impossible to determine, but it has been estimated that as many as five percent of females of high school and college age are afflicted with anorexia or bulimia — mainly the latter. And these are conservative estimates. Four times as many female students do not have full blown cases, but suffer from some of the symptoms such as a morbid preoccupation with body weight, frequent dieting attempts, guilt after eating high calorie foods, low self-esteem, and unrealistically high expectations for themselves. Further, it is believed that 80% of all female college students have self-induced vomiting at least once to lose weight. In other words, there are millions of women with subclinical eating disorders.

Thankfully, not all girls who diet are psychologically predisposed to develop anorexia and bulimia. If they were, the number of victims would be astronomical. A 1988 survey of schoolgirls in San Francisco, for instance, indicated that nearly 90% of the seventeen-year-olds were dieting. Yet, only 20% were overweight according to *current* standard measures—which means that the percentage who were truly overweight was probably much lower. At least 70% of the girls were therefore needlessly subjecting themselves to the tortures and dangers of nutritional deprivation.

Even more incredible was the finding that more than 80% of fourth-grade girls had dieted at least once! Such studies substantiate the claim by Vivian Meehan, president of the National Association of Anorexia Nervosa and Associated Disorders, that dieting is rampant among fourth and fifth graders. The obsession with thinness can so alter the development of girls that the onset of their menstruation can be delayed by two to three years. Such a delay may result in permanent damage to their bones, leading to such problems as curvature of the spine, stress fractures, and early onset osteoporosis.

It is not difficult to understand the girls' anxiety. On top of the pressure exerted by a largely impersonal antifat industry, there are popular female stars like Cher, who in her TV ads for a health spa, told viewers, "If you are not in shape, it is *your* fault." Cher failed to mention that people have different body types, or that she had a thin body type to begin with and that she has spent large sums of money for surgery to "fine tune" that body.

Christina Applegate, the nineteen-year-old actress on *Married. . . With Children*, was more candid in describing her secret to maintaining a svelte, nubile figure. She told *People* magazine, "When I'm doubled over and passing out, then I eat." Hopefully, young women who are interested in being healthy will not follow her example—but you know that many will.

Where does this emulation lead? For a clue one merely needs to consider Tracey Gold, the 22-year-old actress on television's *Growing Pains*. In 1992, after struggling with anorexia for several years, she was dropped indefinitely from the show.

Young girls are also greatly influenced by their parents, usually mothers, who may be distressed by their own bodies. And the attempt to keep girls thin begins even in infancy. As Margo Maine, Ph.D.,

Associate Clinical Director of the Eating Disorder Service at Newington (Connecticut) Children's Hospital, has reported in her hospital's *Eating Disorders in Focus* publication:

> . . . infants and toddlers with impaired physical development are frequently referred to our pediatricians. These cases of nonorganic failure to thrive often are the result of parents who, due to their own eating and body image problems, underfeed their children.

This brings to mind a cartoon in which a very thin young girl of about seven years of age is seated at a table with a few stalks of celery on a plate in front of her. She manages a wan smile while her mother clasps her hands in ecstacy and her father proudly snaps photographs. When this scenario occurs in real life it's not nearly as funny. It is reminiscent of the mother who made her nine-year-old daughter wear a girdle.

Of course, if a daughter does not remain thin, this type of mother will constantly let the daughter know of her displeasure. This was plainly revealed in a *Sally Jessy Raphael* program that aired on November, 18, 1991. It dealt with mothers who were embarrassed and disgusted by their daughters' being fatter than is commonly acceptable in the U.S. Of course, the mothers' spirit-breaking nagging merely resulted in the daughters eating more. Interestingly, without exception the daughters' weight did not matter to their husbands or boyfriends.

It is not only naive children and school girls who suffer from lipophobia and resort to dangerous anorexic and bulimic techniques. In February,1984, *Glamour* magazine revealed the results of its national survey of 33,000 women. It dealt with how they felt about their bodies. Of these, nearly 80% felt they had to be thin for men to find them attractive (a survey of the men would have been revealing). Forty-one percent of the women were moderately or extremely unhappy with their bodies (other studies report much higher figures). Significantly, 30% were *below* current weight norms for their heights. Of these, nearly one-half thought they were too fat! Eighteen percent of the women reported using diuretics and laxatives to lose weight while another 15% engaged in forced vomiting. It is hardly surprising that a million American women are afflicted with anorexia and bulimia *every* year!

The extent of lipophobia in the U.S. was dramatically revealed in a 1989 survey by *Vogue* magazine. It showed that a large majority of the respondents would be willing to give up their husbands/boyfriends, careers, and money for their idea of the ideal figure. Clearly, due to societal pressures to meet thinner standards, women of the U.S. have acquired an irrational and unwholesome preoccupation with losing weight.

And women, bless their hearts, are steadily losing ground — not weight. Standards of fatness/thinness are determined chiefly by such female Olympians as models, movie stars, dancers, Miss Americas, and *Playboy* playmates. In roughly the past twenty-five years, while these standard setters have gotten considerably thinner, the average American woman has been getting fatter. At the beginning of this period, for example, models weighed 8% less than the average woman. In 1990, models weighed 23% less than the average woman! These highly publicized standards of beauty and desirability are driving American women to increasingly greater depths of despair.

Losing an unnatural amount of body fat is an agonizing experience; keeping it off is a chronically agonizing experience. Since, according to the old saying, "misery loves company," these miserable feelings may explain why thin women often have such hostile emotions toward fat women — particularly when the latter are happy with themselves and their lives. When I first started giving talks on the subject of "Fat is *Not* a Four-Letter Word," I was completely taken aback by the intensely hostile comments hurled at me by some of the thin women in the audience. They erroneously viewed my message as being anti-thin. After apologizing for any perceived offensiveness, I explained that even if my message *was* anti-thin, they had to admit it was quite mild compared to the anti-fat insults hurled at fat women. And, of course, I pointed out that my sixty-minute session was a drop in the bucket compared to the continual flood of ridicule and humiliation experienced by fat women — every day of their lives!

A woman who elects to chronically suffer from food deprivation and who regularly exercises to exhaustion to conform to public standards of thinness is understandably not eager to hear that fat women are in reality just as beautiful and probably healthier than women who are unnaturally thin. In addition, it must be a bitter pill for the thin woman whose suffering has not made her happier at all. In fact, studies strongly suggest that her happiness is actually diminished. There is also the nagging thought that perhaps people care more for her thin external shell than for the important attributes that make her the person she really is. An ancient Danish proverb, "The fat sow knows not what the hungry sow suffers," can be applied to today's women. And if a person thinks this figurative statement implies that women are pigs, they are clearly missing the point.

Just as the aim of all treatments for anorexia and bulimia is to first help victims develop a realistic self-image, one of the aims of this book is to help *fat* people develop a realistic self-image. There is a thread that links all three of these groups; it is the great fear of fat. And it certainly is not a natural fear. Most of the world's cultures, even today, would have a difficult time understanding the lipophobia that is rampant in the U.S. and which is rapidly growing in Western Europe.

This fear of fatness, which is unique in history, is often attributed to various factors that promote thinness. Among these are: (1) the medical hazards of obesity, (2) an increased involvement of women in athletics, and (3) the fashion industry's current standards. But there must be more to lipophobia than these three factors. Before the Twentieth Century, the opposite situation existed. Thinness was associated with poor health, motherhood was the women's role, and the full-figured female form was the fashion. Yet, while thinness was generally not admired, there was never an intense, widespread fear of the condition. Scrawniphobia, to coin a term, did not exist.

Why not? Because there was no pack of thinness entrepreneurs equivalent to the teeming mass of MAGGOTS that currently plague our culture. Therefore, people were not constantly exposed to propaganda that proclaimed thin people to be ugly, lazy, stupid, messy, lacking in self-respect, and immoral. Of course, none of these belittling statements would have been true, just as none of them are true for fat people. Fat is unhealthy at excessive levels, but no more so than excessive thinness.

Indeed, the latter is probably far more hazardous, particularly for women, as indicated in the Metropolitan Mortality Table. Besides, even extremely obese people do not die of their condition in their teens and twenties — as do most anorexics and bulimics.

The chief reason pressure is exerted on women to be thin is to make money for the antifat industry. Of course, the latter claim they are merely concerned about the health of fat people. In most cases, however, the antifat hue and cry is actually much ado about nothing. An unnatural physical state of thinness is causing greater health problems than if the fatness issue had never been vomited upon the public. In fact, there is increasing evidence that chronic dieting can, by itself, result in the dangerous disorders of anorexia and bulimia. The national feeling that fat is a four-letter word is in essence a social virus that causes very serious physical and psychological illnesses.

13

DIET AND HEALTH

The intent of this book is not to promote fatness. To suggest that people become as fat as possible is as ridiculous as suggesting they become as thin as possible. What *is* being recommended is that people stop being overly concerned about being fat. After all, fat people are just as attractive, nice, intelligent, neat, clean, graceful, and hardworking as people of different body compositions. As far as health is concerned, most people who are considered to be fat in our society are probably as healthy as thinner people, and in many cases healthier — with the exception of the extremely obese (as with the extremely thin).

People who are emotionally chained to a scale should bear in mind that throughout history people survived quite well without them. In fact, since men and women of old were not forced to live under the uncompromising glare of these currently ubiquitous contraptions, they were very likely happier than the scale-slaves of today.

Advising people to stop worrying about their weight is not to say they should stop being concerned about their health. On the contrary, it is for their health's sake that they should stop worrying about their weight and should start adopting practices that definitely do improve their health and the quality of their lives.

Many of these healthful measures are easily accomplished, including the elimination of drug abuse (including tobacco and alcohol); keeping blood pressure under control through a balanced diet, exercise, and medication; taking afternoon naps; and exchanging a couple of big hugs every day. Not only are sensible exercise and eating most basic to achieving and maintaining good health, they are also the key to helping each person determine and attain his or her own ideal body weight.

Strictly speaking, the word "diet" refers to what a person usually eats. Yet, when people say they are on a diet, it is automatically assumed they are talking about a *weight-reducing* diet. This connotation has developed because so many people have been on such diets. For instance, it is commonly reported that more than one-third of all Americans are overweight. Many millions who are not too fat are included in this number — which adds up to a lot of needless dieting. Actually, about eighty million Americans are dieting at any given time. It's no wonder there is such a massive antifat industry. The obsession to lose weight has even led to the manufacture of diet foods for dogs and cats! You can imagine how people in Third World countries feel when they learn about that.

It has been said that dieting and talking about it has become the national pastime for women — like sports is for men. Because of this interest, the number of diets that allegedly help people lose weight is absolutely mind-boggling. In the latter 1980s it was estimated that more than twenty thousand have been foisted onto the American public since the turn of the century and new diets pop up daily. Each one is touted with the unctuous sincerity of a used car salesman as being "THE ONE!" that produces results where all others have failed.

After a brief heyday, though, every so-called reducing diet inevitably passes into oblivion. The reason for their demise is clear. People soon learn that diets result in, at best, only temporary losses. Of course, permanent reductions are claimed or implied for these diets, but such claims are patently untrue . A five-year study by Dr. Thomas Wadden at the University of Pennsylvania revealed that 98% of all dieters regain their weight within five years. Most regained their weight in a much shorter period. All other independent studies have arrived at similar conclusions. Obviously, if a successful "reducing" diet had ever been devised there would have been no need for subsequent diets to have been concocted. New ones would not be hawked in magazines and tabloids each week. A permanently effective reducing diet would make front page headlines; that has yet to occur.

Since 1960, the diet movement in the U.S. has been gaining momentum steadily. Yet, significantly, during the same period Americans have been getting progressively fatter. This is not mere happenstance. It is a reflection of the fact that reducing diets are not only ineffectual, they generally result in an *increase* in fatness.

The most well-known of these futile, pie-in-the-sky regimens are introduced via books, and there have been thousands published. In 1983 alone about 360 were in print. Typical of such books are *The Complete Scarsdale Medical Diet*, *Beyond Pritikin*, *Dr. Adkins Diet Revolution*, *Fit for Life*, *Medical Makeover*, *The Fat to Muscle Diet*, *The Diet-Type Weight-Loss Diet*, *Thin So Fast*, *Eat To Succeed*, *The 35 Plus Diet*, *The 120-Year Diet*, *The Two-Day Diet*, *The Hilton Head Metabolic Diet*, *The Beverly Hills Diet*, *The I Love New York Diet*, *The Bloomingdale's Eat Healthy Diet*, *The Rice Diet Report*, *The Macrobiotic Diet*, and *Elizabeth Takes Off*. The latter refers to the alluring Elizabeth Taylor and it is easy to envision a lot of men (with excellent taste) shelling-out for a steamy pictorial offering without realizing it deals with dieting. Nearly all of these books have been national best sellers which means absolutely nothing relative to their validity. Indeed, the independent and highly credible Consumers' Union, publishers of the *Consumer's Report*, labels all of the above as, "NOT RECOMMENDED," declaring their dietary advice to be nutritionally unsound and often even dangerous to the health of adherents.

Some diet book authors are out-and-out charlatans. For example, Dr. Stuart Berger, author of *Dr. Berger's Immune Power Diet*, was exposed in 1990 by NBC's *Inside Edition* as grossly falsifying his academic credentials. Even more revealing was the television program's hidden video of Berger's very expensive and highly suspect office practices.

One of the most bizarre diet books was the 1957, *Pray Your Weight Away*. Bordering on the sacrilegious (at least), this book, written by the Reverend Charles W. Shedd, claimed that God intended for everyone to be thin. By equating fat with sin, he sent believers on the holy quest of weight loss. Since 95% to 98% of "fat" people are unable to keep the weight off, a lot of people were apparently letting the Lord down. The chief achievement of the prayer approach must have been a rash of cases of profound guilt.

This religious approach may sound outlandish, but the guilt technique is still popular and effective in the 1990s. If you doubt this, just attend one of the evangelical type meetings used by many weight-watching organizations. If you join, be sure to bring your purse.

On top of all the deceptions, the wasting of consumers' time and money, and the inherent dangers, all of the reducing diets are effective only in the short run. One may wonder, then, why practically every diet manages to attract followers. One reason is that many people are so desperate to lose weight they are willing to try anything. Another is that *any* diet can produce impressive results, initially. It is quite common, in fact, for a person to drop two or three pounds in just the first 24 to 36 hours of a diet. This reduction is possible because glycogen (sugar) stores are quickly exhausted when caloric intake drops. Along with the weight of glycogen, three to four times that weight in associated water is also lost. Taken together, that can easily result in the loss of several pounds.

After the glycogen is depleted, a *much* higher percentage of fat is used for energy. Since about twice as much energy is derived from fat as from an equal weight of sugar, the loss of body weight could be expected to proceed at about half the pace. But because no water is lost when fat is burned, the weight loss actually proceeds at one-eighth to one-tenth the pace! This slowdown after an easy and dramatic beginning can be exceedingly discouraging to a dieter.

Body fat can be lost no matter what the diet, even if it consists of nothing but hog fat (lard) — if more calories are burned than are consumed. Specifically, if a women takes in 500 calories *less* than her body expends during a given period of time, she will burn up 500 calories of stored body fat during that period. This negative energy balance translates to a loss of one-seventh of a pound of body fat. If she maintains a negative balance of 500 calories every day for an entire week, she will lose 3,500 calories — which equals a pound of body fat. If the 3,500 negative energy balance is acquired over a year's time, the person will lose one pound of fat for the year. Time, in other words, is not relevant; calories are. Naturally, when more calories are consumed than are expended, a positive energy balance exists. An excess of 3,500 calories will be stored as a pound of body fat.

In the 1960s a popular weight-loss book, *Calories Don't Count*, was written by an M.D. named Herman Taller. Even though the title was catchy, it was a blatant falsehood. When it comes to losing (or gaining) body fat, calories count very much. The author of the book, incidentally, was convicted of fraud.

Even though calories are of utmost importance when it comes to a positive or negative energy balance, numbers are not everything. As far as gaining body fat is concerned, 500 calories of *dietary* carbohydrates are not the same as 500 calories of *dietary* fat. This is because the body has to expend more energy to digest, transport, store, and reprocess carbohydrates than it expends for similar activities concerning fat. More precisely, 23% of the calories in carbohydrates are used to digest the food, whereas only 3% of the calories in fat are burned up during its digestion. That is, if a person eats 100 excess calories of fat, 97 of those calories can make a bee-line for the hips and thighs — especially if she is a woman. If 100 excess calories of carbohydrates are eaten, only 77 will be available to create potential bulges. In other words, carbohydrates increase a person's metabolic rate much more than does the consumption of dietary fat.

This factor helps to explain why obese women have been known to reduce their caloric intake by 20% while consuming an unlimited amount of complex carbohydrates (fruits vegetables, whole grain products, and legumes). The large amount of fiber in complex carbohydrates also has the effect of filling up subjects with less food.

Once 500 *net* calories are actually in the body, however, their source is irrelevant. Excess calories, whether from carbohydrates or fat (or protein), will be stored as the same amount of fat. With this in mind, one might well ask, "Why worry about what you eat? Why not eat only chocolate, or ice cream, or whatever?" It is because a diet must have diversity to provide all of the nutrients a person needs for health and vitality. Any reducing diet founded upon the principles of eating only a few types of food, such as grapefruit and eggs, is unwholesome. (Grapefruit, by the way, has no special weight-reducing properties as is often claimed.)

What kind of diet is best for a person trying to lose weight? The answer is so simple people find it difficult to believe; it is the same kind that is best for any other person. Such a diet will supply the proteins, fats, carbohydrates, vitamins, minerals, water, and fiber (roughage) necessary for the body and brain to function at their best.

Fiber, which comes from the cell walls of plants, is indigestible. While not a nutrient, fiber is extremely valuable in the diet because it hastens the passage of food through the body. The faster transit helps to prevent constipation and a variety of diseases such as diverticulosis and colon cancer. It also means ingested fats will not linger long enough to be completely absorbed into the body—a circumstance that makes fiber attractive to people trying to lose weight. Some types of fiber also help to remove cholesterol and environmental toxins from the body. In spite of the importance of fiber in the diet, more than 80% of Americans on any given day eat no high-fiber foods at all. For the best health results, the amount of fiber in the diet should be increased gradually and along with it more water should be drunk.

SOME SOURCES OF FIBER

Rich Sources—bran cereals, bran muffins, beans (kidney, lima, pinto), dried prunes, and blackberries.

Moderate Sources—whole wheat bread, popcorn, oatmeal, peas, corn, carrots, broccoli, potato (with skin), apples, and oranges.

Low Sources — white bread, spaghetti, rice, lettuce, grapes.

Water, like fiber, is not generally thought of as being a nutrient. In a sense, though, it is the most vital one. A person can go for many weeks without solid food, but several days without water is the limit. That is not surprising when considering that about 70% of the normal adult body consists of water. The amazing fluid is essential for *every* function of the body yet most people probably do not drink nearly enough for optimal health.

How much water should a person drink? The National Research Council recommends eight 8 oz. glasses a day for an average man (160 lb.) and a little more than 6 glasses for an average woman (120 lb.). But that answer is too simplistic.

Some experts claim an inactive 160 lb. person needs a minimum of 10 glasses of drinking water per day, *over and above* what is acquired in other beverages and foods. Dr. Donald Robertson, Medical Director of the Southwest Bariatric Nutrition Center in Scottsdale, Arizona, thinks people should drink even more if they exercise, eat salty food, live in a hot climate, or are overweight. Robertson believes overweight people should drink an extra glass for every 25 pounds over their ideal weight to adequately metabolize fat — and that this is a dietary key to achieving a weight loss. There is considerable evidence to support his claim.

Some dieters foolishly restrict their water intake because they fear the possibility of becoming bloated by drinking too much water. Paradoxically, it is the intake of too little water that results in water retention. An excess consumption of water merely produces a large quantity of diluted urine — which is very good for the kidneys.

The International Sportsmedicine Institute in Los Angeles provides a tidy formula. It recommends 1/2 ounce of water per pound of body weight for inactive people. This comes to ten 8 oz. glasses for a 160 pound person. For athletes in training it recommends 2/3 ounce of water per pound of body weight; this means thirteen 8 oz. glasses for a 160 pound person. If nothing else, this intake would drastically reduce the incidence of kidney infections and kidney stones. This benefit is extremely important since 20,000,000 Americans are known to have kidney disease, and 80,000 died in 1990 alone.

Such quantities of water may be difficult for most people to consume. It is best to begin by drinking as much water as possible without feeling uncomfortable and to progressively increase the quantity each day. Initially, it will be a good idea to stay within striking distance of a restroom. The bladder will gradually adjust, however, so that a person will have to urinate less often but more copiously. At least that's the theory.

It is much easier to consume sufficient water if caffeine products such as soft drinks, coffee, and tea are omitted. Besides, since they are diuretics, they reduce the amount of water in the body. Alcoholic drinks are also diuretics. In addition, eight ounces of water are required to metabolize a single ounce of alcohol. The consumption of milk, and fruit and vegetable juices should not be reduced due their high vitamin and mineral content. They cannot be counted as a part of one's water intake, however, since their high sugar or salt content increases the body's water requirements. The same is true for sugar-sweetened drinks.

Unfortunately, the purity of water supplies in many American communities is is deteriorating. As this fact becomes more widely known, there will be a tremendous burgeoning of the bottled water industry and the use of home filter systems. The latter, particularly, makes a lot of sense.

The three major classes of food are carbohydrates, fats, and proteins. The average American diet contains about 40% fat, 20% protein, and 40% carbohydrates (half in the form of simple sugars — mainly table sugar) with about 14 grams of fiber. This is a very unhealthy regimen, especially as it relates to cardiovascular disease, cancer, and diabetes. A far more satisfactory, and easily accomplished, diet would contain about 30% fat (or less), 12% protein, and 58% carbohydrates (10% of which should be simple sugars — mainly from fruits) with 30 grams of fiber. A diet with only 20% fat (and more carbohydrates) would be better although it would take a much greater commitment to stick with it.

Planning a sound diet may seem to be a rather complicated endeavor and, in truth, the science of nutrition is incredibly complex — so complex that relatively little is known with certainty. Considerably more research has been conducted on vitamin C than on any of the other vitamins, for example, and a controversy still rages regarding optimal dosages. Even greater uncertainties exist when it comes to other dietary components. Part of the problem is that it's not possible to determine ideal dosages for each individual. Therefore, only averages have been established and even these are highly debatable. In addition, some of the components of a sound diet surely are still unknown.

This nutritional vagueness could understandably lead people to throw up their hands in frustration. Fortunately, there is a very simple plan that meets the needs of everyone. It is the BALANCED DIET. Virtually everyone has heard of the term. Yet, it cannot be avoided when discussing a proper diet; it *is* the proper diet.

The five food groups of a balanced diet are listed in the Eating Right Pyramid below. The shape was selected by the U.S. government's nutritional researchers as being the clearest for educating the public on the dietary guidelines developed by them throughout the 1980s (at considerable taxpayer expense). The nutritional service sent the pyramid and accompanying text to some thirty university and federal nutritionists who judged it to be accurate and useful. The genius of the pyramid is that the shape clearly and simply shows the proper proportion of the various foods in a healthy diet. Notice, too, how the fat and sugar (represented by small circles and triangles) are distributed throughout all of the food groups.

The Eating Right Pyramid

A Guide to Daily Food Choices

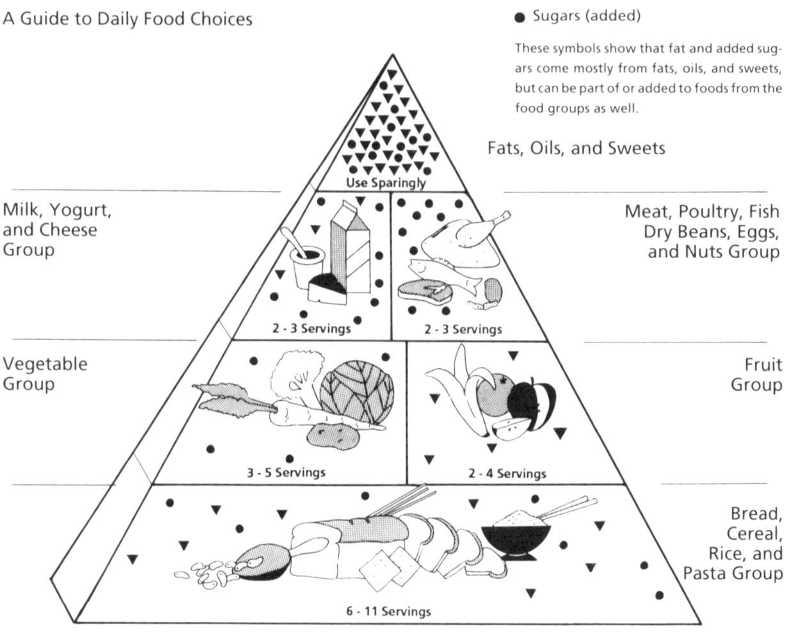

Drawing and text derived from the USDA's, *The Eating Right Pyramid*. 1991.

Unfortunately, the U.S. Department of Agriculture (USDA) halted its distribution of the 32-page booklet, containing the Eating Right Pyramid, shortly after its release in April, 1991. According to *Consumer Reports* (October,1991), the lobbyists for the politically powerful National Cattlemen's Association and American Meat Institute (known collectively as "meatheads") and the National Milk Production Federation opposed the pyramid and had its distribution squelched. The reason being that the pyramid did not give enough emphasis to their products. Of course, it didn't! The chief problem with the typical American diet is that already it contains far too much meat and dairy products — their quantity in the diet *should* be de-emphasized. The meatheads in classic doublespeak tell us that beef is "real food for real people." Well, the fact is, fruits, grains and vegetables are also "real food" — and people who eat them are also "real people."

Condition yourself to thinking of *whole* milk as poison. Seriously. There's a very, very strong relationship between the ingestion of whole milk and deaths due to heart disease. Drink skim milk! If you are a sissy and cannot stomach skim milk, drink milk that's 1/2% fat — not 2%.

The developers of the pyramid's booklet tried not to favor any food group. It is practically impossible to imagine any *certified* nutritionist finding the statement below to be unfair or inaccurate. Happily, on April 28, 1992 rational heads finally prevailed. The pyramid once again was adopted as the nations's primary device for teaching nutrition.

> Each of these food groups provides some, but not all, of the nutrients you need. No one food group is more important than another; for good health, you need them all . . . Just try to pick the lowest-fat choices from the food groups.

The proportion of each nutrient in a diet is very important. For example, some nutrients — such as calcium and vitamin D, and vitamin A and zinc — magnify another's functions. Conversely, some nutrients interfere with the uptake of other nutrients. Too much zinc, for instance, blocks the uptake of copper — too little copper and a body cannot use iron efficiently. On the other hand, too much iron interferes with zinc uptake. An excess of protein flushes calcium out of the body via the kidneys. Too much phosphorus also results in calcium loss — and processed foods are usually high in phosphorus. Fad diets which are based upon eating only a few foods limit beneficial interactions and accentuate the impact of negative ones. Vitamin and mineral pills, especially megadoses, can also play havoc with proper nutrient proportions.

A person can use a computer and devote much time to trying to achieve correct nutritional proportions and still not be successful. A more reliable and simplified method is merely to eat the proper number of servings from each of the five food groups. It is vital to have a lot of *variety* in these groups. The diversity assures the intake of all of the nutrients and the different kinds of fiber a person needs. Fruits are better eaten raw since juices do not provide nearly as much fiber as the whole fruit.

How large should servings be? That depends upon how much a person wants to weigh and such factors as body size, metabolic rate, and activity level. Personal experimentation is required, but one *suggestion* is to start with the sample serving sizes shown in the list below and then adjust them according to personal needs.

ONE SERVING EQUALS:

3 oz. lean cooked meat (not counting bone)

2 eggs

1 cup of cooked dry beans, peas, or lentils

1/2 cup nuts

1 slice of bread (whole grain, please)

1/2 cup cooked cereal

1 oz. ready-to-eat cereal

8 oz. skim milk (cheeses and yogurt are concentrated forms)

A large, extremely active person with a high basal metabolic rate might eat portions that are two times the size of the portions listed above. A small, inactive person with a low BMR may find half-size portions sufficient. To lose weight, foods from *all* of the groups should be eaten in the proper proportions, but the servings should be smaller than he or she is used to having. Some experimentation is, of course, necessary. As long as the diet is balanced, a person can be virtually assured of acquiring all of the necessary nutrients in the proper proportions.

The only time a balanced diet is insufficient is when a person tries to lose weight with a severe restriction of total caloric intake. Any such restriction is called a "crash" diet. Its effects are similar to those associated with total fasting. In either case, the body enters a starvation state. It reacts by attempting to conserve energy, and its fat stores, by lowering its basal metabolic rate — which accounts for 60% to 75% of the energy used by the body. With a stringent reducing diet the BMR can drop 20% within two weeks. This increase in efficiency enables a starving person to survive for a longer period of time so it's a very handy mechanism in times of famine. If a person has a choice, though, starvation diets should be avoided.

During the first day or two on a crash diet, the body uses up all of the glycogen (sugar) stores in its muscles, blood, and liver. It must then rely primarily upon its fat deposits for energy. That sounds fine, but the brain cells need glucose to function. For several days this glucose is produced by the breakdown of protein tissues (mainly muscles). This is not a very efficient source of energy since a lot of protein tissue is needed to make just a small amount of glucose. The extraction of glycerol from fat cells can also be used to produce glucose, but the process is even less efficient. As a result, nearly all of the glucose needed by the brain comes from the sacrifice of muscle tissue during the first several days of a crash diet — and leads to a feeling of weakness.

After that, the flow of fatty acids from the fat cells into the blood stream greatly increases. In the liver the fatty acids are broken down into compounds called ketones. One of the ketones is a sweet smelling liquid, called acetone. Because crash dieters have a very high level of ketones in their blood, their breath will often have the sweet odor of acetone.

The ketones serve as the main energy source in the body during starvation — or any time the body relies almost exclusively upon fat for energy as is the case for untreated diabetics or people on a high-fat diet. Some of the brain cells can even use ketones for energy, but not all have the ability to do so. Therefore, protein tissues continue to be sacrificed for energy. It has been estimated that a person who fasts or goes on a crash diet will lose one pound of protein for every three pounds of fat. Upon resumption of normal eating all of the fat is restored, and generally more — but not nearly as much of the muscle tissue is regained. Cattle farmers make use of this phenomenon when they want to quickly and cheaply increase the fat content of their animals. (That is, they will drastically underfeed the animals for a while before allowing them to feed normally.)

Along with the lowering of the BMR, another major problem with losing weight rapidly concerns lipoprotein lipase. The function of this enzyme is to help deposit fat in fat cells. With large weight losses, the enzyme becomes extremely active and results in fat being stored at a much faster rate than normal when a dieter resumes normal eating. The result is a rapid gain in body fat. Studies indicate the increase in lipoprotein lipase activity remains elevated for years!

Modifications of the fasting approach to losing weight are the liquid protein (or liquid formula) diets. They were developed to keep people from losing muscle tissue while on a very low calorie program of between 420 C. to 800 C. a day — for weeks. That is starvation! During World War II, research showed 900 C. to be the minimum required to maintain bodily functions.

Although liquid protein diets result in rapid short-term weight losses, the diets are extremely risky with at least 60 *known* deaths. Obviously, they must never be attempted without close medical supervision.

Among the programs that use such diets and do provide medical monitoring, the most popular include Optifast and Medifast. Unfortunately, to avoid the high cost of these programs people buy the liquid formulas "under the table" from unscrupulous peddlers, and skip the medical overview.

Because there are unavoidable risks even when adhering to a supervised program, it is recommended even by directors that people who join these programs should be limited to those with medically significant obesity. This is commonly defined as people who are more than 30% (or 50 lb.) greater than their ideal weight — bearing in mind that "ideal" is an ambiguous term.

The liquid diet regimens are not picnics. Even a strong advocate, Vincent Felitti of San Diego's Kaiser Permanente Medical Care (Optifast) Program, has admitted there are relatively few people who are willing to be involved in such an extensive program because it is a big commitment and a lot of work. Dr. C. Wayne Callaway, an associate clinical professor of medicine at Georgetown University, says simply that it's an unrealistic plan.

With weekly clinic appointments, the basic programs cost between $1,400 to $3,000. Movie stars and TV personalities, who are able to afford special treatment, are monitored almost daily by a corps of professionals including a physician, nutritionist, exercise physiologist, and psychologist. No stone is left unturned to ensure that famous clients lose weight — after all, such successes have great public relations value for a diet company. Indeed, some celebrities are paid to act as spokesman. When the celebrities regain their lost weight, their "spots" are simply removed from the air.

Within a few years after the liquid diets started becoming popular, nutrition specialists began witnessing an increase in patients who were trapped in a vicious cycle of fasting and binging. Barry Adler, the president of Diet Fast (a liquid formula diet program), stated that at first everyone knew someone who had lost 100 pounds on a fast, but a year later everyone knew somebody who had lost 100 pounds — and gained back 120. When the liquid diet issue was investigated in 1990 by the House of Representatives' Small Business committee, Rep. Ron Wyden commented, "We are very concerned about the false promises, lack of efficiency . . . and astounding failure rate of liquid diets."

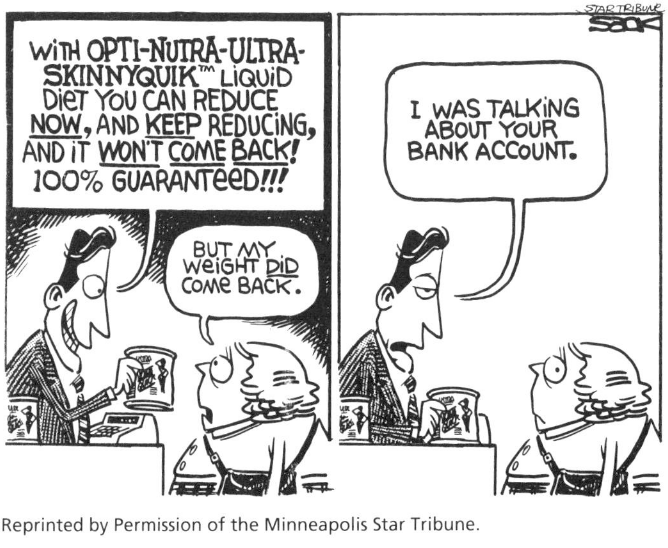

Reprinted by Permission of the Minneapolis Star Tribune.

In October, 1991 the Federal Trade Commission finally caught up with the liquid diet companies. The FTC (I'm really starting to like that crew) accused three companies, Optifast, Medifast, and Ultrafast, of deceiving consumers about the safety and long-term success of their products. Combined, they are a 200 million dollars a year industry. In an agreement with the FTC, the companies are required to "replace unsubstantiated hype with documented facts."

A person might well ask, "What about other weight-loss programs?" Well, the FTC is investigating about a dozen, as yet unnamed, but well-known, over-the-counter products and weight-loss centers. I'll wager that they, too, will all be found guilty of deception. In gambling parlance that is called "easy money."

At what point can a company claim a long-term weight reduction? The FTC is thinking in terms of two years. But that figure is arbitrary — a number picked out of the air. There is absolutely no evidence at all that a two-year period of weight loss is going to have any effect at all on a person's longevity. If a weight loss is going to noticeably improve the health of a person who is truly *excessively* fat, a permanent weight loss is required. That means a lifetime commitment, and that is possible only if a person adopts a lifetime program of exercise and eating a balanced diet with moderate portions — no fads, no "magic."

If there is a "secret" to losing weight, it is probably having six meals of equal size every day. Now, before you get excited, it must be mentioned that that doesn't mean having six big meals. It means spreading the total caloric intake, say, a reasonable 1300, over six meals instead of three — or, far worse, one meal. In a study using "hard core" dieters, it was found that the six-meal-method resulted in a weight loss of as much as 100 pounds. The startling news, though, is that *none* of the subjected complained of hunger at any time!

Because of the lowered metabolic rates that result from *all* rigorous reducing diets, not just liquid protein ones, dieters burn fewer calories at every level of activity. When they go off the diet, which is practically inevitable, they therefore gain weight more easily than before going on the diet. Once a person's BMR has been lowered by stringent dieting, it can only be elevated by *regaining* some weight. This is achieved by increasing the caloric intake toward more normal levels. Although renormalizing the metabolic rate will result in the gain of a few pounds, the gain will level off — with moderate caloric intake.

Large, rapid weight losses of about 20% of body weight produce serious disturbances to the brain's weight control center which results in a*n ov*ercompensation effect, and is another reason a dieter usually gains bac*k mo*re fat than was lost. Still another factor is that dieting merely causes fat cells to shrink, not diminish in number. And with the resumption of normal eating, the depleted fat cells not only rapidly refill, but they multiply — creating as many as twice the "before diet" number. Since the tendency is for fat cells to fill up, the proliferation results not only in a increase in body weight — but a defense of that new body weight through an increase in caloric intake.

Further, with each "yo-yo" cycle, the gain in fat cells tends to be ever greater. Studies suggest that it takes about twice as long to lose fat on the second yo-yo cycle and only 1/3 as long to regain it. One reason for the gain according to Dr. Adam Drenowski, director of Human Nutrition at the University of Michigan, is that cycles of rapid weight loss and gain creates a craving for calorie-rich mixtures of sugar and fat. Most massively obese women are not exaggerating at all when they say, "I dieted my weight up to what it is today." What the diet studios really need are three doors. The usual "hello" and "goodbye" ones, and a third door labeled "hello *again.*" Sadly, every time a woman's weight rebounds after a "reducing" diet, her sense of failure deepens and her self-loathing increases.

Dr. Philip Sinaikin, director of the substance abuse treatment program at Fair Oaks Hospital in Summit, N.J., brought the difficulty of dieting into focus when he stated that a drug addict stands a better chance of recovery than a dieter. However, there is a way to increase the chances for losing weight and keeping it off. The idea is to simply lose it slowly. That way the metabolic rate will not be lowered. It is probably most logical to lose body fat at the same rate at which it was gained. For example, if it took five years to gain twenty pounds, a person should adopt a five-year plan that will slowly but consistently take off twenty pounds. Since most people are too impatient to follow such a suggestion, however, a sensible compromise would be to lose no more than one to two pounds per week — while maintaining a balanced diet. Even then, after every six weeks of losing, a dieter should "plateau" for a few weeks to permit the body's chemical balance to stabilize.

Rapid weight losses may also severely damage the gall bladder. That is why a group of ex-dieters, who had to have their gall bladders removed, in September of 1991 sued the Pennsylvania company that makes the Nutri-System product. The plaintiffs' experts are contending that a rapid weight loss causes cholesterol-saturated bile to collect in the gall bladder and may result in gall stones.

If a balanced diet is all a person needs, why are so many food supplements on the market? Well, vitamin and mineral supplements alone have annual sales of more than 2.6 billion dollars. That kind of money is sure to attract entrepreneurs. Nutritionists generally do not recommend any supplements because long-term effects are unknown and because people tend to overdose. Nevertheless, every year or so a different vitamin, mineral, or other food supplement is spotlighted on the nutritional stage. They range from amino acids to zinc. Scare tactics are far and away the chief advertising technique.

The push to sell a spotlighted food supplement begins with a manufacturer and its imaginative in-house writers. Picking up and elaborating upon the news releases are writers for newspapers and popular magazines. These publications are always searching for new dietary angles since their readers' thirst for such information is unquenchable. Publications surely cannot expect to keep ahead of their competition by extolling the virtues of a balanced diet in every issue. Naturally, once the food supplement propaganda is disseminated by the print and broadcast media it is effectively "legitimatized." The public then accepts it as truth no matter how far-fetched the information.

How accurate is the nutritional information in magazines? It varies widely, but the information below gives some idea. The numbers were compiled by the non-profit American Council on Science and Health (ACSH) after it studied the accuracy of nutritional coverage in nineteen major magazines.

The most reliable magazines, with accuracy ranging from 100% to

93% were *50 Plus*, *Parents*, *Redbook*, *Reader's Digest*, and *Good Housekeeping*. The least reliable, ranging from 46% to 10% accuracy, are also listed in descending order — *Mademoiselle*, *Essence*, *Cosmopolitan*, *Harper's Bazaar*, *Organic Gardening*, and *Prevention*.

Isn't it strange that the least reliable magazine on the list, by far, is Prevention, the nation's highest selling health magazine? Perhaps, it is not so mysterious considering that the magazine's major advertisers are companies that sell food supplements and other "health" products.

With a balanced diet, food supplements are a waste of money. Still, it must be recognized that many people, for one reason or another, are not able consistently to maintain a balanced diet. In these cases, taking a multi-vitamin/mineral pill does make sense — even though the most complete ones do not match a balanced diet's nutritional supply and contain virtually no fiber.

Vitamin megadose regimens continue to have their adherents. One of the major detractions associated with them is that the proper balance between the various vitamins and minerals is disturbed. Another drawback is that every vitamin and mineral can be consumed in harmfully excessive amounts. Indeed, excesses can be as disastrous as deficiencies. This is particularly true for the fat-soluble vitamins, A, D, E, and K. Excessively high intakes of vitamin A, for instance, causes skin rashes, hair loss, fatigue, bone weakness, bone spurs, liver disorders, and blood loss. It is inconceivable that a person can overdose on any vitamin or mineral with a balanced diet.

The American Heart Association recommends that fat should supply less than 30% of the total number of calories in a diet, and that they should be distributed between polyunsaturated, monounsaturated, and saturated fats — with saturated fats being the lowest proportion. How many people have the expertise or patience to keep an accurate account of their fat intake day after day? Surely not many. With a balanced diet you don't need to worry about it.

To further lower the intake of fats, and saturated fats in particular, a few simple steps will ensure success. First, limit the number and size of portions of red meat and trim off as much fat as is feasible. Any butcher should know the leanest brands and cuts. Also, when preparing fowl, its skin should be removed; it contains about half the fat of a dressed bird. Second, use low-fat milk (skim is best), yogurt, cottage cheese, and frozen desserts, as well as skim milk cheeses (not part-skim milk), goat cheese, and low-fat processed cheeses (if the synthetic aftertaste is not too offensive). Third, to reduce saturated fats use vegetable oils such as canola (rape weed oil), corn, safflower, olive, sunflower, sesame, and peanut oils — but use them sparingly since they are all high in calories. As much as possible, eliminate the use of butter, lard, shortenings, and "tropical" oils (palm, palm kernel, and coconut). Liquid or tub margarines are better than "stick" margarines. Sprinkle-on "butter" powders are virtually fat- and cholesterol-free. Holding fried foods to a minimum also helps to reduce dietary fat.

Most people, who are nutritionally aware, probably believe that polyunsaturates are the best kind of fat for lowering blood cholesterol. Research reported in 1985, however, suggested that monounsaturates are much better. No one really knows which is best. All that can said with assurity is that they are both far more healthy than unsaturated fat — particularly, relative to cardiovascular disease.

Adhering to the steps above should reduce fat intake to between 20% and 25% of the total calories in a diet. This level is advisable for people whether they are interested in losing weight or not.

The diet for children up to the age of two, however, should contain at least 35% fat; human milk has a fat content of about 50% fat. Reducing the fat intake of infants can lead to problems since fat is very important to a developing baby. Its maturing nervous system, for instance, needs fat to make myelin, the "insulation" around nerves. For this reason, along with others, the American Academy of Pediatrics advises giving whole milk to infants and toddlers — as opposed to low-fat varieties.

Research by Dr. Brian Morgan of Columbia University's Institute of Human Nutrition shows that low-fat diets for infants predisposes them to adult obesity because it decreases their development of brown adipose tissue (BAT). Some bariatric (obesity) experts now believe the amount of BAT adults have is very important in determining if they will become obese. Those with a relatively high BAT level can burn up an extra 10% of their calories each day.

None of the above information is meant to imply that run-of-the mill fatness — say, ten, twenty, or even forty pounds over one's true ideal — is harmful to the health of adults. In addition to yo-yo dieting, disorders such as cardiovascular disease that are often attributed to a person's being too fat are more than likely the result of too high a percentage of fat in the diet — especially the saturated kinds. Fat people in the Mediterranean area, for example, do not typically die prematurely. This circumstance is believed to be the result of a diet that is low in red meat and high in complex carbohydrates, such as pasta. Highly regarded studies of thousands of Chinese resulted in similar conclusions. Even in America, autopsies on many fat people (300 pounds and over) reveal no significant atherosclerosis. Fatness apparently is not as important to health as how a person becomes fat and stays fat.

A high-fat diet is also related to a variety of cancers according to research supported by the National Cancer Institute. The risk of colon cancer is particularly increased, but there is also an increased incidence of cancers of the breast, colon, and uterus, and prostate.

Even protein, that darling of the weight-reducing and muscle building world, can be consumed in excess. Indeed, the average American consumes approximately twice as much as needed. Excess amounts, whether taken in the form of food, or protein or amino acid supplements, are merely excreted or converted to fat. Excesses, in addition to causing calcium loses from bones and leading to osteoporosis, can result in fluid imbalances and damage to kidneys and liver. Excessive protein, because it raises the level of uric acid in the body, can also result in gout and kidney stones. A high-protein diet has even been linked to various types of cancer including breast cancer.

The large intake of various individual amino acids has also been highly touted. One, lysine, has even been touted as being effective in treating *herpe*s. Another, arginine, is sold as a "growth hormone releaser" that "makes you lose weight as you sleep." There is not a shred of scientific evidence, however, to support these claims. Some amino acids are advertised as making muscles grow faster, but in reality the large consumption of a single amino acid can interfere with the absorption of other amino acids and actually retard the muscle building process — or even be toxic.

The effects of an unsatisfactory diet — deficiencies, excesses, and imbalances — will always reveal themselves in the form of health problems. Symptoms may not appear for many years but eventually they *will* show up. The length of the delay depends largely upon how poor the diet is. In any case, disorders caused by malnutrition can be prevented with a balanced diet.

A major dietary problem has been that canned, packaged, and bottled foods often carry labels that are very misleading — purposely so. One example is "vegetable oil." Many people think all vegetable oils contain only unsaturated fats. Yet, as mentioned previously, coconut oil, which is commonly used in processed foods, is more than twice as high in saturated fats as lard! Most non-dairy coffee creamers consist primarily of coconut oil which means they have much more saturated fat than real cream. Finally, due to the demand of knowledgeable consumers, most of the top makers of cookies, crackers, and cereals are no longer using the tropical oils even though it would be cheaper for them to do so. The graph below shows the approximate amount of cholesterol and the percentages of saturated, monounsaturated, and polyunsaturated fats in common fats and oils.

COMPARISONS OF DIETARY FATS AND OILS

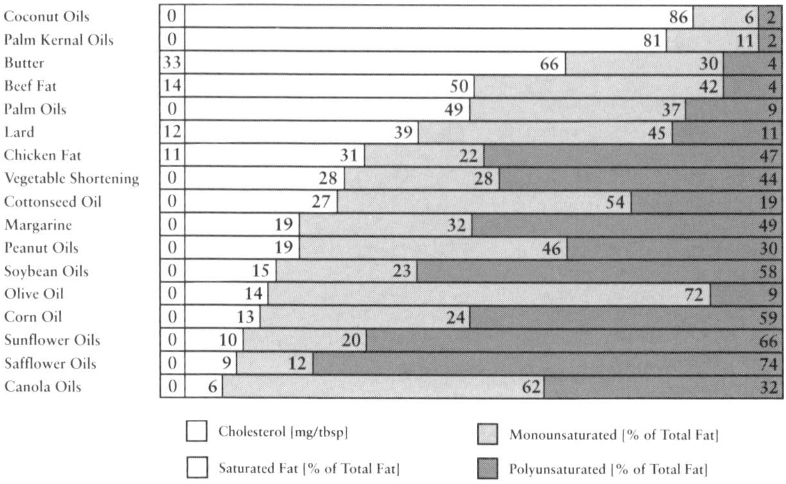

Large, colorful announcements of "No Cholesterol!" and "Low Cholesterol!" proudly embellish many food packages even though their contents may be quite high in saturated fats. And these fats have been proven to have a far greater effect on raising the cholesterol level in the blood than does dietary cholesterol itself!

Another excellent example of doublespeak is the deceptive phrase, "made from pure 100% polyunsaturated corn oil" that is emblazoned on the label of some products — then among the list of ingredients in the tiny print on the back of the package is the seemingly innocuous term, "hydrogenated corn oil." How many people know that when a vegetable oil is hydrogenated, its unsaturated fats are converted to saturated fats? The advertisers are hoping *not many*. Partially hydrogenated vegetable oils are not as bad as the totally hydrogenated ones but the consumer has no way of knowing their degree of hydrogenation. The oils are hydrogenated because the process helps reduce the oils' tendency to turn rancid, but it also reduces the oils' biological value. As a rule of thumb, the more saturated a fat is the more solid it will be at room temperature. Butter and lard, for instance, will be solid (though soft) while corn oil and olive oil will be liquid.

Amazingly, oils from fatty fish such as salmon, tuna, mackerel, and sardines are much less saturated than the least saturated vegetable oils and fifty *times* less saturated than beef fat! These fish oils are also high in fatty acids called omega-3s which have a strong influence on the lowering of blood cholesterol and triglyceride levels.

Some researchers believe the pervasive food processing that exists in our culture has stripped a vital type of omega-3 fatty acid, linolenic acid, from our diet. This fatty acid is one of the three essential ones and is unique in that it plays a key role in the formation of hormone-like substances that control a number of important functions in muscle contraction, nerve-impulse transmissions, blood pressure, and *metabolism*. The latter gives rise to the thought that the great reliance upon processed and commercially prepared foods in the last few decades may have lowered the metabolic rate of Americans in general — thus contributing to the increasing body fat levels that have been well-documented during the same period.

Sometimes highly processed meats, such as hot dogs and bologna (including turkey bologna), are advertised as being something like "80% fat-free." This figure may be true when the total weight of such products is considered, but 55% of that weight is water, which adds no calories whatsoever. When the weight of the water is discounted, about 60% of the meat's weight consists of fat. And since fat has about twice as many calories for its weight than either carbohydrates or protein, about 80% of the total calories in the meat comes from fat — mainly saturated.

This same ploy is commonly used to advertise any product that has a high water content. A company can claim, truthfully, and deceptively, that its whole milk contains only 3.25% fat (by weight) even though that fat — which is mainly saturated — provides about 48% of the milk's calories. Two-percent and 1% milk contain about 37% and 18% fat, respectively. Skim milk and powdered milk contain practically no fat; they are the only kinds of milk adults should drink.

Many other confusing, and often purposely misleading, terms are featured on food packages. "Natural," for instance, has no legal meaning (except when applied to meat) and foods so labeled may in reality be highly processed and contain large amounts of preservatives and artificial flavorings. "Light" (or "lite") may just mean a product is light in color, texture, or taste. Other deceptive terms include "organic," "sugar free," "naturally sweetened," "low calorie," "reduced calorie," "dietetic," "cholesterol reduced," "sodium free," "reduced sodium," "low sodium," and "very low sodium." Sodium, by the way, comes in many sources other than sodium chloride (table salt). Sugar, too, comes in many forms other than sucrose (table sugar) including glucose, fructose, corn syrup, honey, and molasses. A product can also be labeled sugar-free and contain many calories from sugar alcohols such as mannitol, sorbitol, and Xylitol.

While sugar is not the villain it is often decried as being, foods that are high in sugar and have *no other* nutrients should be strictly limited because they merely provide a lot of "empty calories." The average American consumes 133 pounds or sugar per year and that is astronomically excessive. Much of it is hidden in products like ketchup, soups, canned vegetables and fruits, and, of course, cereals and soft drinks.

People will get plenty of "empty calories" even if they try to avoid them.

That is not to say people should use substitute sweeteners. At least we know what happens to the sugar we consume. Mainly, it is stored in the liver until needed. Then, it is sent to cells to be burned for energy. The substitutes are not burned for energy. What happens to the stuff? How does it effect the body in the long run? No one knows. And the people who use the substitutes to cut calories are probably fooling themselves anyway. For example, it has been found that when people substitute low-calorie soft drinks for the "real thing," their *total* sugar consumption remains the same. Obviously, they just increase their sugar intake in other ways.

It is also important to know each packager's definition of "serving size." For example, the FDA is considering forcing meat packagers to list nutrients on meat labels — based upon serving size. The FDA wants the serving sizes to be realistic, to be based upon amounts that are typically consumed. The USDA, influenced by the meat people, are considering using *one-ounce* serving sizes! Why? Labeling on such small amounts would give the impression that the product is much lower in fat and total calories. My goodness, who do you think would want that?

The term "lean" is also misleading. The USDA (a crew that I'm liking less and less) defines "lean" as beef or poultry that has no more than 10% fat. Ground beef is apparently exempt from the rules, despite the fact that it is beef. In 1988 the Center of Science in the Public Interest conducted a survey and found that ground beef labeled "lean" actually contained anywhere from 20% to 30% fat! A series of studies by the USDA itself revealed that "extra lean" ground beef only had slightly less fat than its "lean" counterpart. "Lean" frozen dinners can, similarly, contain high levels of fat.

Food labels with such enticing adjectives as "dietetic," "low calorie," and "reduced calorie" are pretty tricky also. Foods so labeled are required to contain one-third fewer calories than their regular counterparts. But the actual calorie count is allowed to be within 20% of the number stated on the label. In other words, the label may read 100 calories while the actual count is 120 calories. Besides, the regular foods may be very low in calories to begin with. Confusion also arises because some dietetic foods are allowed to contain as many calories as the regular version *if* they have a reduced sodium level.

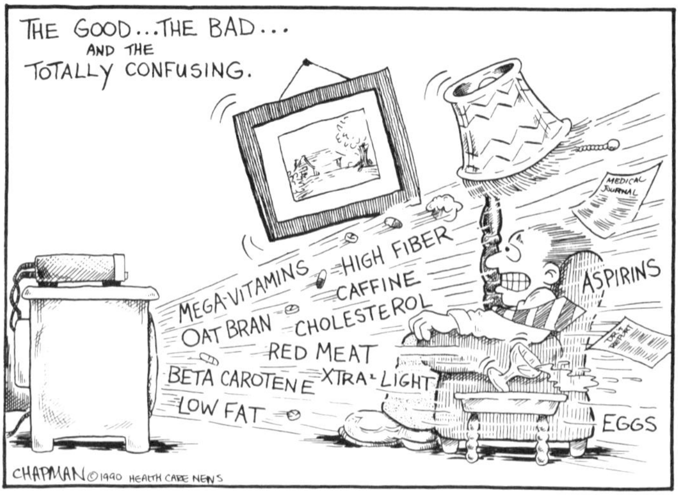

Copyright © 1990 by *Health Care News.*

To eliminate the confusion that exists in the labeling of food packages, the Nutrition Labeling and Education Act (NLEA) was passed in 1990. It mandated that the FDA would reform food labeling in a three phase program. The first phase would require food manufacturers to identify on labels all ingredients including color additives. The ingredients would appear in descending order by percent of content by weight. This would include all sweeteners, protein hydrolysates, flavor enhancers, milk derivatives, and sulfiting agents. It is also proposed that retailers eventually would have to provide nutrition information on the 20 most frequently consumed raw fruits, vegetables, and fish. Another proposal requires manufacturers to state the actual percentages of fruit and vegetable juice in beverages. Labels on multi-juice beverages will have to list the exact percentage of each juice in the drink.

In the second phase, the FDA will propose regulations on label format, nutrient content, and serving size. Using a simplified format, labels will have to provide nutrient information on protein, fat, carbohydrates, fiber, vitamins, minerals, and sodium.

Phase three deals with health claims that food manufacturers often make. The FDA proposals will limit health claims to those in which valid scientific evidence exists. Especially targeted are such terms as "light," "fresh," "no cholesterol," and fat percentage claims.

The FDA intends to publish its final regulations by November 8, 1992. Manufacturers will have until May, 1993, to implement the label changes. The labeling will be a great aid to consumers — *if* they become nutritionally knowledgeable. Presumably the FDA will also distribute pamphlets to the public to help educate them.

Although labels on processed food are often deceptive, at least the knowledgeable consumer has some idea of the contents. Lord only knows what most restaurants put in their dishes. I recall once asking a waitress if the "chef" used unsaturated oil for cooking since that was the "only kind my doctor allowed me to eat." She returned a moment later and assured me that was the kind they used for everything. About a month later I stopped at the same place and went through the same routine with the same waitress — but substituted the term "saturated oil." That time she returned and with an angelic look said, "That's all the cook ever uses." Being an extraordinarily perceptive fellow, it dawned on me that perhaps other restaurants were also capable of being less than candid with their customers.

A COMPARISON OF TURKEY PRODUCTS (3 OZ. SERVINGS)

Product	calories	fat (g)	sodium (mg)
turkey breast, meat only (roasted)	119	1	44
turkey breast, meat and skin	160	6	57
Louis Rich Turkey Frank	195	16	922
Butterball Turkey Bologna	210	18	1110

The surest way of adhering to sound nutritional rules, and knowing what you are putting in your stomach, is to cook everything from scratch. In case you have never tried it, "home cookin'" is also the tastiest method; the words alone almost make the mouth water. A number of excellent cookbooks contain healthy, low-fat recipes. My wife has prepared hundreds of them and I can attest to their exciting, gourmet tastes — even some of the tofu recipes — if you keep an open mind. The list above from the *Tufts University Diet and Nutrition Letter* (March, 1990) compares home prepared turkey with some processed turkey products and gives some idea of the value of home preparation of food.

A 3 oz. serving of Weight Watcher's Chicken Nuggets, incidentally, contains 180 C., 11 g. of fat, and 360 mg. of sodium. A 3 oz. serving of home-roasted chicken breast contains only about 119 C., 1 g. of fat, and 644 mg. of sodium — and costs about *one-fourth* as much as the Weight Watcher's Nuggets. The number of calories derived from a gram of fat can be determined by multiplying the number of grams by 9.

For years there has been a progressively intensifying campaign against the consumption of cholesterol. One almost expected the nation's president to appoint an anticholesterol czar. Just as the furor reached fever pitch, another side of the story came out. Anyone with a cholesterol anxiety is well-advised to read *Heart Failure*, a book by Thomas Moore. It provides some balance to the flood of cholesterol-damning articles. Basically, what the author has done is to take existing research and show how it has been purposefully misinterpreted to create a national cholesterol phobia — to the massive financial advantage of the medical profession.

The position taken in *Heart Failure* has been supported by the American Council on Science and Health. In September, 1989, this organization issued a report based on the findings of a panel of medical experts which stated that cholesterol's role in heart disease has been exaggerated and is worrying the public unnecessarily. The president of ACSH, Dr. Elizabeth Whelan, concluded there was no need to alarm the entire population about cholesterol.

The public certainly has been alarmed. Food manufacturers, *ad nauseum*, have jumped on the anticholesterol bandwagon. By 1988 oat bran, for instance, had been acclaimed as a miracle food that lowered blood cholesterol. A grandfatherly actor confided to television viewers that eating oatmeal was, "The right thing to do." I have to admit I rushed out and bought a box before the shelves were emptied. Stock in oat companies skyrocketed. A mere two years later, however, a report in the *New England Journal of Medicine* (January, 1990) concluded that oat bran has no special powers to reduce cholesterol after all — and that it is no more effective than low-fiber grains and causes more bloating and diarrhea. Oat stock plummeted back to Earth. In reality, any type of grain has the effect of lowering blood cholesterol when it replaces foods that are high in saturated fat (such as bacon and pork sausage). Oat bran may have lost its favored status but, as with other grains, it is still a valuable part of a balanced diet.

It cannot be denied that a high level of cholesterol in the *blood* is a definite risk factor for heart disease. The problem is the propaganda that states everyone must stringently lower *dietary* cholesterol. Studies reveal that a large majority of people do not need to worry about their cholesterol intake — and many of those who should be concerned could not significantly lower their blood cholesterol through a reduction of dietary cholesterol anyway. In some people, when a high amount of cholesterol is consumed, the liver just produces less from carbohydrates; in other people an excess intake is merely shunted into the bile by the liver and then excreted via the intestines. In either case, a person's genetic "set-point" for blood cholesterol remains about the same.

A small proportion of the population does have a genetic predisposition for hypercholesterolemia. For these people, drug therapy, coupled with an extremely low-cholesterol, low-saturated fat diet (especially the latter), can lower the risk of heart disease. It does not make sense, though, for *everyone* to be driven into a cholesterol paranoia because of an abnormal minority.

A simple, logical way has been suggested to determine whether your blood cholesterol can be lowered through diet. Call the local American Heart Association chapter (AHA) for a suitable testing center. If a test shows your level to be high, get on a low-saturated fat, low-cholesterol diet. The AHA will provide specific information for this. After about eight weeks have another test taken. If your blood cholesterol drops at least 10% to 15%, dietary adjustments may be beneficial — for you. This approach, unfortunately, is far from being foolproof since cholesterol levels (like heart rate and blood pressure) can fluctuate considerably. The level varies with stress, weight change, menstrual cycle, illness, and medication. Other variables include the season, time of day, the position a person is in during the testing, and the length of time it takes to test the sample — along with the common and often substantial human error. When all of these factors are taken into account, the findings of a cholesterol test can be inaccurate to the point of being meaningless.

Even the most ardent anticholesterol people admit that dietary cholesterol is only one of many factors that are associated with an increased risk of cardiovascular disease, and is a relatively minor one at that — for most people. Some factors, such as heredity, cannot be controlled. Most risk factors, however, can be. Positive measures include reducing saturated fat in the diet, reducing stress, exercising, and giving vent to feelings of anxiety. Cigarette smoking is the single most important risk factor for heart disease.

The cholesterol controversy is not unique. Until very recently, for instance, everyone was advised to stringently restrict their intake of salt. Why? Because in some people, even a small excess can result in high blood pressure or exacerbate an existing condition. Now, however, it is recognized that not everyone has this supersensitivity. In fact, some advocates of salt reduction even admit that it's nearly impossible to maintain a low enough level (500 mg/day or less) to lower blood pressure significantly. Amazingly, research conducted by Dr. Brent Egan of the Medical College of Wisconsin, Milwaukee showed that in some people a low-salt diet actually *raised* blood pressure. In some cases, the low-salt regimen also resulted in an increase in blood cholesterol and the hormones associated with diabetes, poor kidney function, and gout.

Dr. John Laragh, Director of the Cardiovascular Center of New York University-Cornell University Medical Center has stated that the whole thing has gone too far, that it's a classic example of extremists coming in and stretching the truth. The exaggeration of the dangers of salt has led health professionals to advise salt restriction for everyone. This "cattle herd" approach should not be surprising; it is merely an example of bureaucratic mentality transferred to the medical/nutritional arena.

The above discussion, however, must not be construed as a green light for people to consume as much cholesterol or salt as they want — or any other nutrient. If there is evidence that high levels of any nutritional substance may be harmful, and a person does not know whether he or she is supersensitive or not, logic suggests that its intake be restricted at least a bit. Such a reduction is not likely to be harmful and it might do some good. MODERATION is really the key. And moderation, along with VARIETY, is the distinctive characteristic of a balanced diet.

Today, many women are so concerned about their weight that it interferes with their enjoyment of a balanced diet. This was unheard of until well into the twentieth century. People ate until they intuitively figured they had eaten enough and then stopped — except at occasional bashes such as wedding celebrations. It turns out that the old-timers were right on target. The current belief is that every individual has a "set-point" relative to fatness. That is, the body has a regulatory system designed to maintain body fat, within narrow limits, at a fixed level — and the body feels most comfortable at this level.

According to this theory, a part of the brain called the hypothalamus, which controls body temperature, hunger, thirst, and the pituitary gland, is believed to also have the primary role in determining the body's set-point for fatness. Influencing the "fat-stat" in the hypothalamus are input from such organs as the brain, thyroid gland, liver, and gastrointestinal tract. One's genetic make-up and number of fat cells also affect the set-point. In some people the set-point for fatness may be lower than 5%, while in others it may be higher than 45%. No one knows the exact range — or even the average.

A negative energy balance caused by a reduced caloric intake causes body fat levels to drop below the fat set-point. The body, however, vigorously resists the drop. It perceives itself as starving and makes adjustments to cope with the condition. One adjustment, as discussed previously, is the lowering of the metabolic rate. Of course, people find starvation to be extremely unpleasant.

As body fat continues to fall below the set-point, the metabolic rate also continues to decline. As it does so, a person finds it increasingly more difficult to lose fat. And as long as a body's fat level is below its set-point, a person will experience the distress of food deprivation. After losing sixty-seven pounds, Oprah Winfrey admitted on her television program that every day for the rest of her life it would be sheer torture to keep the fat off. That agonizing feeling was her body talking and its message was loud and clear. Compared to her fat set-point, her body's fat level was abnormally low and it was pitifully pleading, "Help! I've fallen and I can't get up." The way to get up, naturally, is to eat more food. To help prevent an eating overcompensation from occurring with the resumption of normal eating, the increase in calories should be acquired primarily in the form of carbohydrates — not fat.

It would obviously be much easier for people to lose weight if they could lower their set-points. But is this possible? Surgery to the hypothalamus can definitely produce a change but that's an extremely drastic step. Since the risks far outweigh its benefits, brain surgery for weight control is not performed on humans. A more practical question is whether the set-point can be controlled by changes in a person's lifestyle.

Research suggests that a long-term exposure to high-fat diet will result in an elevation of the set-point. This is still another reason why a person who desires to lose fat is advised to stick to a low-fat diet. The most effective way to lower the set-point, however, is through regular participation in a suitable exercise program.

According to set-point theorists, many cases of excessive fatness are due to some disorder in heredity or any of the other factors that help to determine the set-point. That would explain why all "reducing" diets have such pitifully low rates of success. The diets have to overcome a powerful and complex physiological condition that is natural for a person. That natural condition *may* be abnormal or unhealthy, but it is a deep-seated part of one's make-up and, as such, is extremely resistant to change. For short periods of time a person may have the will power to force the fat level to drop considerably below the set-point. To keep it there permanently, however, is another story. Superhuman willpower is needed to endure the persistent feelings of distress resulting from the body's constant, strident demands, and there are not many superhumans around. In the large majority of cases, a lower weight probably would not result in a significantly healthier or longer life anyway. Even *if* it would, one has to wonder if the few extra years of additional existence on Earth would be worth the lifetime of self-inflicted torture required to achieve it.

There are, of course, people who are so massively obese that it has a significantly adverse affect on their physical well-being, enjoyment of life, and longevity. The underlying problem may be due to any number of reasons ranging from physiological abnormalities to behavioral disorders that cause them to eat too much. These people in terms of health should, of course, lose weight. Although this is a not a "diet book," it was felt that some sound advice had to be offered on the subject.

Although there is no simple, single answer, to losing weight, it is safe to say that people are not going to reduce body fat unless they sincerely want to. And if they do not want to, that is their decision. The only suggestion to these people is to at least follow the dietary advice given in this chapter. Since it addresses the subject of diet solely from the standpoint of good health, the advice applies to everyone.

14

EXERCISE AND HEALTH

Proper exercise, along with a balanced diet and rest, is one of the three foundations of good health. Exercise is also the key to reducing body fat — should a person desire to do so. Studies show that fat people, in general, eat no more than others — but they are less active. Since exercise is such a vital requirement in attaining and maintaining one's ideal weight, this chapter is devoted to the topic.

It is commonly known that calories are burned at a faster rate when people are active than when they are sedentary. What is not so well-known is that the metabolic rate remains significantly higher for several hours after exercise ceases, and may remain at least slightly elevated for as long as twenty-four hours. Further, while a sedentary person's metabolic rate increases by about 30% shortly after a meal is eaten, the post-meal metabolism of a person who exercises regularly increases by as much as 110%. Exercise is also important in a fat-reduction program because it helps prevent the loss of muscle tissue that occurs with dieting alone.

Not only does exercise burn off fat, it is nearly always the only healthy thing that makes a permanent reduction possible — for a person of any age. A major reason is that exercise is the only way people can significantly lower their bodies' set-point for fat. As explained previously, if a woman's fat set-point is 40% of her body weight, dropping to 25% (or whatever) causes her body to plead continually to get back to 40%. Food, in essence, becomes addictive. However, when the set-point is lowered to 25% through exercise, the body feels satisfied at that level; it does not continually cry out for more food.

If weight loss is beneficial to health, it follows that exercise is also beneficial to health. But even when the weight-loss aspect is eliminated, exercise has many healthful benefits. In Chapter Five it was briefly mentioned that cholesterol is carried in the bloodstream in combination with proteins to form lipoproteins. Of the several categories of lipoproteins — the low-density lipoproteins (LDLs) and high-density lipoproteins (HDLs) are the ones most associated with the risk of coronary heart disease. LDLs are commonly called the "bad" carriers and for good reason. They carry cholesterol from the liver to the walls of the arteries where the gunk accumulates, along with other particles such as fat, and results in a condition called atherosclerosis — or hardening of the arteries. Eventually this plaque can so narrow the diameter of an artery that even a small clot can plug the passage and stop the flow of blood through it. This is bad news no matter where it occurs in the body, but when the blockage takes place in the heart or brain, it can be disastrous.

HDLs are the "good guys" because they collect the cholesterol from arterial walls and transport it to the liver where it is broken down and excreted with the feces. A very small percentage of people are lucky since they are genetically programmed to have a lot of HDLs. People not so blessed need not despair, however. Aerobic activities, such as brisk walking, jogging, and swimming, can increase the HDLs to a level that is on par with the inheritors.

Incidentally, people who use anabolic steroids to increase their muscles mass and decrease body fat, put themselves at extreme risk for coronary heart disease since these drugs severely decrease a user's HDLs. An average man has an HDL level of about 45 mg/dl; anything less than 35 is considered to be a major risk factor for coronary disease. In one study, the HDLs of steroid users averaged 15 mg/dl and one of subjects measured a mere 1 mg/dl.

Different kinds of programs are used to improve different components of physical fitness, such as endurance, strength, speed, and flexibility. Aerobic (endurance building) programs, however, have the greatest positive effect on health. In addition to lowering body fat setpoints and increasing HDL levels, the long list of changes attributed to aerobic exercise have to do chiefly with cardiovascular benefits. An increase in the number of capillaries in the heart musculature is responsible for enhanced cardiac circulation and is one reason why aerobically trained people tend to have fewer and less severe heart attacks than sedentary ones. Also, because a trained heart contracts more forcefully than a weak one, it pumps more blood with each beat. This permits the heart to beat more slowly at every level of activity except at near-maximal levels. With its slower beat a strong heart has more time to rest between beats and is therefore more efficient than a weaker one..

High blood pressure, a most insidious killer, is reduced with physical training — not tremendously so, but certainly enough to lower the risk of heart attacks, stroke, and kidney damage. Exercise also has preventative and therapeutic effects for a wide variety of other diseases, including diabetes and cancer. This is not to say that exercise is a panacea, but it does have potentials of which most medical practitioners are not aware. Some physicians do have an inkling of the potential, but do not have the expertise to prescribe exercise. Besides, it is much easier and far less time consuming to just prescribe drugs.

Along with the heart muscle, the muscles that move the skeleton and those involved in breathing are strengthened through exercise. Their capillaries also proliferate thus permitting greater quantities of blood (and nutrients) to be delivered to these tissues so they can work at a higher level — which is especially useful in emergency situations.

Sexual activity is not an emergency situation — generally speaking — but it is nice to know that an exercise program does heighten an interest in sex. Unfortunately, a greater interest in sex does not promise increased opportunity. Engaging in sex once or twice a week helps to lower one's blood cholesterol and clear up the skin. Not only does exercise make for better sex, according to Dr. Peter Wood, Co-Director of Stanford University's Heart Disease program, sex can be regarded as a pleasant athletic diversion. Of course, its fitness value depends upon how vigorously it is performed. Wood recommends the standard pelvic thrust to strengthen abdominal muscles and to loosen those of the lower back. With characteristic prudence, I will decline further comment on this subject.

A less exciting result of regular exercise is an increase in the density, and therefore strength, of bones. Weak, brittle bones cause a condition known as osteoporosis. Twenty-four million Americans, chiefly women, are currently afflicted. Related to this statistic is the fact that each year over 1.3 million people over age forty-four break their hips; for many the result is death within a year. A woman can swallow highly touted calcium pills by the dozen every day and wash them down with a gallon of milk and it will not do much to prevent osteoporosis unless she also exercises. Weight-bearing activities such as walking are especially recommended both for prevention and treatment of the disorder.

As is bone loss, the loss of muscle tissue is also greatly accelerated after menopause. And for both conditions the first three years appear to be the worst. Exercise also helps tremendously in reducing the decline of muscle tissue.

Premenstrual syndrome (PMS) is a disorder that also plagues many women. Caused by hormonal changes, PMS results in the body retaining five to ten pounds more water than usual. Much of the excess fluid collects in the muscles while some accumulates in the lungs and reduces their oxygen intake capacity. These effects naturally tend to make a woman feel tired and sluggish. Brisk rhythmic exercise relieves PMS by reducing excess body fluid. As the fluid is reduced, exercise also becomes easier.

In addition, women who exercise tend to have less severe dysmenorrhea than their sedentary sisters. Strong abdominal muscles also make childbirth much easier. With all of these factors in mind, it would seem that exercise programs are even more beneficial for women than for men. Contrary to the fears of many women, exercise will not transform them into masculine creatures with massive muscles. It is difficult enough for men to "bulk up," and they average about fifty times more testosterone than women. Actually, exercise for women is feminizing since it increases their production of female hormones. It's no wonder nearly all beauty queens and actresses known for their physical charms do engage in exercise — in ways ranging from weight training to various forms of dancing.

Some people avoid exercising because they do not believe they have enough energy for it. Unless the fatigue is a symptom of a disease, these people should at least give exercise a try. They will find that a ten- to fifteen-minute walk can result in an energy boost that lasts for as long as two hours. Eating a candy bar (a supposed "energy booster"), on the other hand, raises the blood sugar level only briefly before the insulin output increases to lower the sugar level — and diminish vitality.

By starting at a very low level of exercise and gradually increasing the intensity and duration with each session, people will soon find they have more and more energy to expend. At the same time, due to more efficient movement they will waste less energy. This increased efficiency can be attributed chiefly to the learning of more skillful movement patterns and partly to improved flexibility. Greater flexibility translates to fewer aches and pains, especially as one ages.

Physical activity pays still another dividend for older people — a feeling of youthfulness. We all get old, with luck, but we don't have to be in a hurry to look or feel old. Since skin appearance is a primary barometer of age, it should be mentioned that exercise, particularly aerobics, retards wrinkling. The heightened blood flow to the skin improves its supply of nutrients and the removal of its cellular wastes, thereby resulting in an increased depositing of collagen and elastin fibers in the skin which makes it more elastic and youthful.

Most of the diminishing physical capabilities commonly blamed on aging are in reality the result of a sedentary lifestyle. The admonition, "use it or lose it," is not a frivolous one. Like all animals, human have evolved to be active. Whenever we move, therefore, we are merely giving expression to a biological need. Suppression of that need cannot possibly be healthy — physically, mentally, or emotionally.

Not only can much of the physical deterioration commonly linked to aging be dramatically slowed down with proper exercise, it is never too late to start exercising, assuming one has no medical condition that would suggest otherwise. Again, mental as well as physical improvement can occur. One study, for example, showed that people who began exercising in their seventies improved their problem-solving abilities, short-term memories, and concentration. Women, especially, were discovered to have less anxiety and depression when they exercised, thus confirming similar studies using younger subjects.

It is becoming increasing clear that exercise leads to increased longevity. It has been estimated that the average life-span of Americans would be increased by about two-and-a-half years if they all engaged in sufficient physical activity. That is the same increase that would result if cancer were completely eradicated.

But even if increased longevity were not an outcome of exercise, the fact that one can be healthy and active in his or her advanced years is reward enough for a lifetime of regular exercise. Some people may clutch their chests and gasp, "A lifetime! You mean I have to exercise my entire life?" The answer is "yes." And why should that be surprising? We eat and sleep at regular intervals throughout our entire lives. We should also exercise at regular intervals. Physical activity should not be viewed as a life sentence anyway, but as a privilege. Ask a person who has that privilege restricted in some way, say, by paraplegia or a severe heart condition.

It cannot be overemphasized that the benefits of exercise are not limited solely to the physical realm. In exercise classes, the first obvious improvement in the students is evidence of increased self-confidence, self-esteem, and a sense of well-being. The outward signs include better posture, more smiling, and more extroverted behavior. These signs often occur dramatically — sometimes after only one or two sessions. For people suffering from depression and anxiety, the improvement can exceed that achieved through drugs or psychotherapy. The behavioral changes resulting from exercise can be more dramatic and exciting than the physical ones.

Perhaps the most benefit of exercise is stress reduction. Even five minutes of stair climbing reduces stress dramatically for several hours. If an activity is enjoyable, it is even better at decreasing stress. In *Psychology Today* (May, 1984) Robert G. McMurray (University of North Carolina at Chapel Hill) said that the euphoria associated with aerobic activity very likely comes from the release of stress. He further suggested that the "high" feeling was psychological. The exercise reduced stress so effectively that some high-stress sufferers begin to feel they cannot get by without the exercise.

For improving health in general, and cardiovascular fitness in particular, aerobic exercises are supreme. These exercises refer to activities during which people are able to supply their bodies with sufficient oxygen to meet their energy needs. As a result, they can engage in such activities for extended periods of time without becoming exhausted. Practically everything the average person does from sleeping to moderately paced running is aerobic. But when the term "aerobic exercise" is used, it usually refers to prolonged activities characterized by heavy breathing. Among the more common aerobic activities are jogging, running, rope jumping, aerobic dancing, bicycling, rowing, skating, walking, cross-country skiing, and swimming. All of these activities can improve the fitness of the heart and help stop the build-up of plaque in the arteries — and perhaps even reverse the process.

Of course, before engaging in any exercise program see a physician for a physical examination. This is especially important for older people and those who have been sedentary.

To achieve the benefits of aerobic exercise three questions logically arise. How often? How hard? How long? To improve fitness and health, exercise must be done regularly and that does not mean once a month. In fact, exercising once a week does more harm than good; all that results is an increased chance for injuries. Twice a week will only barely maintain your level of fitness. For significant improvement at least three exercise sessions per week are necessary — with about two days between sessions.

The most subjective, but easiest, technique for determining the required intensity and duration of exercise is based upon your perception of your exertion. The list below provides some guidance.

RATING SCALE OF PERCEIVED EXERTION
very, very easy
very easy
fairly easy
somewhat hard
hard
very hard
very, very hard

When entering any exercise program, a sedentary person should begin with very easy exertions and progress to more intense levels. How rapidly? Listen to your body. Being slightly stiff the next day, although not harmful, means you are on the borderline of doing too much. Muscular soreness on the day after an exercise session is a definite sign to slack off a bit. A regular session should never be started if muscles are sore. Very mild activity is okay to hasten the restoration process, however, and stretching the sore muscles is especially helpful. Common sense is the best guide for determining progression. It is always more sensible to be conservative in increasing the intensity of the effort than to be excessively enthusiastic.

Before long, an average person should be able to exercise safely for a minimum of twenty minutes at an intensity that is perceived as being at least "somewhat hard." Such activity is sufficient for small physical improvements. For greater improvements, the intensity of exercise (walking, for example) should be increased gradually to at least the "hard" level, and the duration increased to thirty minutes or more. To simplify, the three words to be kept in mind when devising an exercise program are "regular," "overload," and "progressive."

A proper progression serves to eliminate pain and soreness. The adage, "no pain, no gain," must have been invented by a sadist. Pain, either during or after an exercise session, is not at all necessary for improvement to occur. It is, however, a signal that the body is doing too much. Unfortunately, beginners often use post-exercise soreness as an excuse to stop exercising entirely.

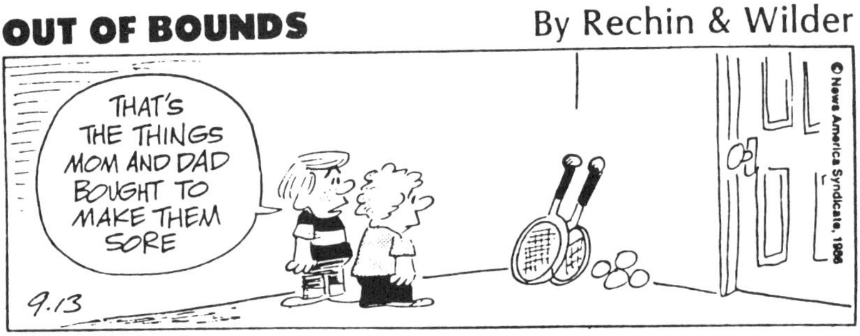

Reprinted with Special Permission of North American Syndicate.

Surprisingly little time and effort is required to achieve a substantial improvement in fitness and health, compared to the sedentary population. Greater benefits can be attained by increasing the time and effort devoted to training, but the returns will be markedly diminished relative to the expenditure of time and effort. This finding was revealed by research from the prestigious Institute for Aerobic Research and the Cooper Clinic in Dallas. The study was the most extensive and finely controlled analysis ever done on the effects of exercise on longevity. It followed more than 13,000 Americans over eighteen years of age for an average of eight years, and was one of the few large studies that included women as well as men. The chief finding was that sedentary people can add years to their lives with just moderate involvement in exercising programs such as brisk walking.

In fact, it seems as if the exercise requirement for good health is decreasing with each study. The latest suggests that strolling for three miles (five days a week) is nearly as beneficial as brisk walking.

If you find that you begin to really enjoy exercising, a very likely occurrence if you do not progress too rapidly, and want to exercise more often, that's fine. From the standpoint of health and fitness it is most desirable to progress to four workouts a week and perhaps even five. The duration of each session can also be increased to forty-five minutes or an hour. In these cases, though, the intensity should be reduced to prevent overtraining and decrease the chances for injury. If the training sessions are mild you can even exercise every day without fear of injury.

Each exercise session should be preceded by a warm-up period to gradually increase the body temperature and heart rate. A light sweat is indicative of a sufficient warm-up. A person won't start sweating immediately, though. The exercising body does immediately produce more heat, but the brain "tells" it to store the heat. With the resulting increase in body temperature, the muscles perform more efficiently. After about ten minutes (the precise length depends upon the ambient temperature and the intensity of the activity) the heat production reaches excess levels; the body attempts to lose it by sweating. Some people seem to believe that sweating is proof that they are allergic to exercise, but there is no scientific evidence for this.

Stretching movements that are similar to the exercise activity should also be done before exercising in earnest. Then, at the cesssation of exercise, gradually cool down. Five minutes of easy walking is usually enough to allow the heart rate to approach resting levels

When the times for warming-up and cooling-down are added to exercise sessions, a person engaged in a regular exercise program will be devoting from two to six hours per week to physical activity. While this may seem like a lot of time, people can almost always find time for activities that are most important to them — and what is more important than being and feeling healthy and fit?

Although the perceived effort method is a very simple guide to exercise intensity and duration, a much more objective and accurate guide to determining exercise intensity involves measuring your heart rate (HR). Of the various formulae, the one below is the simplest. It uses a percentage of your maximal HR to determine how fast your heart must beat in order to achieve a training effect. The maximal heart rate must first be obtained by subtracting your age from 220. For example, the maximal HR for a thirty-year old would be 220 - 30, or 190 beats per minute.

To obtain a training effect for the cardiovascular system the HR of a person of average fitness must increase to at least 60% of the maximum. That is, multiply the maximum HR by .60. For a woman of thirty this is an HR of 114. If it goes higher than that, she will obtain even greater training effects but for safety purposes it should not exceed 75% of maximum (or 142 beats per minute).

It is important to know that the percentage varies according to such factors as a person's age and fitness level. People who have a low fitness level due to an inactive lifestyle and those who are above sixty years of age need only raise their heart rates to about 45% of their maximal HR to begin achieving a training effect. People who are very fit, on the other hand, will need to increase their HR to between 75% and 90% of maximum to improve their fitness.

This method of guiding the intensity and duration of an exercise session naturally requires the accurate measuring of a person's heart rate. The pulse can be taken at a number of locations on the body. Since the pulse seems strongest at the throat, as shown below, most people choose this location. Unfortunately, pressure on the artery at this point can, by reflex action, lower the HR as much as twelve beats per minute. As a result, the HR may be measured at 135 and actually be 147 — and that may be dangerously high. The trick is to press the fingers against the artery just hard enough to detect the pulse.

A pulse taken at the wrist will not result in a reflex lowering of the HR and therefore tends to be more accurate. Since the pulse is sometimes difficult to find, it helps to find it before exercising and to mark the spot with a small circle. When exercising, it is usually necessary to stop in order to take a measurement. To reduce the rest period and obtain a more accurate measurement, the HR should be counted for ten seconds and then multiplied by 6 to obtain the HR per minute. Counting should begin with "zero" for the first heart beat. This procedure may sound complicated, but it gets easy after a few times. Besides, with a little experience most people will be able to estimate their HR rather accurately merely from perceived efforts.

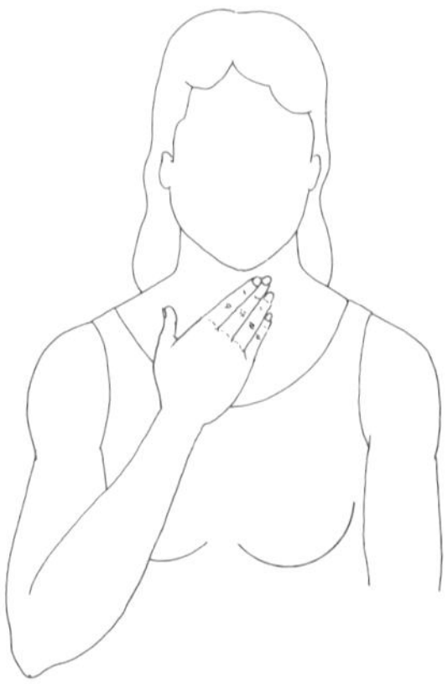

Neck (carotid) pulse

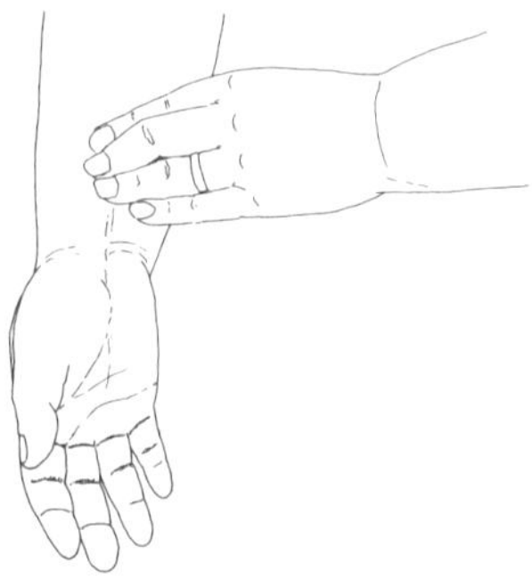

Wrist (radial) pulse

Since aerobic sessions consist of continuous, or near continuous activity, their intensity levels must be considerably less than maximal. For a person trying to lose body fat this is ideal because during mild and moderate exercise, most of the body's energy comes from the burning of fat. With exercise above 70% of maximal intensity, sugar becomes the primary source of energy.

Although any of the aerobic activities mentioned previously will allow a person to persist at these relatively low levels of exertion, they are not all equally recommended. The ones that consist of high-impact movements, such as jogging, running, and jumping rope put considerable stress on the joints of the feet, ankles, hips, lower back, and knees — particularly the latter. On level ground, for instance, the force on a runner's heel upon impact is typically about 5,000 pounds per square inch. A reasonable amount of stress is desirable to strengthen bones, but high impact activities tend to produce excessive stresses which causes injuries to the joints.

High-impact aerobic dance with its jolting, wrenching movements would seem to have have the highest injury potential, particularly when performed on hard surfaces. Not surprisingly, most aerobic instructors themselves suffer from impact injuries. An additionally hazardous, and absolutely unnecessary, aspect of aerobic dancing is the apparently obligatory playing of music at literally deafening levels. Music is fine when kept at reasonable levels, but prolonged exposure to loud sounds always causes damage to the hearing apparatus. The harmful effect is multiplied when accompanied by strenuous exercise because, in addition to diverting blood to the active muscle tissue, such activity triggers the release of adrenaline. Both events result in a reduced supply of blood to the inner ear. Since that causes the thousands of tiny hair cells in the inner ear to swell and begin falling out, the result is a permanent hearing loss. If an instructor is reluctant to significantly lower the decibels, a smart student will wear ear plugs.

Low-impact aerobic activities are definitely preferable to the high impact types. This is true for everyone, but the heavier a person is the more it applies. In low-impact aerobics, a part of a participant's body is always on the ground — or on a supporting surface. Walking, bicycling, rowing, and swimming are excellent low-impact aerobic activities. Walking is especially recommended. It has about one-half the impact of jogging, does not require special skills, and it can be done virtually anywhere. To derive the most benefit, though, it has to be done briskly. As Thomas Jefferson advised, "Habituate yourself to walking fast without fatigue." Such walking lowers total blood cholesterol and increases the HDLs as much as running at two to three times the pace, provided the same distance is covered. Both activities are equally effective in reducing body fat since approximately the same number of calories are expended per mile. The most dramatic health benefits occur when a person walks or runs at least twelve miles per week — in three or four sessions.

If you absolutely hate any kind of serious exercise such as brisk walking or swimming, don't do it! And you should not feel guilty about not doing it. Life is too short to be miserable three times a week for half-hour periods. And anticipating the workouts only multiplies the unpleasantness. But there must be some activity you enjoy doing such a stroll in the park with a friend, splashing around in a pool, bicycling, or gardening. How can you hate those kinds of activities? They're relaxing and fun. Okay, admittedly, deep down inside I hope you will gradually want to indulge in more strenuous exercise — and enjoy it. And the change may occur more quickly than you might imagine. If you don't progress, however, even mild exercise such as strolling has considerable health benefits, especially psychological. Just moving, even playing golf, beats being "couched" in front of a television set, downing a bowlful of munchies.

Incidentally, "health" and "physical fitness" are not synonymous. Although a physically fit person generally may tend to be healthier than an unfit person, it certainly does not automatically follow. Health can be improved greatly without a great increase in fitness.

Since walking is a very popular activity, and deservedly so, a few comments are required here. When walking, avoid ankle weights; when enough weight is used to increase the effort of walking, the incidence of groin injuries soars. To increase the energy expenditure of walking, merely walk faster or walk up a hill or stairs. Climbing stairs, incidentally, especially two steps at a time, is excellent for exercising the buttocks.

Hand weights, tend to quickly tire the arms and interfere with a walker's stride. They can also injure the arm and shoulder joints. If you are determined to use hand weights, though, start slowly with very light poundages and gradually increase the weight over a period of time.

Social dances, including square dances, are not usually mentioned as being aerobic events, but they are just modified forms of walking and running. Perhaps they are just too much fun to be taken seriously. An evening of dancing, however, does have considerable aerobic benefit, particularly when they include the faster dances. All of the non-partnered social dances are also fine. Twisting, assuming you've heard of the dance, is a wonderful exercise for the mid-section and it takes just a few seconds to learn the basic movement. Tap, modern, jazz, and ballet exercises are also excellent for developing fitness.

Swimming has been extolled as being the best all-around exercise and it has to rank near the top. Unlike most aerobic exercises it strongly involves the upper body, and the wearing of swim fins makes the activity even better because of the added resistance to leg motion. Swimming is excellent for obese people because it permits them to exercise without putting great stress on the joints of the lower body.

Aerobic exercises done in the water are also excellent for the same reason. If you exercise in the water, however, do not expect to lose body fat nearly as rapidly as those who expend the same amount of energy exercising on land. Apparently the coldness of the water causes the body to maintain more fat for insulation. Exercising in tepid water probably would not have that effect and a larger weight loss may occur.

Many aerobic exercise machines are now on the market. They include rowing, stair climbing, and cross-country skiing simulators, as well as treadmills and stationary bikes. The electronic machines, with programmed routines, heart rate feedback, and fitness scores are more interesting to use — and are much more expensive. If you've ever seen a person jogging grimly in the rain, snow, or slush — or in 100° weather — you have a clue to the chief advantage of exercise machines. Moreover, outdoor space limitations often make it impossible to jog, bike, or ski. Exercising indoors also allows a person to escape much of the air pollution that is so prevalent in most cities. It is true that indoor exercising will deprive the neighborhood dogs of considerable sport; they delight so in nipping at the heels of intrepid joggers and bicyclers. But humans have a propensity for being more concerned with maintaining the integrity of their ankles and nerves than in providing merriment for canine antagonists.

It is not easy for a neophyte to decide which aerobic machine will be the most enjoyable to use over the long run. Though it is not generally feasible, it helps to exercise at least several times on one of each type. Common sense, and research, suggests that a machine that exercises both the upper and lower body is preferable to one that involves only one region. No matter which you finally decide upon, however, it is of utmost importance to buy a quality machine. It will cost a lot more initially, but will provide good service for years instead of falling apart after a few weeks or months. In addition, high quality machines are quieter and smoother, and therefore are more enjoyable to use than cheap ones.

Not all exercises produce aerobic benefits. The main object of many exercises is to increase the strength and size of muscles by requiring them to contract against greater resistance than usual. Weight training is the most well-known example of these developmental programs — which are now more commonly known as bodybuilding.

For years the role of such training in a weight reduction program was overlooked or even denigrated. Bodybuilding was a "closet" activity; people who engaged in the activity did not readily admit it. Now, participants proudly wear shirts emblazoned with the "Gold's Gym" logo. And, for the first time, the prestigious American College of Sports Medicine is saying that building muscle mass is as important as increasing aerobic capacity. This is true for everyone. A study at Tufts University in 1990 found that an eight-week training program helped ninety-year olds build more muscle mass and become more mobile and self-sufficient. And Dr. Michael Pollock of the University of Florida's cardiology and physiology division recommends larger muscles even for "little old ladies."

Strength training does not necessarily mean using massive weight and building huge muscles. Exercising with light dumbbells, for instance, can help strengthen the back, improve posture, and help women avoid bone loss.

In addition, enlarged muscles consume more energy, even at rest, than when they were smaller. Specifically, every pound of increased muscle mass uses about 50 calories a day. Because enlarged muscles burn more calories, they are more useful in helping a person lose weight.

Since resistance exercises build muscle tissue, they are excellent for sculpting the body if a person so desires. No, a Woody Allen can never have the physique of an Arnold Schwartzeneggar, or a Cher the contours of a Dolly Parton; we are all born with a specific body type. Everyone, however, does have a considerable potential for variation. If a person desires the physical, psychological, and cosmetic benefits of bodybuilding exercises, it is recommended that they do a group of about ten exercises designed to reach every muscle group. They should be performed two or three times a week — with aerobics on three alternate days. Typically, that would amount to about forty-five minutes a day — less time than people devote to eating.

Women who bodybuild need not fear looking like Schwartzeneggar. Not many men can approach his massiveness even with appropriate genetics, years of incredibly heavy resistance training, and the use of anabolic steroids. Besides, if a woman finds she is getting larger muscles than she prefers, all she has to do is use lighter weights and do more repetitions.

There are many kinds of bona fide muscle building machines. It is impossible to say which type is best since each has its good and bad points. They are all effective, though, when used properly. Whether any of these machines are superior to a simple set of "free weights" (barbells and dumbbells) is highly doubtful when all factors are considered. In fact, after publishing a series of articles, the Journal of American National Strength and Conditioning in Feb./Mar. 1982 concluded that free weight training better meets the requirements of training and have numerous advantages over machines. In addressing the often-raised "safety issue," the article states that not a single study comparing the incidence of injuries has ever been published.

Free weights also take up much less space and are far less expensive than machines. A hundred-pound set of weights is more than enough for most women to work all the major muscle groups. Consisting of a barbell and two dumbbells, a basic set usually costs less than $100 new, and it is often possible to buy a set for around $10 at a garage sale. Machines are sometimes outrageously expensive. Before the Nautilus company went out of business, for example, it charged thousands of dollars for each of its machines and about eight were needed for a basic workout. In addition, a very large room was necessary to contain the machines.

It is not within the scope of this book to provide exercises for developing every muscle group in the body but the abdominals are so important to a person's general health and well-being, they in good conscience cannot be ignored. Next to the heart and the "breathing muscles," the abdominals are the most important muscles of the body. In addition to being basic to good posture, the twisting and bending actions of abdominal exercises have a beneficial massaging effect on the internal organs. As a result, constipation is virtually eliminated. Although this common disorder is often a source of jocularity, it is no laughing matter. Unfortunately, constipation is generally treated with laxatives which only tend to worsen the condition.

When discussing abdominal development, it must be understood that there are four groups of such muscles involved. Each, as shown below, has different points of attachment, and fibers that run in a different direction. Since each abdominal group therefore produces different movements, different exercises must be performed to develop each muscle group.

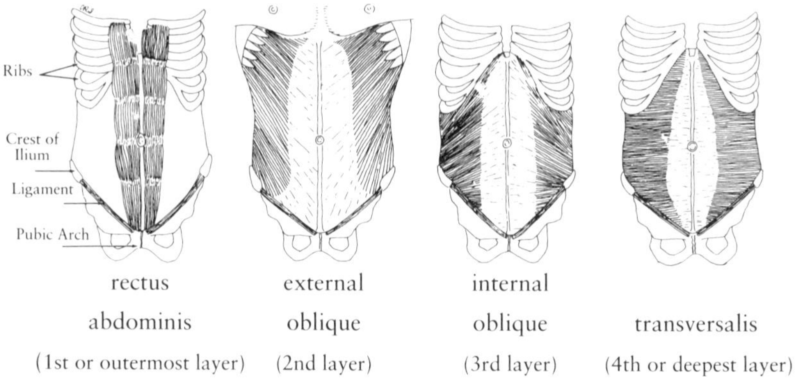

Four Layers of Abdominal Muscles

The rectus abdominis is the potentially prominent "washboard" muscle at the front of the abdomen. To develop this muscle many people do sit-ups, but an infinitely better exercise is "curl-ups." Although, there is no sacred basic position for curl-ups, the one shown below was chosen

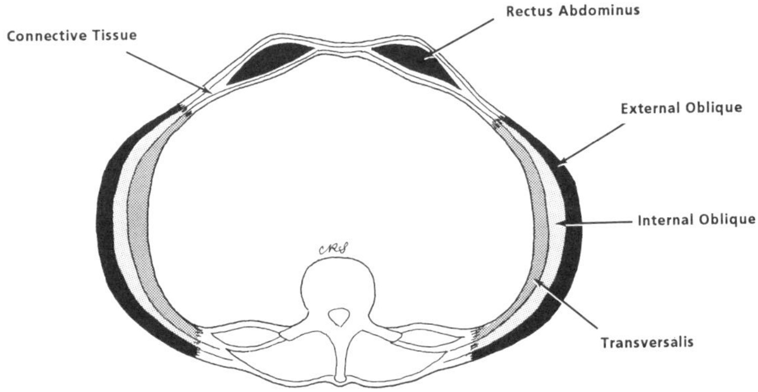

Cross-Section of the Abdomen (showing the layers of muscle groups)

because it ensures that the lower back (pelvis and lumbar section) will remain immobile and flat on the floor throughout the entire exercise. That is imperative!

For beginners, the shoulder blades do not even have to leave the floor for the "abs" to be strengthened; it's the effort that counts. As the muscles get stronger, a person will be able to curl the body higher. Usually an inch or two will be the maximum depending upon the flexibility of the spine. But if you never get them off the floor that's okay. Put your hands were they feel most comfortable. You can fold them across the chest. If you

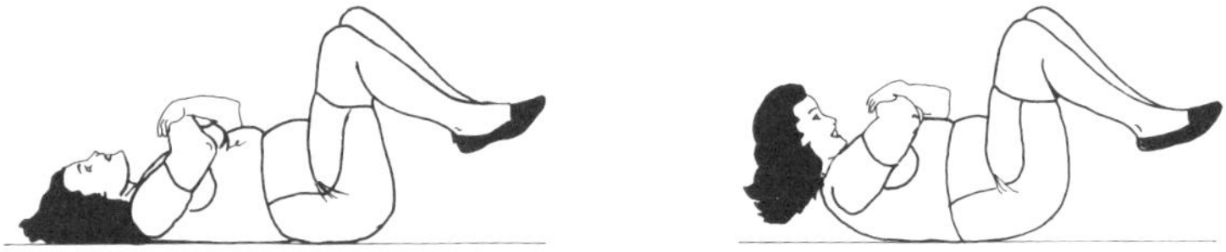

A "Crunch."

clasp them behind the head, be careful not to pull against the head; that can injure the neck. In any case, always do curl-ups slowly and smoothly — no faster than, say, three or four seconds per curl-up. After a number of repetitions, change leg positions and do the same number. To do "crunches" keep both legs raised. Other excellent variations can be created with the addition of twisting motions. The number of repetitions should be gradually increased.

If your legs have to be held down, it is proof that curl-ups are being done incorrectly. Yet "sit-up bars" that attach to the bottom of interior doors to hold down an exerciser's feet are usually on the market. I was stunned once to hear fitness guru Jack LaLanne tell his television audience that the feet had to be held down for sit-ups to be properly done. Although this is absolutely incorrect advice, most viewers put their faith in LaLanne since he is delightfully charismatic and has an exceptional physique.

This basis for expertise, invalid as it is, also explains why so many exercise books and videos feature actresses and models. Producers are well aware that most viewers believe a well-formed body is proof of exercise knowledge. *Sports Illustrated*, for instance, used four shapely, well-known models in their 1990 exercise videos. Calling the women "fitness experts," the commercials promised viewers, "The body you want in just eight weeks . . . firm, slim, and trim." Whether the women were fitness experts or not depends upon how the term is defined. But to expect an average person (much less an obese one) to achieve the body he or she wants in eight weeks is patently absurd. Viewers who would fall for that could not be expected to realize that such charmers have genetic advantages — and sometimes surgical ones. The models could achieve superior physiques in spite of inefficient programs. Programs should be tailored with an individual's goals and potentials in mind — and based upon the best scientific evidence. Such programs are not likely to be developed by people whose chief credentials are the ability to assume fetching poses. Because these "fitness experts" typically lack even the most basic academic credentials, such as a bachelor's degree in physical education, they often spew out information that can result in serious health problems or chronically painful injuries.

Low-back pain, for instance, will afflict 80% of American adults at some time during their lives. Paradoxically, a large percentage of cases are caused by the muscles of the lower back being, not too weak but, too strong compared to the opposing abdominal muscles. Sit-ups actually cause this muscle imbalance because they strengthen the iliopsoas (ill-eeoo-so´-us) muscles of the lower back much more than they strengthen the abdominals.

The iliopsoas muscle group flexes the body at the hip joint. As shown below, it is the primary mover for sit-ups; abdominal muscles are secondary. Since the iliopsoas does the strongest contracting, it becomes the strongest muscle group. The prime mover for curl-ups, on the other hand, is the rectus abdominis; the iliopsoas is not involved at all — which is why curl-ups are so effective for strengthening the "rectus." By

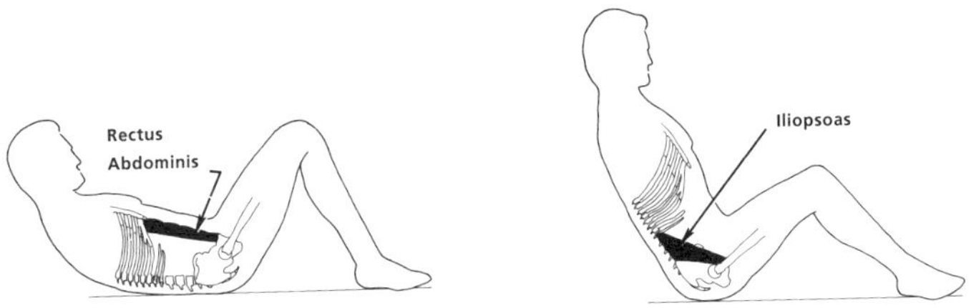

Prime Movers for Curl-ups and Sit-ups.

eliminating iliopsoas involvement, the exercise can prevent and treat cases of lower back injuries caused by the lower back muscles being too strong. A person with low-back pain, however, must always see a physician before exercising in case the condition has another cause which can be aggravated by bending and twisting the trunk.

Many people, especially women, wish to strengthen the muscles of their lower abdomen. Leg raises are most effective for this, but not the old-fashioned, straight-legged kind. Like sit-ups, they lead to low-back pain. It is best to keep the knees drawn up to the chest while lifting the lower part of the body off the floor. If the muscles are not strong enough to produce movement, that is okay; just trying will strengthen the muscles.

The external and internal oblique muscles assist the rectus abdominis in doing curl-ups, but their primary function is to produce twisting motions of the trunk. Therefore, to strengthen the oblique muscles (which work in unison) twisting at the waist — either the upper body or the lower body — is required. A lot of people have trouble performing

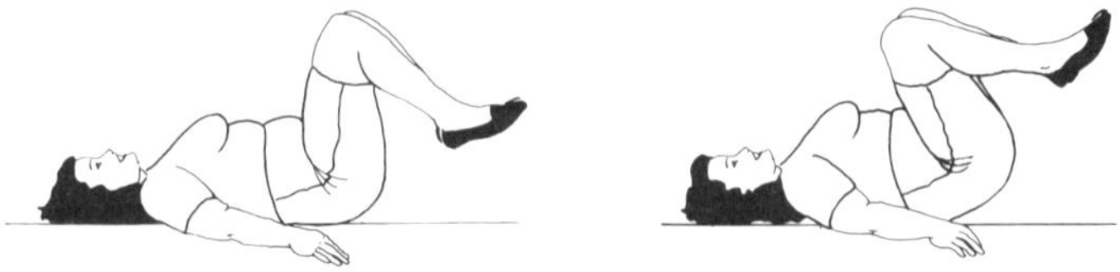

Bent-leg Raises.

these movements properly. Sitting while turning from side-to-side is the most foolproof method. Putting a broomstick across the shoulders and resting the arms on it offers a little more resistance to movement. Doing the twisting motions slowly prevents overdoing.

The transversalis is usually the least exercised muscle of the abdominal group. Relatively few people are even aware of its existence. To

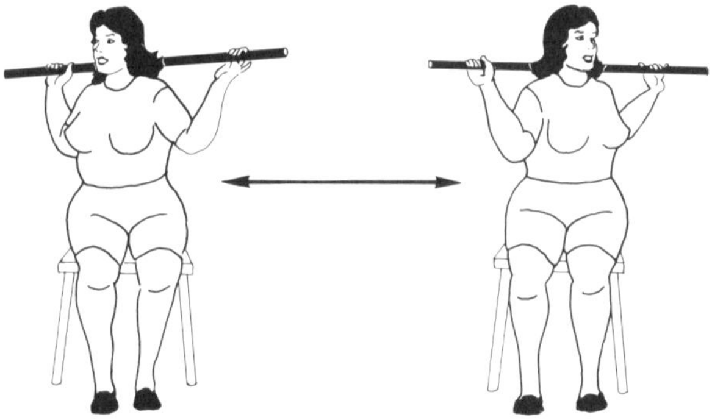

Trunk Twisting Exercise for the Abdominal Oblique Muscles.

exercise it, merely "suck in your stomach" forcefully and hold the contraction for a few seconds. Just ten to fifteen contractions a day will significantly decrease the girth of the waist — and the more "suck-ins" the better. They can be done practically anywhere and anytime.

One of the very best practices for strengthening the abdominals is to consistently maintain a properly erect posture with the "stomach" held in a bit. Although the posture will initially require some concentration to maintain, before long it will feel natural. Besides giving the appearance of being vital and self-confident, studies suggest that good posture will actually tend to instill these traits.

The exercises presented here strengthen the abdominal muscles and thereby tend to reduce the dimensions of the midsection. No amount of any exercise, however, will reduce body fat if more calories are consumed than are expended. With this positive energy balance, the excess calories are stored as fat on the body. The percentage of the total that is stored on each body part, including the abdomen, depends upon one's genetics. Conversely, no matter what part of the body is exercised, if there is a negative energy balance, fat will be lost from the entire body. And the specific percentage lost from each part also depends upon one's heredity. Abdominal exercises will not burn-off more fat from the midsection than if the same number of calories are burned-off by doing arm exercises. In other words there is no such thing as "spot reducing" when it comes to losing fat. The most dramatic proof for this assertion is the fact that the fat percentage of the preferred arms of tennis players is the same as that of their non-preferred arms.

The abdominal exercises described in these pages do not require any apparatus and they are superb ways to exercise these major muscles. Each exercise also permits many variations to work the abdominal muscles in a variety of ways and to reduce the chances of boredom. Of course, consumers are led to believe by manufacturers of abdominal reducing devices that their products must be used to achieve the best results. Their advertisements are replete with the typical MAGGOTY techniques such as testimonials (often by famous people) and jargon including — "a brilliant device," "as seen on TV," "hailed as a scientific breakthrough," "no risk guarantee," "you must see a flat-as-a-pancake stomach or return it within 30 days for a full refund," "beware of cheap and inferior imitations," and "in accord with the latest scientific knowledge of human anatomy and biomechanics."

Could anyone be naive enough to fall for such rubbish? Well, millions upon millions of these worthless devices have been sold. The price is usually $19.95 plus several dollars for shipping and handling. Apparently, the industry assumes that hordes of people will take a chance on any product, no matter how hair-brained, as long as it costs less than twenty dollars. The industry is obviously accurate in that assumption. The slicker companies will have another MAGGOTY device to foist onto the market after its current one has sucked all of the money it can from the pockets of a gullible public.

The most flagrant deceptions in the exercise market are those devices which allegedly produce the benefits of exercise, including weight reduction, with no effort at all on the user's part. When it comes to exercise, however, nothing is gained without muscular exertion.

Granted, some very fancy machines are available and none is as impressive looking as the electric muscle stimulators (EMS) with their knobs and flashing lights. The machines function by sending volleys of low-intensity electrical pulses to muscles via electrodes. The "sales-pitch" is that the impulses cause muscles to contract and burn-up calories — thereby leading to decreases in body fat. In reality, the contractions are so mild that people expend more calories by scratching their rumps, literally — and the scratching feels a lot better. In fact, a 1990 study at Northeastern University in Boston found that EMS users only burned about 6 calories in 36 minutes when the electrodes were simultaneously attached to the abdominal, buttocks, and thigh muscles. At that rate it would take more than two weeks of continuous EMS to burn 3500 calories (one pound of fat).

If the machines could deliver high-intensity electrical pulses, the stimulated muscles would contract more forcefully and therefore expend more calories. The potential for disaster, however, would also soar. People with cardiac problems, of which there are about 63 million in the U.S., certainly do not want strong electrical impulses surging throughout the thoracic cavity and interfering with the natural impulses that cause the heart to beat. In fact, a person with a healthy heart would be wise to avoid any external electrical stimulation. Strong electrical impulses may also trigger the growth of dormant tumors that many people have scattered throughout their bodies. These tumors, like sleeping dogs, are best left alone. Wisely, since these high-intensity devices have various medical uses, most are available only for use by qualified practitioners.

Other devices that are attractive to people who want fitness without effort are the so-called "exercise" tables. These motorized sectional tables raise, lower, rotate, and vibrate various areas of a body that are reclining on them. The passive exercise devices are usually so expensive they are found chiefly in health spas and figure salons although Sears does sell one for $1,276.35. Its ad trumpets, "Exercise the EASY way!" and, "Our toning table does all the work for you!" The same ad features a stationary bicycle with a "Power toning cycle" that "propels you through a great workout — WITHOUT THE WORK!" Now, that is a classic contradiction. Many people are fooled by such deceptions, but the fact is — for muscles to become stronger and body fat to be burned, the user must do the work, not the machine.

Although many worthless exercise products are being sold, there are also many fine products for both aerobic fitness and bodybuilding. These make exercising more fun for some people; however, it must be emphasized that machines are not necessary. Walking is quite sufficient for aerobic improvement, as are jogging and running. For bodybuilding a person can do heavy resistance exercises such as push-ups, lunges, and chin-ups. These can be modified to meet the capabilities of people at any level of fitness.

Instead of buying equipment — which usually rusts out instead wearing out — it makes much better sense to hire a personal trainer with a degree in physical education (preferably fitness management). By far the best recommendation, though, is to join a fitness and wellness center at a university if there is one nearby that has such a facility. They are always staffed by highly qualified personnel. This situation contrasts sharply with commercial emporiums that are staffed primarily with salespeople.

What has been recommended in this chapter — relative to the intensity, duration, and frequency of exercise — is not the fastest way to become physically fit, but is the most sensible way in order to reduce the chances of damage to the body. The medical maxim, "first, do no harm" applies equally as well to exercise.

It is not difficult to exercise too much, too long, or too often. Amusingly, sports figures often talk about "giving 110%," or whatever. The highest I've ever heard, 200%, was offered by Roger Craig, manager of the San Francisco Giants baseball team — 200% may be a world record. In reality, the most physical effort anyone can give is 100%.

People who exceed this level, by definition, have entered "Injury City." And those who approach 100% are knocking at the gate.

It is easy to understand why athletes in an effort to triumph would push themselves to their limits during competition, but why would a recreational athlete do so — or a person merely trying to become healthier and more fit? Since intense efforts greatly increase the chances for injury, they simply do not make sense. Besides bringing training to a screeching and sometimes prolonged halt, injuries interfere with normal activities and cause a lot of pain and discomfort.

Although moderation makes sense to the average person, some people become so obsessed with training that rationality is lost. The most likely explanation for this obsession is that prolonged, intense exercise (in highly trained people) results in the release of endorphins by the brain. These chemicals, two hundred times more potent than morphine, reduce pain and produce a feeling of euphoria. For some people this "high" becomes a virtual addiction. For example, the lyrics from Ray Steven's Joggin' (MCA Records) are absolutely hilarious, but they express precisely how many joggers feel about the activity. The song tells of a jogger who in spite of foul weather, galled thighs, a severe inflammation of the Achilles' heel, Doberman dogs biting his buns, muscle cramps, and runner's knee (and that's just part of the first stanza!) keeps on joggin'. The poor devil admits he's a "fool for pain" and that no amount of sufferin' will ever stop him from joggin'. Most significantly he asks if that's the way a healthy person is supposed to feel. It's a good question. The answer should be obvious.

Exercise may seem like a "good" addiction, but excessive levels, in addition to its many physical problems, lead to depression, anxiety, and uncharacteristic outbursts of anger. Women, especially, are prone to become anorectic.

A Reebok shoe advertisement in 1991 said, "Life is short. Play hard." Somehow those sentences seem discordant. The combination, "Life is short. Relax and enjoy it." seems to make a lot more sense.

While it is true that some people exercise too much, the vast majority of people exercise too little. More than 80% of Americans say they exercise, but The Center for Disease Control in Atlanta reports that only

10% do enough to obtain significant health benefits. The vast majority of people simply do not "stick with it." Something must be done to increase drastically the percentage of people involved in activity programs in terms of sufficient intensity, duration and frequency — but what?

A first step would be to learn why Americans who do exercise do so. According to a survey reported in *American Health* (March, 1985), nearly 90% of all Americans who did any kind of exercise did so to improve their health, for weight control, to feel good, for fitness, or to improve their appearance. That is, they viewed exercise as medicine. This view is substantiated by the term "exercise prescription" which is commonly used by the medical and fitness professionals when discussing an individualized exercise program. Exercise can indeed be superb medicine. Along with a balanced diet, exercise is the supreme kind of medicine — both prophylactic and therapeutive.

Unfortunately, from infancy it is deeply ingrained in our minds that medicines taste bad — that is, they are unpleasant experiences. If people exercise merely because it is a form of medicine, the odds of their "swallowing it" for thirty-minutes three or four times a week for the rest of their lives are infinitesimally slim.

To increase these odds people must view exercise as being a pleasurable experience. Moreover, people who enjoy exercising obtain more of the benefits than those who view their workouts as drudgery. Yet, the *American Health* survey found that only about 10% of the respondents exercised because they enjoyed it. The traditional way for making physical activity fun is to wrap it in a game situation. Since a "little bit of sugar makes the medicine go down," play would seemingly be an excellent solution. The problem, however, is that most adult sports, such as golf, bowling, and even tennis the way it's usually played, do not require a sufficiently sustained intensity to produce aerobic benefits. Besides, these games which are supposed to be recreational usually end up being stressful, competitive encounters. This is hardly appealing in the long run in a world that is already too "high powered."

Logically, the most successful approach to developing an active lifestyle would be for people to learn to enjoy the kinesthetic sensations associated with exercise. These feelings are invoked by movement and muscular contractions, and originate at sensory receptors located in muscles, joints, and tendons. The delightful sensations of an exaggerated, uninhibited yawn is an example of a kinesthetic event that practically everyone has experienced. All physical activities can produce equally sensual and exciting sensations; indeed, most have a far greater potential for doing so since they consist of more complex and prolonged kinesthetic patterns. The first step to getting "high" on the kinesthesia of exercise is to concentrate on the sensations.

Concentration is the key to maximizing sensory appreciation. In a revealing statement the authors of *Pumping Iron: The Art and Sport of Bodybuilding*, describe a Mr. Universe while he performed arm curls exercises as, ". . . staring at the sheath of his biceps fill and empty, his face as remote and as rapt as a yogi's, his mind somewhere down inside the fibers of that arm." He was clearly in intimate communication with the kinesthetic sensations evoked by the exercise. Although this communication is probably most easily developed in bodybuilding exercises, it can be cultivated for any physical activity.

Some people develop kinesthetic appreciation by chance. Most, however, are only vaguely aware that the sensations even exist. Physical education (PE) classes are the obvious places for kinesthetic appreciation to be developed, but instructors typically are too concerned with developing physical fitness. That goal is, of course, highly desirable. Deplorably, however, studies show that in the typical PE class lasting fifty minutes, students are only active for five to ten minutes and, of that brief period, their heart rates were above 150 for only one to two minutes. In other words, the fitness benefits are not achieved even when students are enrolled in a PE class — which is far too seldom to begin with.

Small wonder that, according to a letter from the President's Council on Physical Fitness and Sports, the scores on youth fitness tests have not improved since 1965. And the council points out that the scores were very low at that time.

The competitiveness that is stressed in most PE classes generally "turns-off" all but the most highly skilled students. Ironically, by helping students to develop an appreciation of their kinesthetic sensations, an instructor can practically guarantee they will be active during their entire lives — and thereby acquire and maintain satisfactory levels of physical fitness.

An article in *Parade Magazine* (December 4, 1988) entitled, "Start Exercising — and Stick with It," advised readers, "To make exercise a habit for life, avoid discomfort and aches; do it for pleasure." This excellent advice was reiterated in large print. Then, at the end of the article the author contradicted the statement by saying, "You can give yourself 'thought' rewards and try to think of something pleasant, rather than thinking about your effort." I could hardly believe my eyes. The implication was that people should subordinate, ignore, or even reject, what is potentially the most appealing aspect of exercise — the kinesthetic sensations.

Sadly, the author of that article does not stand alone in this attitude; he is in the mainstream. Aerobic dance instructors play loud music for the same reason — to distract their students' minds from the physical activity. Modern exercise emporiums go even further with music, conditioned air, carpeted floors, hot tubs, and fancy decor to make exercise a pleasant experience. Practically every sense is taken into consideration except the one that is most directly associated with physical activity — namely, kinesthesia.

Exercise — like sex — should be a delightful, sensual experience. One has to wonder if aerobic and gymnasium instructors believe music must be played to make sex endurable. If so, they are not doing it right. And they are not doing exercise right, either, if they need music for distraction. This is not to imply that music cannot or should not be used to enhance either of these vital activities.

People are advised to concentrate on the sensations of their muscular efforts because there is so much pleasure to be found in them. It may take awhile for some people to appreciate fully the sensations. One of the best ways to get started is to use dumbbells since the resistance can be widely varied to a level that each individual will find most pleasurable. Dumbbells should be used slowly to allow a person time to grasp fully the subtleties of kinesthetic sensations. Wine connoisseurs, to use an analogy, do not gulp down champagne. They swish it slowly around the mouth while concentrating on the subtleties of its taste and aromatic sensations.

That brings to mind a cartoon showing an elderly man raking leaves. His younger neighbor was using a new-fangled leaf blower and tauntingly suggested he buy one, too, because it took the work out of gathering leaves. The old fellow shook his head in disagreement, and with a gentle smile said that the blower just took the all of the fun out of the chore.

That is the right idea when it comes to exercise. Enjoy it! Physical exertions associated with chores or occupational activities can be appreciated just as much as recreational ones. In fact, physical work, including those that are usually considered laborious or tedious, can actually become recreational. When exercise, of all kinds, is viewed in this context, the prospect of a lifetime of physical activity is no longer dreaded. It is looked forward to as a source of pleasure. And that is THE secret, the only secret, to a lifelong commitment to exercise.

15

THE RIGHT TO BE FAT

It should be clear by now that much of the poor health attributed to being overweight is actually the result of poor dietary and exercise habits. For fat people who are concerned about their health, and everyone should be, Chapters Thirteen and Fourteen have been offered as safe, effective guidance. General dietary and exercise rules are presented, but the weight-loss aspect is occasionally touched upon since it is assumed that many readers of this book might be interested in losing weight — safely and permanently.

That is not to say that everyone who wants to lose fat actually needs to. There is a wide diversity of body types and a healthy range of fatness for each of the types. Of course, there *are* many people who are fat to the extent that it is hazardous. For some, excessive fatness may be due to a physiological or psychological disorder. Other people may not care about how fat they are — or if they do care, it is of minor importance. It must be emphasized that a lack of interest in losing body fat is no reflection upon a person's character or intelligence. Whether or not anyone wants to lose weight is a very personal decision. People have different priorities in life. And people have the right to be fat if they wish, without suffering ridicule and insults.

Even if a person is excessively fat due to eating too much, is that really so awful? Assume for a moment that being fat actually does shorten a person's life by a few years. Would that person be better off if, through a lifetime of stringent dieting, he or she managed to be thin? Would the years of gnawing hunger be worth it? Remember, too, that the years of life that might be lost are not at the young or middle-age period, but at the old-age end. These are the years that many people are not too excited about enduring anyway. As an articulate, "robust" friend of mine explained, "I don't want to give up the certainty of culinary delights to increase my chances for being a nonagenarian — a wrinkled, bedridden prune, who doesn't recognize his children, and has to have someone change his diapers."

Compared to many dangerous and unhealthy lifestyles, overeating is really quite tame and inoffensive. Besides, the inclination to overeat is understandable since, like exercise, eating can be an extremely delightful sensory event.

Human beings engage in countless activities that endanger their health but which do not draw the ire and condemnation of others. One of the unhealthiest situations imaginable occurs when a parachutist's equipment malfunctions. Yet people who engage in this dangerous enterprise are usually viewed as being heroic. Okay, some of the uninitiated may have doubts about the intelligence of parachutists, but their character is not assailed. The same can be said of mountain climbers and boxers; people who race horses, automobiles, powerboats, and motorcycles; and professional football players (who die, on the average, about thirteen years before the average man). Many non-sport occupations that people choose are also dangerous. Police work, firefighting, and the military come immediately to mind. Presidents of the U.S. probably have the most dangerous occupation in America. It seems grossly inconsistent that people who engage in these and other hazardous activities are held in high esteem while those who are, or are assumed to be, unhealthily fat are hassled and defiled.

Many antifat articles subtly suggest it is the fault of fat people that they are consistently discriminated against in employment, promotion and public acceptance; that they are more likely to suffer from anxiety, depression, loneliness, unhappiness, and low self-esteem than are thinner people; and that society has stereotyped them as being gluttonous, lazy, etc. The implication is that if fat people want to reverse this situation, they should merely lose weight. This is like telling African Americans that racism is their fault — that if they want to eliminate discrimination they should bleach their skin. That is, of course, a ridiculous proposal. Whenever stereotyping exists, it is society's responsibility to change *its* attitudes and prejudices. People who do not conform to an arbitrary standard should not have to change; they have the right to be different. That's what the United States of America is supposed to be all about.

Too often fat people have allowed themselves to be badgered into thinking they do not have the right to be fat. The fact is, they do have the right to be fat. If they truly feel that a lifetime of delectable gustatory fulfillment is preferable to a lifetime of what they consider to be torturous abstinence — even at the possible sacrifice of several years of life — they have the right to act accordingly. It is unrealistic to expect everyone to have the same priorities in life. Fat people should not feel unworthy and incompetent as human beings even if they are morbidly obese — any more than other people who vary from any norm should have such negative feelings.

Many fat people, however, particularly women, have been driven to low self-esteem, and that deficiency has an extremely destructive effect upon their lives. Mark Twain expressed this feeling in his introduction to *Pudd'nhead Wilson.*

> There is no character, howsoever good and fine, but it can be destroyed by ridicule, howsoever poor and witless. Observe the ass, for instance; his character is about perfect, he is the choicest spirit among all the humbler animals, yet see what ridicule has brought him to. Instead of feeling complimented when we are called an ass, we are left in doubt.

In a more scientific vein, the noted psychologist Nathaniel Branden wrote on the first page of his book *How to Raise Your Self-Esteem*:

> How we feel about ourselves crucially affects virtually every aspect of our experience, from the way we function at work, in love, in sex, to the way we operate as parents, to how high in life we are likely to rise. Our responses to events are shaped by who and what we think we are. The dramas of our lives are the reflections of our most private visions of ourselves. Thus self-esteem is the key to success or failure.
>
> It is also the key to understanding ourselves and others. Apart from problems that are biological in origin, I cannot think of a single psychological difficulty — from anxiety and depression, to fear of intimacy or of success, to alcohol or drug abuse, to underachievement at school, to sexual dysfunction or emotional immaturity, to suicide or

> crimes of violence — that is not traceable to poor self-esteem. Of all the judgments we pass, none is as important as the one we pass on ourselves. Positive self-esteem is a cardinal requirement of a fulfilling life.

With this passage in mind it is easy to see why it is so despicable for FATISTS and MAGGOTS to goad the general public into ripping tenaciously at the self-esteem of fat people. Again, though, it must be admitted that fat people have to accept part of the blame. They have passively allowed the money-grubbing antifat forces to foist a sense of guilt upon them. Wearing a hair shirt in the expectation of achieving a glorious hereafter is one thing, but for fat people to torture themselves through unreasonable dieting to please other people, primarily insignificant others, is quite another matter. It is totally foolish and absurd.

People do not have to allow themselves to be oppressed. As proof, one need only to look at the overthrowing of communist governments in Eastern Europe and the Soviet Union. Closer to home, African Americans offer the most successful example of fighting oppression. For one hundred years after being freed from slavery, they permitted themselves to suffer at the hands of intolerance and bigotry. Then they decided they had had enough, that they indeed did have rights. Led by such visionaries as Martin Luther King Jr., they demanded those rights and the end of unfair treatment. Their rallying cry was, "Black is beautiful." Far more than referring merely to physical appearance, the statement was an assertion of self-esteem. They were proclaiming to the world — and more importantly to themselves — that they had value and potential. Without such positive feelings, people will always be plagued with self-doubt, inadequacy, guilt, and a fear of full participation in life.

These are the feelings that have been instilled in fat people. If the African Americans, who were about 11% of the population, were able to fight the system and throw off the yoke of low self-esteem, so can fat people. In fact, it should be a lot easier for them since, according to some estimates, they comprise up to 40% of the population.

Too many fat people adapt by being deferential to other people. The obsequious, "jolly fat person" behavior, however, is no more effective in attaining self-worth than the servile, "Step 'n Fetchit" behavior was for African Americans. Both approaches are counterproductive to achieving respect. If our society is to change its negative attitudes toward fat people, fat people will first have to view themselves in a more positive light. To achieve this increased self-esteem Dr. Branden recommends focusing on (1) a *greater awareness* of one's feelings, desires, thoughts, and abilities; (2) *self-acceptance* or learning not to be in an adversarial relationship with one's self; and (3) *self-expression* or self-assertion.

Paradoxically, to increase awareness and self-acceptance it might help a fat person to assume the ridiculous — namely, that being fat or obese *is* indicative of a character flaw. The next step is to develop a "so what" attitude since no one is perfect anyway. Even if fatness is indicative of a character flaw, it is an infinitesimally minor one as far as a person's total value is concerned. People who lack self-esteem because of fatness might well study the partial list of character traits below. It should help them realize there are many qualities that are incomparably more important than the percentage of body fat in determining one's worth.

adventurous	ambitious	artistic
calm	capable	charitable
cheerful	clean	compassionate
congenial	considerate	cooperative
courageous	creative	dependable
enthusiastic	forgiving	friendly
generous	gentle	helpful
honest	intelligent	interested
interesting	kind	likable
loving	moral	neat
optimistic	polite	practical
reliable	respectful	responsible
sensitive	self-reliant	studious
sympathetic	talented	thoughtful
tolerant	trustworthy	warm

No one is perfect. If, indeed, being fat makes a person imperfect, FATISTS are infinitely more imperfect. Fat people should give themselves credit for their good traits and the many wonderful things they have to offer instead of dwelling on what they have been led to believe is a bad trait.

As psychologist Rita Freedman expressed in her book *Body Love*, as far as looks are concerned, a woman's mental health is as important as her physical health. Each woman must learn to appreciate her special, individual characteristics and accept what she cannot change. When a woman has a realistic self-image, she can feel beautiful no matter what she looks like. Incidentally, losing weight has never been found to improve a woman's intelligence, talent, compassion, etc. Oprah Winfrey is a perfect example; she did not become a smarter, more talented, better person with her much publicized weight loss. And when she regained the weight her I.Q. did not drop. She was still beautiful and lovable. She would be so at any weight because of her warmth, personality, and intelligence. This can be true for practically every person.

If a fat person, a truly excessively fat person, wants to lose weight, it is certainly not the intent of this book to discourage her (or him). If that is *her* decision, she should be encouraged. But if she loses weight merely to please another person, that is nonsense. There are multitudes of people who will find fault with others, no matter how they look. If you conform to that person's idea of "ideal" weight, assuming it is humanly possible, they will probably hassle you about something else — your hair style, skin, the way you laugh, *ad nauseam*. These are not loving people. They are not the kind of people who are accepting of others. You do not need them for friends; they are deadly to your self-esteem.

The monumental social disapproval directed toward fatness in our culture contributes heavily to the constant stress suffered by people who are considered to be fat. Since excessive stress adversely affects human behavior and ability to function, it is amazing that fat people are as mentally and psychologically robust as they are and are able to perform as well as they do in a hostile, fatist society.

Self-assertion by fat people involves responding to FATISTS whenever they make deprecating comments. A defense of fatness is not called for since the condition needs no defense. But there are countless other ways of handling insults. In an eye-to-eye situation, sweetly pointing out to a boor that his or her comment was rude and ignorant will be sufficient to convey a message of disapproval. Such enlightenment should cause a thoughtful person to reflect before making similar statements in the future. For FATISTS who are exceptionally dull-witted or insensitive, however, it may be necessary to point out that they are as reprehensible as racists or sexists, and that every case of intolerance and stereotyping merely reveals an offender's ignorance and lack of character.

Before getting too instructional, though, a fat person should realize that some bigots may react with violence when the true nature of their ego-boosting prejudices are exposed. Since discretion is sometimes the better part of valor, it might behoove a fat person to avoid some face-to-face encounters and to concentrate on self-assertion on a more global scale. The latter is far more efficient and effective than face-to-face confrontations anyway. Insights into effective global techniques can be obtained by studying methods used in fighting racism and sexism. The most devastating attacks are on the soft underbelly of FATISTS — their wallets. Tactics include employee strikes against companies that practice fatism, boycotts against businesses that sell MAGGOTY products, and letter-writing campaigns to companies that sponsor television programs that contain slurs against fat people or portray them in stereotypical ways. Revealing letters to the editors of newspapers can also communicate dissatisfaction with a fatist culture. These and other forms of self-assertion can help change our society's bigoted attitudes.

An example of what one person can do in the struggle against fatism was revealed on the *20/20* television program (November 16, 1991) on a segment entitled, "Being Fat — is It Such a Crime?" It featured a lovely young nurse, Sharon Russell, who finally decided she had had enough of being discriminating against because she was fat. She courageously sued a nursing school that had dropped her from their program because she was "too fat." And she won! She received her degree at another institution and currently works as a nurse in St. Petersburg, Florida.

Some of the most blatant public examples of fatism are seen in comic strips and children's shows. These circumstances are particularly reprehensible since they start molding children's minds at a very impressionable age — and pass on prejudices to a new generation. This early stereotyping is not a recent phenomenon. For decades Popeye's obese friend, Wimpy, was portrayed as being outrageously gluttonous. But Wimpy was at least a gentle, inoffensive person.

The same cannot be said of character called "the fat broad" in the nationally syndicated "B.C." comic strip. The cartoon below is an example of its incredible insensitivity to fat people. Because of the character's name, face and hair, her manner of eating, and her poor grammar, the cartoonist has contributed to perpetuating the myth that fat people are unattractive, gluttonous and stupid — and that it is permissible and funny to insult them with the implication that they are "cows."

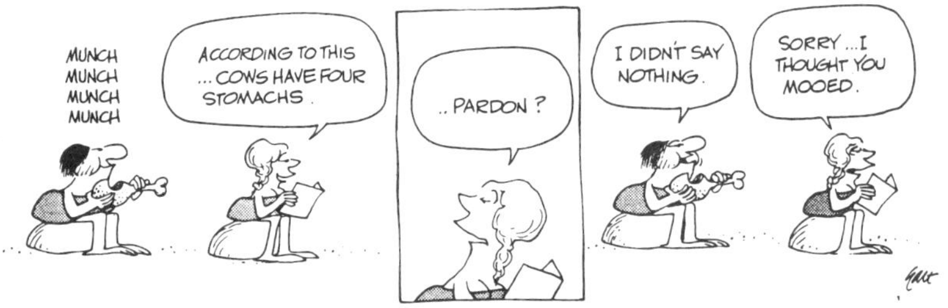

By Permission of Johnny Hart and Creators Syndicate, Inc.

That fat people are permissible targets for ridicule is clear proof that fatism is okay. With insight on the subject that one would expect from a fat person, actress Conchata Ferrell, a regular on NBC's *L.A.Law*, observed that, "Fat people are the last minority it's okay to treat badly." A very good point! Conchata also observed that in our culture, "What is admired is girls with the bodies of fourteen-year-old boys." That's true, and it's a far cry from previous centuries where women were admired for having womanly shapes — with cushiony breasts, abdomens, hips, and thighs.

In a supposedly advanced culture such as ours, it is incredible that such a fatist (and sexist) term as "fat broad" can be used in a popular comic strip that is avidly read by millions of impressionable youngsters — and adults. It is even more astounding that no one has challenged the use of the denigrating term. Can you imagine the highly justified uproar that would result if a black person in the strip was named "the fat nigger?" Today's African Americans have acquired too much self-esteem to remain meekly quiet.

I was extremely reluctant to use the B.C. cartoon because, in other areas of life, the cartoonist is a compassionate and generous person. In the first place he allowed me to use his work and, secondly, he requested that I send the permission fee to the Syracuse Cancer Research Institute. Clearly, he is not a bad person. And I suspect a lot of FATISTS are not either, even though in general I have not dealt gently with them in this book. Many of them are probably just ignorant of the hurt they cause fat people when they act and speak thoughtlessly. Nothing, however, shall be said to soften the well-deserved comments directed toward MAGGOTS.

That is not to say that fatness cannot be an acceptable source of humor. Every group (and person) should be able to laugh at itself. Unfortunately, this trait is rapidly diminishing. There are jokes and cartoons based on fatness that are funny and *inoffensive* just as there are racial, religious, age, gender, and nationality jokes that are humorous and benign.

It is when a joke is clearly malicious, that it is patently objectionable. And the poison of mean jokes is grotesquely intensified when the same theme is repeated over and over. This constant reinforcement can create stereotypes that have absolutely no validity. Fat jokes, like the once ubiquitous "Polack" jokes, are proof that this can occur. Even benign jokes become vicious through repetition.

A lot of people need to disparage others to bolster their own insecure egos. Using jokes to belittle vulnerable targets is not the only way to gain this support but it is usually a very easy and safe way — a cowardly way. By wrapping hateful feelings and intentions in humor, bigots can present themselves to the world as jovial, good-natured people instead of revealing themselves as the mean-spirited bullies they in truth are.

People, who feel immoral because they have more body fat than society arbitrarily deems appropriate, might ask themselves which is worse, a person who is fat or one who cruelly makes fun of fat people? If both of these people were to knock on the Pearly Gates and face the Being who answers, which person do you think would be standing on "thin clouds?"

It is difficult to understand the inordinate concern of our society towards fat people. There are so many issues facing the people of the U.S., and the world, that are vastly more important than a person's percentage of body fat. Indeed, fatness can only be considered a problem in one aspect — health. Even then, in most cases the problem is either minor or nonexistent.

If people want to alleviate health problems, there is no end of really momentous ones to which they can devote their efforts. About one million Americans are stricken with cancer each year; half will die. One American in ten has a sexually transmitted disease; more than one and a half million are infected with the HIV (AIDS) virus. Mental illness also has its share of victims. More people are disabled by depression alone than any other physical disorder except cardiovascular disease. Suicide is the end result of many cases. Each year 400,000 American teenagers attempt to end their lives; 13,000 are successful. The list of serious illnesses that are truly deserving of attention is a lengthy one, yet our society devotes an inordinate amount of time and energy to "worrying" about the health of people who are merely overweight — and most of those are not excessively so.

Then there is the enormous drug problem. Nearly fifteen million Americans are regularly taking illegal drugs. Two-thirds of our teenagers have experimented with them and the abuse of all drugs is moving into elementary schools. One out of ten babies are born drug-damaged, often permanently. We are losing the war on illegal drugs and is there is no indication that victory is possible.

Legal drugs are abused by even more people. The number includes prescription and over-the-counter varieties along with alcohol and tobacco. Eighteen million Americans have an alcohol problem. The National Institute on Alcohol Abuse and Alcoholism estimates that at least 25% of patients in general hospital beds are being treated for conditions related to alcohol use, including illnesses, accidents, violent acts, and dysfunctional families. In addition to the $117 *billion* drained out of the economy in lost productivity due to alcohol abuse, the cost of health care for everyone is tremendously inflated. With a $52 billion tab, tobacco smoking is not as costly to our economy as alcohol, but it causes many more deaths each year. More than 420,000 Americans died in 1991 from the addiction (compared to 57,000 during the United States' eleven year involvement in the Viet Nam war). A study reported in the May, 1990 issue of the *Journal of the American Academy of Actuaries* showed that men who smoke cigarettes throughout their lives will die nearly *fifteen* years earlier than men who never start. The number of patients in hospital beds would be halved if people did not smoke! Not all are direct smokers; some are non-smokers who have been victimized by "second-hand" smoke. Indeed, is has been estimated that passive smoking is the third leading cause of preventable deaths (50,000 annually), behind smoking and alcohol.

FATISTS should consider that fat people do not harm others by shoving "second-hand" substances down their throats—as do smokers. Overindulging on food does not dull a person's mind—as does alcohol — or cause tens of thousands of traffic fatalities a year. Nor do food abusers commit the majority of crime in this country to support their habits — as do users of illicit drugs. If 10% of our people have personalities that lead to addictions, as is often estimated, it seems as if our country would far fewer problems if it encouraged food abusers instead of vilifying them.

Many of our social problems can be attributed to the steady disintegration of the American family. The U.S. has the highest divorce rate (60%) of all the developed countries. Six million women are battered each year. Two-thirds of our children live in single family homes. Eight million American teenagers get pregnant each year, most of them unmarried. This leads to one million teenage abortions during the same period. They are not the only ones having abortions; one of every three pregnancies in the U.S. is so terminated. Our infant mortality rate, with 40,000 such deaths yearly, is one of the worst among developed countries. Old people have their problems, too. Seventy-three thousand die annually due to excessively prescribed drugs. Nursing homes are often little more than "snake pits." And only 2% of physicians are trained in geriatrics even though the percentage of oldsters in our population is rapidly increasing.

Our society has plenty of other social ills beginning with three million homeless people. Thirty-five million adult Americans (about 1 out of 7) are functionally illiterate — a reflection of the fact that nearly one-third of our 40 million school-aged children never graduate from high school. How do many of these people make a living? Our astronomical crime rate is a major clue. In 1989 a record number of men and women (627,402) were incarcerated in federal and state prisons. The number would be much higher but inmates are being released early because the institutions are bulging at the seams. Handguns are used in the commission of many crimes and for good reason — they can be obtained so easily. More Americans were killed by firearms in 1984 and 1985 than in the entire time years we were embroiled in the Viet Nam war. Not all violent crimes involve guns. More than 90,000 rapes are reported each year. It is estimated that there are many times more *unreported* cases.

In addition to the real violence there is the staged variety. The National Coalition on Television Violence estimates that by the age of eighteen the average child (without VCR or cable) has witnessed 26,000 murders on TV. Further, 750 studies have found that television violence has a harmful effect on viewers. It is no wonder that our nation is far and away the most violent on Earth. Yet FATISTS are spending their time ridiculing people who *they*, the FATISTS, have judged as being too fat.

The U.S. does not have a monopoly on the problem market. Internationally, nearly fifteen million children die each year of starvation related diseases. And the prospect is not going to improve as long as the Earth's population continues to increase by 240,000 people each *day*. Of all the world's problems, the most serious have to do with the environment because they can severely affect, and even destroy, all life on our planet. Because the list of dangers is unimaginably long, only a few representative examples can be mentioned here. Sewage, human and animal, fouls the Earth's water. In the U.S. alone the Environmental Protection Agency estimates that $83 billion in new treatment facilities are required merely to keep up with current needs. We are also rapidly running out of landfills. Every *day* Americans throw away 200,000 tons of food, 20,000 cars, and 4,000 trucks. Trash has reached mind-boggling amounts. An eighteen months' stack of disposable diapers alone can reach to the moon — data which, hopefully, will not give ideas to the artist, Christo.

Even nastier than used diapers, although some would say that it's close, are the 700,000 tons of toxic wastes that are spewed into the environment each day in the U.S. The more malignant refuse includes the hundreds of trainloads of atomic waste products sitting on tracks waiting for "government geniuses" (an oxymoron if there ever was one) to figure out a safe disposal method. It's not an easy problem since the radioactive stuff will be emitting its deadly rays for many thousands of years. When your grandchildren and great-grandchildren reprovingly ask for an explanation — and you come up with a valid answer — please enlighten the rest of us.

Many chemicals are less dramatic but may be just as deadly in the long run. Included are pesticides, herbicides and industrial wastes. Of the latter, ozone destroying chemicals, called chlorofluorocarbons (CFCs) are just one category. In just one year, 1987, 200 million tons of CFCs were released into the atmosphere. The current rate of ozone depletion is leading to a global catastrophe in the form of skin cancer, plant and animal destruction, and a disastrous warming effect on the Earth's temperature. The plant destroying effect of CFCs is exacerbated by acid rain. This insidious rain is the result of 27 million tons of sulfur dioxides being expelled yearly into the atmosphere from chimneys and exhaust pipes in the U.S. alone. But nothing fells trees at a faster rate than saws and bulldozers. The Brazilian rain forests, for instance, are being decimated at the rate of an acre per second, or thirty-one million acres each year. Not only do these trees help keep the Earth cool, they consume carbon dioxide and pump vast quantities of oxygen back into the atmosphere.

An even more important source of oxygen, however, is oceanic phytoplankton. These tiny plants also provide the basis of the marine food chain. It is no secret that the fragile oceans are being strangled with sewage, pesticides, industrial effluents, and oil spills. Some experts fear the oceans are already in their death throes. Many animal and plant species are becoming extinct — *daily*. More have vanished in our lifetime than disappeared previously since the dawn of Man! And most humans are blithely closing their minds to the fact that eventually their turn will come. They do not understand that every time a species is "lost" a rivet pops loose from Spaceship Earth.

We are not aware of all the forces threatening to destroy our cultures and our planet, but just the ones mentioned above are staggering to contemplate. The most dangerous problem, however, may be mankind's inability to "get along" with each other. If the gross insensitivity continues, the already monstrous number of victims will only increase — and it is all totally unnecessary. The difficulty arises any time one segment of a population is unable to except others, who are different, as being worthy of respect and value. Much evil has been, and is being, generated simply because of intolerance toward such differences as race, religion, gender, and nationality.

Basing a person's value upon such meaningless factors is ludicrous, but using fatness as a determiner of value is incomprehensibly asinine. Many of our own loved ones, including grandmothers, mothers, wives, and daughters are often fat, and negative stereotyping only serves to harm them in profoundly painful, long-lasting ways. How a FATIST can play a part in subjecting loved ones to this senseless torture is unfathomable. Fatism is particularly severe and harmful in our country because the standards for "ideal" body fat percentages are so abnormally low.

With the abundance of really serious health issues, it does not make sense to dwell on the health issue of fatness — especially since in the large majority of cases, people who are considered to be fat in our society have no significant physical health problems caused by fatness anyway. Many fat people may have crippling psychological problems but these are not due to being fat. As evidence, the people in fat-tolerant regions of the world have absolutely no psychological illnesses associated with fatness.

The psychological problems in the United States are caused by mercenary MAGGOTS who have created a nasty antifat atmosphere. If the denigrating behavior of FATISTS is altruistically motivated, as they often claim, they might consider devoting their energies to far more worthy endeavors such as lobbying against smoking, joining Mothers Against Drunk Drivers (MADD), or doing volunteer work at a geriatric center. Closer to home they can plant a tree, pick up litter, or recycle trash.

A by-product of becoming involved in these and other truly altruistic activities is a maturation that logically might lead to tolerance for individual differences. A socially sensitive, tolerant person is sure to feel that others have the right to be fat without suffering the hassles of a fatist society.

Yes, many people have been known to advise a woman to lose weight "for her own good." A bit of advice for this presumably well-meaning segment is to simply, "stop the nagging!" Such harassment, no matter how well-intended, increases a woman's anxiety — which generally only leads to her gaining more weight. Besides, if person does not know the fat person, or is not close to her, her weight is absolutely none of his business. Any unsolicited comment is merely a reflection of his (or her) insensitivity.

Assuming that fatness is an imperfection, why should fat people feel like failures because they are imperfect? No one else is perfect. Further, it is the height of arrogance for a person to badger fat people to lose weight simply because he or she considers fatness an imperfection. When a fat woman is harrassed, instead of defending that which needs no defense, she might respond by asking, "Pardon me, are you perfect?"

There are men who say, "I love my wife. She's a wonderful woman, but her fat turns me off." On October 18, 1991, the *Sally Jessy Raphael* TV talk show dealt with the topic of husbands who force their wives to lose weight. There were a few moments of hilarity, but anger and sadness were the chief emotions aroused. All three of the guest couples were about thirty-years of age. The first husband threatened his wife (on the air) with philandering and divorce if she did not regain the size she had on their wedding day. In fact, he imposed a weekly ritual that required her to attempt to struggle into a size seven pair of jeans. His wife, incidentally, had given birth to four of his children!

The second husband humiliated his wife with "oink, oink" sounds, in public, when he thought she was eating too much. In his infinite wisdom, for a period each day since their baby had been born, he had been sitting on his wife's hips in a misguided effort to push them back to their pre-pregnancy dimensions. He also told her he wished she would become anorexic or bulimic. A really loving husband, that one.

The third husband claimed that having a baby was merely an excuse that women use to get fat. He was the one who complained it was embarrassing to be seen with a fat wife. Poor fellow. His 5'7" wife had "ballooned" up to 125 pounds! The other two wives were also "real porkers." One was a size seven, and the mother of four was a size nine. Incredibly, not only were the women physically beautiful, they were intelligent, articulate and seemed to be very nice. Such husbands as theirs should count their blessings and stop harping on something so irrelevant as weight.

The husbands' attitudes are easy to understand in a society where people have learned through overwhelming antifat propaganda that fat is ugly. If a man cares deeply about a woman, though, her weight should have negligible bearings on those feelings. A man is a fool if he lets society's narrow-minded beliefs interfere with his love — or if he permits a bunch of MAGGOTS and their FATIST lackeys to dictate what he finds appealing. He would do well to relax and enjoy the lushness of a traditional female body.

Of course, a man who is attracted to fat women will need a lot of self-confidence to buck the dictates of society. Simone de Beauvoir, in her book *The Second Sex*, was right on target when she wrote that no man is truly free to love a fat women. A major reason for the truth of this observation is the activity of people like antifat magnate Richard Simmons who on his television show warns his devotees to beware of "fat lovers." Keep in mind that such admonitions come from people who are members of the antifat industry who, like Simmons, make their living by convincing the public that fat is ugly, disgusting, and that fat people are rushing to an early grave.

A man who is a fat lover might also keep in mind that fat women were considered to be attractive throughout history and that only recently has fat been considered to be a disfiguration. Even if fatness were, in truth, disfiguring — and a wife got fat — should that affect her husband's love for her? One might also ask if a mastectomy, or loss of a limb, or scarring of her skin should diminish his feelings for her. An affirmative response would expose a basic immaturity and a gross lack of feeling. Any mature person realizes that "inner" beauty ultimately is what counts; the outer shell is not only superfluous but transitory — fleetingly transitory.

Shakespeare beautifully expressed this in his Sonnet 116.

> Let me not to the marriage of true minds
> Admit impediments. Love is not love
> Which alters when it alteration finds,
> Or bends with the remover to remove.
> O no, it is an ever-fixed mark
> That looks on tempests and is never shaken;
> It is the star to every wand'ring bark,
> Whose worth's unknown, although his height be taken.
> Love's not Time's fool, though rosy lips and cheeks
> Within his bending sickle's compass come.
> Love alters not with his brief hours and weeks.
> But bears it out even to the edge of doom.
> If this be error and upon me proved,
> I never writ, nor no man ever lived.
>
> (The "bark" in line six refers to a type of boat.)

What passes for physical beauty in any culture is fleeting. If a person does not develop a more mature concept of beauty based primarily upon character, kindness, and personality, he or she can become ugly very quickly. Indeed, without these universally recognized positive traits a reigning matinee idol or beauty queen can be quite repulsive.

Women do not need cosmetics and contrivances, and starvation and exhaustion, to be attractive and sensual. Femaleness by its very nature is beautiful — and that includes outer-beauty as well as inner-beauty. Unfortunately, feminine beauty in our culture is usually defined in terms of whatever the industry happens to be peddling.

If a man has a problem with his lady being too fat, the couple should consider counseling to help them — mainly him — deal with that problem. Ideally, whatever the outcome, both will come to understand that fat is not a four-letter word. If enough individuals arrive at this conclusion, fatism will decline in spite of the efforts of the antifat industry.

16

SUMMARY, CONCLUSIONS, AND OUTLOOK FOR FATNESS

Since about 1960, fat has increasingly become a de facto four-letter word in our society. Because of this, a number of negative traits have been attached to fat people, including gluttony, sloth, stupidity, ugliness — and even immorality. This denigration has been focused most intensely on women, a circumstance that is blatantly unfair since females are genetically programmed to have a considerably higher percentage of body fat than males.

What FATISTS think would not be so important, but by unceasingly vomiting the same message, the bigots have bullied fat people into actually believing they are less worthy and less desirable than other people. The stupidity of this belief is obvious; throughout history fat people have usually had the highest status within their cultures. Fat men tended to be the most respected and admired by others because they were, visibly, able providers. Fat women, on the other hand, were generally highly valued for their attractiveness, beauty, and sensuality. The location of fat on the body and the degree of fatness that was most prized varied according to the vagaries of fashion.

In the "Roarin' Twenties" very thin women, for the first time, became the standard for beauty. Even then, however, fat women were not and ridiculed and insulted. Around 1950 the push to loss weight begun in earnest. About ten years later the antifat industry was hatched. Its MAGGOTY entrepreneurs quickly surmised that by propagandizing the public into believing fat people were undesirable in nearly every way imaginable, fat people would beat a path to their doors and purchase their worthless "weight-loss" products. The antifat scheme was successful beyond its originators' wildest dreams. At first, the victims of the scams probably consisted chiefly of very fat people. Before long they would be joined by people who were only mildly overweight. With increasing speed, the ranks were swollen by hordes of people who were not fat at all, including many who were distinctly, even morbidly, underweight. The continual infusion of massive amounts of advertising money whipped the population into an antifat hysteria. As a result, in less than thirty years the antifat industry had mushroomed into a thirty-three-billion-dollars-a-year operation — and it continues to climb.

The financial ripoffs, massive as they have been, are secondary to the physical and psychological ills caused by the industry. Although some of the products and schemes are merely worthless, many produce harmful side-effects. Even worse is the fat paranoia that has resulted in the epidemic of anorexia and bulimia that exists today. The most widespread damage, however, has been the loss of self-esteem of untold millions of people — mainly women.

One of the chief points upon which the antifat industry harps is the supposedly unhealthy aspects of fatness. It is true that being excessively fat is a health hazard (as is excessive thinness), but the point at which any *individual* becomes overly fat has never been established. Various "ideal" body weights and percentages of body fat are confidently bandied about; in reality, though, the arbitrary figures are meaningless. At most they represent averages, but "average"is not synonymous with "ideal." Ideal indicates perfection. For instance, the average height for American women is about 5 feet 5 inches, but it does not mean her size is any better (or worse) than those of women who happen to be taller or shorter.

Even *if* an average "ideal" body fat percentage could be determined for each gender, the figures could not be construed as being ideal for everyone. The percentage of body fat that is most appropriate for any specific individual is based upon his or her body type. These types, which are genetically determined, range from very thin to very fat.

Each person's ideal body fat percentage obviously has to be determined on an individual basis. Unfortunately, no measurement or method of assessment has ever been been devised that can accurately reveal these figures. It was promised earlier that a practical and logical method for achieving an ideal body fatness would be revealed in this book (except for those whose fatness is due to a pathological condition). The method is so simple you may cheated when you hear it, but the truth often is simple. Quite simply, all a person has to do is adhere to a balanced diet (with moderate caloric intake and a lot of water) — while engaging in an exercise (preferably brisk) program on a regular basis, say, at least 30 minutes three or four times a week. The chapters dealing with diet and exercise provide considerable information in these areas for guidance — which explains why those chapters needed to be so long. If the advice is followed, a person's fat percentage will gradually shift toward his or her ideal level — and the process is normally quite easy and painless.

This healthy and effective long-term approach is being proved by Oprah Winfrey and Roseanne Arnold. After trying many unsuccessful "reducing" diets they are now losing weight the proper way. If they do not get impatient and try to speed up the process with "rapid-loss" diets, they will eventually achieve their ideal weight. They may already be there; it is unlikely that they have the same body type as Barbara Mandrell.

How gradually should people lose weight? It depends upon how far a person is from his or her ideal range. It may already have been achieved. If a person is fifty pounds overweight, it may take a year or more. Most people would like to be told how they can lose a large amount of weight in a short period of time with little or no effort — and there are plenty of MAGGOTS who are willing to sell them a "magic" product to assist them. The truth is, there is no magic product. A multitude of studies show that a steady fat loss of one or two pounds per week, with periodic plateaus, is a rate that's most likely to be maintained and to result in a permanent reduction without resulting in unhealthy side-effects. A *lifelong* commitment to a healthy lifestyle is absolutely basic for a lifetime of good health. There is no getting around that fact.

There are excessively fat people who do not place a high priority on losing weight. They will probably continue to be fat and that decision is their prerogative. But two vital questions arise. One, will our society continue to vilify and ridicule fat people? And, two, will fat people continue to allow themselves to be victimized into suffering low self-esteem? There are many signs which happily give hope for a negative response to both questions.

For the first time in several decades, women's magazines are beginning to soften their hard line against fatness. *Cosmopolitan* magazine, which prides itself as being at the forefront of change, ran an article in its August, 1989, issue entitled, "The Return of the Female Form." It advised women to stop dieting to distraction and exercising to exhaustion. Further, it urged women learn to love their curves — as men always have! The article tells women to be glad they really look like a women; it is their "time" because after decades of being told they could never be too thin, the femininely contoured form once again is being appreciated.

Even *Playboy*, in a December, 1988, article, "The Bod for '90," predicted the "welcome return of the well-rounded women." Whether that type will be reflected in their centerfold models remains to be seen. Being a dedicated researcher, I was afraid I would have to peruse the issues each month for the entire decade, but my wife graciously volunteered to assume that task for me.

The September, 1989, edition of *Woman* magazine carried an article entitled, "Curves are Back!" It declared that the thin look is out and the big, voluptuous, curvy look is back in. Two months later an article in *Woman*, "Learning to Love Your Body at Last," pointed out that most women who think they are fat are actually healthy, exciting women who look great. Instead of needlessly worrying about losing weight, the author wisely advises self-acceptance — and offers a thirty-day plan to shape up self-esteem.

The latter is especially sound advice when considering that in the 1984 *Glamour* survey the respondents claimed that losing ten to fifteen pounds was more important than success in work or love. Ten to fifteen pounds! Okay, admittedly, if a women is a hundred pounds over recommended standards, it is likely that she is excessively fat in terms of health — not a certainty, but very likely. But if she is a measly ten to fifteen pounds over the current standards, it is extremely unlikely that her health is the least bit adversely affected. Indeed she is probably healthier with the "extra" weight.

As R. Paul Abernathy, head of Purdue University's Department of Food and Nutrition said in September of 1991, it is actually more dangerous to be too thin than to be twenty percent overweight. He added that, according to statistics, people who are obese, by the government's definition, are living longer than people whose weight is lower than what the government recommends. This corroborates the data in the Metropolitan Life Insurance Mortality Tables. Clearly, it appears as if the vast majority of the *Glamour* respondents, as well as the public in general, are making much ado about nothing when it comes to typical degrees of fatness..

The respondents to the *Glamour* survey were a special group; the fact that they purchased the magazine and answered the survey suggests that they had a greater than average interest in their appearances. It is also probably true that other women are not as concerned. The latter women are the ones who are beginning to refuse to numbly conform to unreasonable standards of fatness.

The launching pad for the positive changes in attitude toward fatness lies with the baby boomers, those born between 1946 and 1964. Millions are "coming of age" — middle-age to be exact. With the maturity that is characteristic of this period of life, people are beginning to see the value of *moderation* and *common sense*. They are becoming less interested in conforming to unrealistic expectations regarding appearances.

Realizing that a perfect-looking body is virtually unattainable no matter how much effort and time is devoted to it, most middle-agers are far more concerned with achieving good health. Starvation diets and torturous exercise programs to lose weight — that are doomed to failure — are already starting to be replaced with life-long commitments to moderate and sensible lifestyle changes. At the same time, as indicated by magazine articles and television talk shows, there are glimmers of a greater acceptance of individual differences, including fatness. Since the baby boomers comprise a large segment of the population, their attitudes are already beginning to reshape the views of society as a whole.

The transition, however, has a long way to go before it is complete. The typical woman who feels she is overweight still exudes anxiety and a lack of confidence. Of course, if she does not think she has value, it is difficult for others to do so. She senses their lack of respect and feels even more worthless, thus falling into a vicious cycle. Her self-effacing mannerisms merely draw attention to a physical condition that many people may otherwise not even notice. Or if they do notice her fatness, it may not strike them as being unattractive anyway; they may well find it alluring.

An article in *Cosmopolitan* (October, 1989) entitled, "Thoughts on Thighs," gives one such viewpoint. Its author, a man, writes of a lady friend's thighs:

> Wonderfully lush, reasonably toned pillars (though not according to *her* strict criteria), warm and huggable. Many's the night, my pillow out of order, I've snuggled against them, taking dreamy, cozy comfort in their softness, like two teddybears — constantly reassuring her that the goddess of thighs had been kind.
>
> Women, brainwashed by the Workout Cult, have tragically succumbed to the myth that leaner is sexier. Misguided, they believe that thighs should be a cross between copper tubing and bridge cables or like the upper legs of female bodybuilders, off of which bullets bounce.
>
> What an unpleasant idea — just ask any man who truly loves and appreciates women . . . He'll also cite the scientific connection between her bountiful thighs and his heightened enjoyment of lovemaking.

Accompanying the article was an illustration showing a voluptuous woman with large, curvaceous legs stretched out languidly on the beach. In the background was a bevy of fashionably skinny women peering down forlornly at their own pencil-thin appendages.

Lushness of other body parts, such as buttocks and breasts, is also often highly prized by many men. *Cosmopolitan's* (November, 1989) article, "Breasts are Here to Stay," was hardly an earthshaking revelation. And men are starting to speak out in favor of women, who in our society are thought to be fat in general. The letter to Ann Landers (Jan. 30, 1990) which follows is particularly eloquent.

> DEAR ANN: I cannot rest until I respond to the New York woman whose boyfriend keeps encouraging her to gain weight. Since his former wife was a slender bride who had become quite heavy, N.Y wondered

> if perhaps her boyfriend is trying to relive his marriage.
>
> This kind of psychoanalytic gobbledygook is a good example of the extent to which people have become brainwashed in this age when "thin is in." Had the opposite been true and the guy had insisted that she lose weight, no one would have thought a thing about it, much less assigned hidden motives. My own guess is that the gent (like many others) simply prefers women who have a little meat on their bones.
>
> It's incredible how difficult it is to convince people that it is quite possible for a man to prefer plump to petite. I should know, Ann, because I have had this preference all my life. I've told my family and friends repeatedly that heavy women are fine with me, but they insist on fixing me up with hollow-cheeked females who are as flat as a board in front and in back.
>
> No one ever bats an eye at a preference for blond over brunette, or olive skin over fair, but as soon as someone prefers chubby over skinny, it's time to invoke Freud. Considering how many of the Old Masters painted women with voluptuous bosoms, heavy thighs and buxom backsides, it's difficult to understand today's worship of the bag of bones and the hank of hair. Call me a maverick, but make mine fleshy.
> — Baltimore
>
> DEAR BALTIMORE: You've made a lot of women happy today. Bless you for writing.

Ann may have added that there are a *lot* of mavericks out there. And they are coming out of the closet in increasing numbers. In 1989, a Phil Donahue program was devoted to men who were attracted to fat women. The men, who were of average weight or less, appeared with their wives — some of whom tipped the scales at about four hundred pounds. Whether viewers thought the women were beautiful or not depends upon individual tastes and is therefore irrelevant, but all were clearly intelligent and loving, had delightful personalities and senses of humor, and felt good about themselves. In other words, they were attractive women.

A more recent Donahue show, September 12, 1991, dealt with the same issue. One caller said she thought men who preferred fat women were "not normal." If Phil had asked her if she thought it was normal for *every* man to prefer women with the same color hair, or shade of lipstick she probably would have thought he was crazy for asking such a stupid question. Most of the callers and the studio audience seem to support the concept of individual preferences—and respecting everyone's right to make them. That's a good sign. The program, incidentally, revealed a new publication, *Mirage*, which contains the names, autobiographical material, and telephone numbers of men who want to meet very fat women.

Many fat-fancying fellows do not have the ego strength to swim against society's fatist current and give public vent to their hidden desires. Some of those faint-hearted lovers have to resort to pornographic magazines whose pages are devoted solely to featuring fat and obese models.

In addition to the talk shows, other television programs are addressing the issue of fatism. The most hard-hitting of these was an episode of *Designing Women* in 1990 called, "They Shoot Fat Women, Don't They?" In it, a gorgeous fat woman was played by Delta Burke, who in real-life has herself been the target of fatists in tabloids and of jokes by mean-spirited comedians. In her television role, Delta attended her high school reunion and was treated with shameful insensitivity. Later, her sister in the show (Dixie Carter) noted that people seem to love it when rich people lose their money and beautiful women get fat. The initial script reportedly had Delta asking why, and Dixie replying, "I don't know, Darlin'. I guess it just sort of props them up." Unfortunately, that sage observation was cut from the show.

Helping to change the general attitude toward fatness is the immensely popular situation comedy, *Roseanne*. Its Emmy award-winning star, Roseanne Arnold, is fat—and her screen husband, played by John Goodman, is a tad rotund himself. They portray a lower-middle class married couple who give vent to such typical expressions as affection, anger, warmth, and testiness — and who find each other sexually desirable. Viewers may recognize that Roseanne and John are fat, but the trait is incidental to the program's humor and story line. The fact that the two are generally accepted as being typical people, who just happen to be fat, is a sign that the pillars of fatism, rotten to begin with, may be starting to crumble.

Another sign was the crowning of the 1992 Miss Big and Beautiful on the Sally Jessy Raphael television show with the contestants averaging about three hundred pounds. Although the affair was a far cry from the hype and scope of the Miss America contest, the contestants and audience took it quite seriously — maybe because the contestants were indeed beautiful.

Perhaps the strongest indication of growing fat acceptance was the addition of Conchata Ferrell as a regular on *L.A. Law*. This was probably the first time a fat woman was a regular on a popular television series in something other than a comedic role.

Apparently people are starting to realize that even *if* fatness has negative aspects, they are nothing compared to the evil of bigotry and to the vultures who prey on vulnerable people to enhance their own weak egos. There seems to be a growing opinion that fat people have as much right to dignity as everyone else. As yet it is not a massive reversal in opinion, but at least it is in the right direction.

The pendulum swing from ultra-slim bodies to the more natural female form doubtlessly would have begun a long time ago, except for the intense bombardment of propaganda from the antifat industry. Even though the MAGGOT'S odious grip on our culture is being pried loose by the forces of common sense and moderation that is starting to sweep the country, it is a slow process. For example, the occasional positive article about fatness in women's magazines in still far overbalanced by antifat propaganda in the form of articles, fashion layouts, and advertisements. A perfect example of this imbalance appeared in *Cosmopolitan* (April, 1989). It was a very fine article by Rita Freedman entitled, "Learning to Love your Body." Its premise was that a woman's self-image has little to do with reality; it is the image she *project*s that determines how others will view her. Yet, the lingerie model in the accompanying picture had a "playmate" body that practically every women in American would kill for — as would a goodly number of men. The editor obviously had no feeling of what the article was about. Too often, anti-antifat progress seems to be one step forward and two steps back.

CATHY By Cathy Guisewite

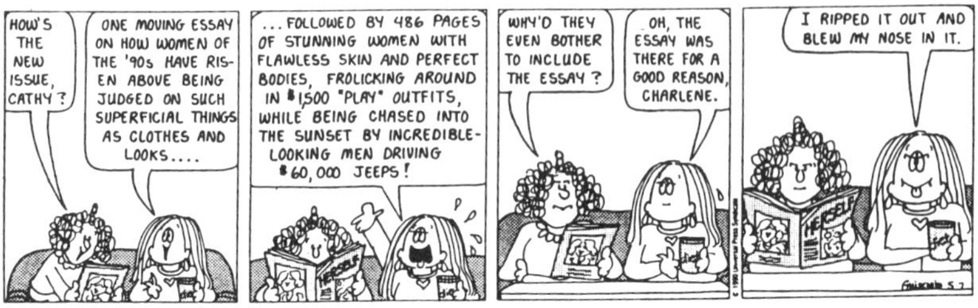

How can the downfall of fatism be accelerated? For starters, it must be understood that the dollar is all-powerful in our country. If any type of "ism" is to be defeated, therefore, the flow of dollars must be the chief consideration. Refrains such as "black is beautiful" or "fat is beautiful," and appeals to fairness and sensitivity fall upon deaf entrepreneurial ears. Those organs are attuned to the cry of, "Green is beautiful" — and the melodic crinkling of banknotes. Nothing spurs the business sector into action with greater alacrity than realizing that money can be harvested from a situation or group.

Even though capitalism shows an ugly side when it reaches runaway proportions, the struggle against the evils of fatism is most effective when it uses the system. A breaching of MAGGOTY ramparts, therefore, will be achieved only when entrepreneurs in general find they can make money by catering to fat people. A subtle but powerful weapon is fashion. Large numbers of women, for instance, did not take to exercising in vast numbers until the clothing industry produced more colorful, stylish exercise apparel. By the same token, scuba diving did not catch on as a sport among women until the paraphernalia (fins, masks, suits, tanks, bags, etc.) were manufactured in a wide range of colors and styles. The same is true for snow skiing. Most people want to look stylish.

For many decades, fashionable clothes were not being designed for fat women. They had to wear anything that was available — and what was available was distinctly uninspiring and did nothing to enhance the "full-figured" form. Most fat women knew they did not look very appealing in the available garb; no type of body could have. The lack of fashionable clothes further eroded their self-confidence.

Eventually, a few stores that specialized in clothes for fat women opened for business. Some, including Catherine's Stout Shop and Sweet Sixteen, became national chains. Then, in 1980 Carole Shaw began publishing a magazine, *Big Beautiful Women* (or as it is usually known, *BBW*), that became very influential in helping to establish a new, positive image for large women. In keeping with its name, *BBW* uses only big, beautiful women as models to display clothing fashions that are flattering to them. Several pages of the magazine is devoted to mail order sources. *Radiance* is another magazine that caters to large size women.

A few years later, Shaw joined forces with Hank Nuwer and wrote, *Come Out, Come Out, Wherever You Are*. Stressing fashions, the book contained a profile of big, beautiful women that included salary ranges, life styles, education, occupation, and type of activities they enjoy. The profiles revealed BBWs to be an interesting group of people — who had at least their share of money. Money! That must have attracted some attention and spurred clothing moguls into action, especially since one out of very three adult American women (more than 30 million) is a size 16 or above. It did not take an entrepreneurial genius to realize that a vast, affluent market was being ignored. One could almost hear panting businessmen saying, "Fat, ugly? No, no, my dear! Come, let me hug you." And if the men gave physical expression to their comment, the experience probably would have given them considerable insight to the statement, "Try it. You'll like it."

The rest is history. Large, well-known clothing outlets such as J.C Penney and Lane Bryant are now offering stylish apparel that is designed strictly for large sizes. And the number of such outlets is certain to multiply. Already, Catherine's, which sells large-size women's clothing, has 233 stores in 35 states. Their sales in 1991 was about 130 million dollars. While the economy was going down, their sales were going up. Capitalism, can be beautiful; it just depends upon how it is used. The scent of green ink in the "fat market" is clearly beginning to set entrepreneurial nostrils aquiver.

Attractive undergarments for larger women are also becoming commonly available. One brand of pantyhose, "Just My Size" by L'Eggs, for example, comes immediately to mind because of their extensive advertising. The models who wear them are ample proof that women who are considered to be fat can indeed have very shapely, pretty legs—and walk in a sprightly manner. It is difficult for any woman, thin or fat, to walk jauntily when she feels dowdy because of unflattering clothing.

The clearest evidence, however, that fat women are once more being considered beautiful and sexy is the increased offering of erotic lingerie in large sizes by such companies as Frederick's of Hollywood. Larger sizes (up to size 24) and greater variety are offered through catalogs by Spiegel, Queen's Lace, Mature Legance, Oh! Such Style, V-Fashions, and

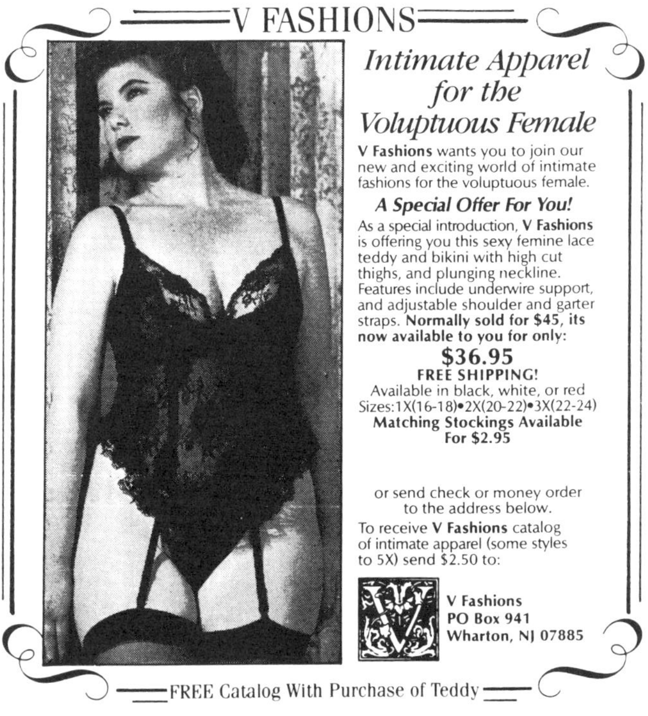

A Lingerie Offering From the V-Fashions Catalog.

Lane Bryant. It seems very contradictory, though, that the bathing suit and lingerie models in Lane Bryant's catalog are thin! If their clothes are supposed to look attractive on large women why not use fat women? Not using fat women for models is a slap in the face to them — not the most intelligent marketing technique.

Clothes are also now being designed especially for overweight children. In the mid-1980s Copie Lilien and Kim Runyon interviewed a number of childhood obesity experts. Clothing was an issue that kept coming up as having a tremendous impact on the self-esteem of fat children. Since there was a scarcity of fashionable apparel that was cut with the fat child in mind, the two women decided to start a company, named At Last, Inc., to fill that void. Sales, predictably, have soared.

The most significant, and refreshing, sign of change occurred with the August, 1991 announcement that "Barbie," (with unattainable equivalent measurements of 36-18-33) is going to have some competition. A new fuller-figured doll (with reasonable equivalent measurements of 36-27-38 and a shorter neck and larger feet) is designed to offer young, impressionable girls a more realistic female body image. Called the "Happy to be Me Doll," it is being sold by High Self-Esteem Toys Corp. in Minneapolis. Hopefully "fuller figured" dolls, fat as well as plump, will also be on the shelves before long. Never in my life did I think I would be recommending dolls; my sailing buddies are going to have a field day. But the value of this product is worth the ribbing I'm sure to get.

Ironically, when women do come close to looking like Barbie, she is ridiculed and called such names as "bimbo" and "air head." As a female friend said, "You *know* Barbie's not going to be a neurosurgeon." That's not really fair either. When it come to being fat, it seems that women are often damned if they are and damned if they aren't.

A designer, Jean de La Bruyère, observed that there are no ugly women, only those who do not know how to be pretty. Presumably, he is suggesting that conforming to society's tastes regarding clothing, hair styles, and cosmetics helps a woman to be prettier. He may be right, but a woman doesn't have to be a slave to the glamour industry to be attractive. There are more universal standards of attractiveness than mere prettiness. Cleanliness, neatness, and good posture, for instance, are always in style. All of these traits are visual manifestations of a positive self-image. Most attractive, however, are the messages that come from within. If a woman exudes such characteristics as confidence, a sense of humor, warmth, and caring, discerning people will always find her appealing.

I've always had a sneaking suspicion that God made a mistake when he (or she) came up with the menstrual cycle. Or maybe it was a practical joke. But he sure knew what he was doing when he invented the smile. I will never forget walking into a large office reception room with a glib, extroverted male friend and noticing a fat, plain woman in her early thirties sitting in a chair. My friend asked the woman if she was being assisted. She nodded blandly and mumbled that she was waiting to see the personnel director. My friend raised his arms dramatically and expostulated, "Damn, he gets all the pretty gals!" In an instant the woman's body straightened and her face broke into one of the most radiant smiles I have ever seen. The transformation of her appearance was astounding. She was not just pretty, she was absolutely stunning! It is amazing what a smile can do to improve a person's looks. Since that day, I've been more observant and have concluded that all people immediately become beautiful when they smile — a sincere smile. And it's tragic that feelings of shame and guilt, due to being fat, can suppress such smiles. Incidentally, when the woman was called into the director's office a few minutes later, she was still smiling and her stride was confident. Her bright demeanor had to have had a powerfully positive effect on her chances for being hired.

Fatism certainly appears to be on the way out; merely recognizing its existence is a big step in the right direction. It would help, of course, if the term "fatism" was listed in dictionaries along with the equally sinful traits of racism, sexism, and ageism.

As fatism declines, the reduction of social pressures to lose weight will diminish the "fat anxiety" in our culture. Since this decrease will assuredly result in a decrease of compulsive eating, the amount of body fat on the average American can be expected to also decrease. When weight loss is no longer an obsession, most overweight people will lose weight without even trying — and reach *their* ideal body fat percentage.

There will always be people who, for some reason or another, are heavier than average. But as the public becomes less weight conscious and more accepting of body type variations, the negative traits that have been attached to fat people, through ignorance and meanness, will gradually fade away. There is indeed a glimmer of hope for the plight of fat people in our society.

With a substantial decline of fatism, fat people can logically be expected to experience of great sense of freedom. No longer will they feel pilloried because of their fatness. For that matter, the specter of fatness will be exorcised from the minds and spirits of women in general. It may be that an even greater sense of liberation will be felt by women who by years of tremendous effort, expense, and effort have managed to maintain an unrealistically and painfully low amount of body fat.

Practically speaking, some degree of fatism will continue to plague our culture for a long time. The impetus for this evil will be provided chiefly by an antifat industry that will persist in spewing out its demeaning propaganda as long as it can rake in dollars. Such propaganda will always find fertile soil among bigots who are unwilling, or too naive, to see through its totally mercenary motivations. Hopefully, the exposure of the FATIST and MAGGOTY villains will help to achieve the primary goal of this book — to help people understand that fat is NOT a four-letter word.

CREDITS

A wide variety of books, articles, photographs, and cartoons were used in the production of this book. The author and publisher wish to express their deep appreciation for permissions to use all of the source material. In all cases, every effort was made to contact copyright holders. If there is any oversight, we will be eager to update our information.

There is no uniformity in the credit lines because different companies require different forms when giving permission. Most of the credits, particularly for art and cartoons, are given in the text near the works. Some companies require a credit line in both the text and in this section.

Page 18. Excerpted from the *Playboy* column, "Women: Hollywood Women," by Cynthia Heimel. *Playboy* Magazine (October 1990), Copyright© 1990 by *Playboy*. Used with permission.

Page 25. Albrecht Durer, *Adam and Eve,* The Metropolitan Museum of Art, Fletcher Fund, 1919, (19.73.1). All rights reserved, The Metropolitan Museum of Art.

Page 25. Peter Paul Rubens, *Venus and Adonis,* The Metropolitan Museum of Art, Gift of Harry Payne Bingham, 1937, (37.162). All rights reserved, The Metropolitan Museum of Art.

Page 26. Francois Boucher, *The Toilet of Venus,* The Metropolitan Museum of Art, Bequest of William K. Vanderbilt, 1920. (20.155.9). All rights reserved, The Metropolitan Museum of Art.

Page 32. Grand Wood, American, 1891-1942, *American Gothic*, oil on beaverboard, 1930, 76 x 63.3 cm. Friends of American Art Collection, 1930-1934. Photograph © 1991, The Art Institute of Chicago, all rights reserved.

Page 33. Pablo Picasso, *Seated Nude.* Photograph National Museum of Modern Art, George Pompidou Center, Paris.

Page 36. Michelangelo Buonarroti (Caprese 1475-Roma 1564), *The Fall,* Fresco, Sistine Chapel, Vatican City.

Page 36. *The Decorated Body* by Robert Brain. Copyright © by Robert Brain, Courtesy of HaperCollins Publishers.

Page 44. From *Shakespeare Alive* by Joseph Papp and Elizabeth Kirklan. Published 1988 by Bantam Books.

Page 46. Warshaw Collection of Business Americana. Archives Center. National Museum of American History, Smithsonian Institution.

Page 52. *Advertising in America* by Charles Goodrum and Helen Dalyrymple. Harry N. Abrams, Inc., New York, 1990. All rights reserved.

Page 52. Coca-Cola is a registered trademark of the Coca-Cola Company owned and used with permission of the Coca-Cola Company.

Page 57. From *Pumping Iron II.* Copyright © 1984 by Charles Gaines and George Butler. Pumping Iron is a trademark of Pumping Iron, Inc.

Page 88. Stephen K. Campbell, *Flaws and Fallacies in Statistical Thinking,* © 1974, vii-viii. Reprinted by permission of Prentice-Hall, Inc., Englewood Cliffs, N.J.

Page 95. Reprinted from *How to Tell the Liars from the Statisticians* by Robert Hook, pp. 20-21 by courtesy of Marcel Dekker, Inc., New York, 1983.

Pages 108-110. Drawing produced from photographs in *Varieties of Human Physique* by William H. Sheldon. Reprinted by permission of William H. Sheldon Trust.

Pages 120 and 121. Permission granted by Ann Landers and Creators Syndicate.

Page 127. Father Andrew M. Greeley, National Opinion Research Center, University of Chicago.

Page 149. Excerpt from *Doublespeak* by William Lutz, Copyright © 1989 by Blonde Bear, Inc.

Page 172. Reprinted with the permission of Merrill, an imprint of Macmilliam Publishing Company, from *Health* by Michael H. Hamrick, David J. Anspaugh, and Gene Ezell. Copyright © 1986 by Bell and Howell.

Page 177. Statistical Bulletin and Metropolitan Mortality Table, reprinted with the permission of the Metropolitan Life Insurance Company.

Page 181. *Don't Diet.* Copyright © 1988 by Dale Ahrens. By permission of William Morrow and Company, Inc.

Page 264. Reprinted with permission from *Parade,* copyright © 1988.

Page 269. *How to Raise Your Self-Esteem* by Nathaniel Brandon, © 1987, Reprinted by permission of Bantam Books, Inc.,

Page 290. Permission granted by Ann Landers and Creators Syndicate.

FOOTNOTES

1. Larsson, B., Björntorp, P., and Tibblin, G. "The Health Consequences of Moderate Obesity," *International Journal of Obesity*, Vol. 5:97-116 (1981).

2. Hubert, H.B., Feinleib, M., and McNamara, P.M. "Obesity as an Independent Risk Factor for Cardiovascular Disease: A Twenty-six Year Follow-up of Framingham Heart Study Participants," *Circulation*, Vol. 67:968-977 (1983).

3. Kaplan, Jay R., Manuck, Stephen B., and Shively, Carol. "The Effects of Fat and Cholesterol on Social Behavior in Monkeys," *Psychosomatic Medicine*, in press (1991).

4. Virkkunen, M. "Serum Cholesterol in Antisocial Personality," *Neuropsychobiology*, Vol. 5: 27-30 (1979).

5. Virkkunen, M. "Serum Cholesterol Levels in Homicidal Offenders," *Neuropsychobiology*, Vol. 10: 65-69 (1983).

6. Virkkunen, M. and Penttinen, M. "Serum Cholesterol in Aggressive Conduct Disorder," *Biological Psychiatry*, Vol. 19: 435-439 (1984).

7. Virkkunen, M., DeJong, J., Barko, J., Goodwin, F.K., Linnoila, M. "Relationship of Psychological Variables to Recidivism in Violent Offenders and Impulsive Fire Setters," *Archives of General Psychiatry*, Vol. 46: 600-603 (1989).

8. Muldoon, M.F., Kaplan, J.R., Manuck, S.B., Mann, J.J. "Effects of Dietary Fat on Central Nervous System Serotonergic Activity (abstract)," *Psychosomatic Medicine*, Vol. 53: 216 (1991).

9. Muldoon, M.F., Manuck, S.B., Matthews, K.A. "Lowering Cholesterol Concentrations and Mortality: A Quantitative Review of Primary Preventative Trials," *British Medical Journal*, Vol. 301: 309-314 (1990).

10. Chiang, B.N., Perlman, L.V., and Epstein, F.H, "Overweight and hypertension: A review," *Circulation*, Vol. 39:403-421 (1969).

11. Messerli, F.H., et al., "Disparate cardiovascular effects of obesity and arterial-hypertension," *American Journal of Medicine*, Vol. 74:808-812 (1983).

12. Tuck, M.L., et al. "The Effect of Weight Reduction on Blood Pressure, Plasma Renin Activity, and Plasma Aldosterone Levels in Obese Patients," *New England Journal of Medicine*, Vol. 304:930-933 (1981).

13. Data from P. Berchtold, V. Jorgens, C. Finke, and M. Berger (1981), In G.A. Brooks and T.D. Fahey, *Exercise Physiology: Human Bioenergetics and its Applications*. New York: Macmillan. 1984.

14. Maxwell, M.H., et al., "Error in Blood Pressure Due to Incorrect Cuff Size in Obese Patients," *Lancet*, Vol. 2:33-36 (1982).

15. Berger, M., Muller, W.A., and Renold, A.E., "Relationship of Obesity to Diabetes: Some Facts, Many Questions," In *Diabetes, Obesity, and Vascular Disease*, ed. H.M. Katzen and R.J. Mahler, pp 211-228. Washington, D.C.: Hemisphere Publishing. 1978.

16. Keen, H., Jarrett, R.J., Thomas, B.J., and Fuller, J.H., "Diabetes, obesity and Nutrition: Epidemiological Aspects," In *Diabetes and Obesity*, ed. J. Vague and F.J.G. Ebling, pp 91-103. International Congress Series no. 454. Amsterdam: Excerpta Medica. 1979.

17. Saville, P.D., and Dickson, J., "Age and Weight in Osteoarthritis of the Hip," *Arthritis and Rheumatism*, Vol.11:635-643 (1968).

SELECTED BIBLIOGRAPHY

Space limitation prevents the author from listing all of the publications that provided information in the preparation of *Fat is NOT a Four-Letter Word*. The publications selected below were most useful and interesting, and are suggested for the reader who wishes to do more reading on the topics covered in this book.

BOOKS

American Heart Association Cookbook (4th Edition). David McKay Co. Inc., 1984.

Ahrens, Dale M. *Don't Diet*. New York: William Morrow and Company, 1988. Pg. 247.

Edited by Barnett C. Rosalind, Biener, Lois, and Baruch, Grace K. *Gender and Stress*. New York: The Free Press (Macmillan), 1987.

Bennett, Wiliam and Gurin, Joel. *The Dieter's Dilemma*. New York: Basic Books. 1982.

Black, J. Anderson and Garland, Madge. *A History of Fashion*. New York: Willaim Morrow and Company, Inc, 1975.

Brain, Robert. *The Decorated Body*. New York: Harper and Row, Publishers, 1979.

Broad, William and Wade, Nicholas. *Betrayers of the Truth: Fraud and Deceit in the Halls of Science*. New York: Simon and Schuster, 1983.

Edited by Brownell, K.D. and Foreyt, J. P. *Handbook of Eating Disorders*. New York: Basic Books, Inc. Publishers, 1986.

Campbell, Stephen K. *Flaws and Fallacies in Statistical Thinking*. Englewood Cliffs, NY: Prentice-Hall, Inc., 1974. pg. 195.

Cooper, Kenneth H. and Cooper, Mildred. *The New Aerobics for Women*. New York: Bantam, 1988.

de Beauvoir, Simone. *The Second Sex*. New York: Penquin, 1986 (1949).

Frankel, Reva T. and Yang, Mei-Uih. *Obesity and Weight Control*. Rockville, Maryland: Aspen Publishers, Inc., 1988.

Freedman, Rita J. *Bodylove*. New York: Harper and Row, 1989.

Fussell, Samuel Wilson. *Muscle: Confessions of an Unlikely Bodybuilder*. New York: Poseidon Press, 1991.

Gaines, Charles and Butler, George. *Pumping Iron: The Art and Sport of Bodybuilding*. New York: Simon and Schuster, 1974

Gaines, Charles and Butler, George. *Pumping Iron II: The Unprecedented Woman*. New York: Simon and Schuster, Inc., 1984.

Goldman, Robert, Bush, Patricia, and Klatz, Ronald. *Death in the Locker Room:Steroids and Sports*. South Bend, Indiana: Icarus Press, 1984.

Goodrum, Charles and Dalrymple, Helen. *Advertising in America*. New York: Harry N. Abrams, Publishers, 1990.

Graveeter, Frederick J. and Wallnau, Larry B. *Statistics for the Behavioral Sciences* (second edition). St. Paul, Minnesota: West Publishing Co., 1988

Hooke, Robert. *How to Tell the Liars from the Statisticians*. New York: Marcel Dekker, Inc., 1983. pg. 168.

Lyons, Pat and Debbie Burgard. *Great Shape*. Bull Publishing, 1990.

Lutz, Wiliam. *Doublespeak*. New York: Harper and Row, Publishers: New York, 1989. Pg. 278.

McCarter, William and Gilbert, Rita. *Living with Art*. New York: Alfred A Knopf, 1985

Papp, Joseph and Kirkland, Elizabeth. *Shakespeare Alive*! New York: Bantam Books, 1988.

Rudofsky, Bernard. *The Unfashionable Body*. London: Rupert Hart-Davis, 1972.

Shaw, Carole and Nuwer, Hank. *Come out, Come out, Wherever You Are*! Los Angeles: American R.R. Publishing Company. 1982.

Sheldon, William H., with Dupertuis, C.W. and McDermott, E. *Atlas of Men*. New York: Harper and Brothers, Publishers, 1954.

Sheldon, William, with Stevens, S.S. and Tucker W.B. *The Varieties of Human Physique*. New York: Harper and Row Publishers, 1940.

Wolf, Naomi. *The Beauty Myth: How Images of Beauty are Used Against Women*. New York: William Morrow and Company, 1991. 291p.

Wood-Allen, Mary. *What Every Young Woman Ought to Know*. London and Philadelphia: VIR Publishing Co. 1905.

PERIODICALS

American Health, P.O. Box 3016, Harlan, Iowa 51593-2107.

In Health (formerly *Hippocrates*) P.O. Box 52431, Boulder, CO 80321

Mayo Clinic Health Letter, P.O. Box 53889, Boulder, CO 80322-3889.

The Harvard Medical School Health Letter, P.O. Box 10944, Des Moines, IA 50340.

The Health Letter, P.O. Box 19622, Irvine, CA 92713.

National Association to Advance Fat Acceptance (NAAFA) *Newsletter*, P.O. Box 188620, Sacramento, CA 95818.

Radiance, P.O. Box 30426, Oakland, CA 94604.

Tufts University Diet and Nutrition Letter, 53 Park Place, New York, NY 10007.

University of California, Berkeley Wellness letter, P.O. Box 420148, Palm Coast, FL 32142.

ORGANIZATIONS

Anorexia Nervosa. Box 7, Highland Park, Ill. 60035

National Association to Advance Fat Acceptance (NAAFA). P.O. Box 188620, Sacramento, CA. 95818 (916) 433-0303.

National Council Against Health Fraud. P.O. Box 33008, Kansas City, MO 64114. (816) 444-8615).

Overeaters' Anonymous. 4025 Spencer Street, No. 203, Torrance, CA 90503. (213) 542-8363.

Rockport Walking Institute. P.O. Box 480, Marlboro MA 01752.

Walkers Club of America, 445 E. 86th St., New York, NY 10128 (SASE). (212-722-WALK).

INDEX

A

Abernathy, R. Paul, 288
Academy Awards, 46
acetabulum, 9
acetone, 216
Achilles, 262
acid rain, 279
acne, 57, 142
acromegaly, 98
acupressure, 158
Acutrim II, 138
Adam and Eve, 25, 27
adenosine triphosphate, 67
adipocytes, 71
adipose tissue, 71, 72, 74, 75, 76
Adler, Barry, 218
Advertising in America, 52
aerobic dance, 248
aerobic exercise, 238, 243
Ahrens, Dr. Dale, 180
AIDS, 197
Alka-Seltzer Plus, 138
Allen, Woody, 252
Alsop, Joseph, 127
Amazon, 41
amenorrhea, 57
American Academy of Pediatrics, 223
American Anorexia and Bulimia Association, 197
American Beauty, 49
American College of Sports Medicine, 251
American Council on Science and Health, 221, 231
American Gothic, 33
American Health, 186, 262, 263
American Heart Association, 222, 232
American Journal of Medicine, 183
American Meat Institute, 213
American Medical Association, 128, 149
American Scientist, 83
American Society of Plastic and Reconstructive Surgeons, 160, 161
amino acids, 69, 70, 143, 144, 221
amobarbital, 147
Amores, 27
amphetamines, 137
anabolic steroids, 56, 141, 142, 144, 238, 252
Anabolic Mega-Pak, 151
Anderson, Julie, 190
Andres, Dr. Reubin, 175
Animal Farm, 127
anorexia nervosa, 191, 193, 194, 195, 197, 198, 199, 201, 202, 203, 282, 286
anti-rejection drugs, 84
Appedrine, 138
appetite suppressants, 137
Applegate, Christina, 199
Aqua-Ban, 140
Archaeological Museum, Ankara, 24
arginine, 224
Aristotle, 127
Arnold, Roseanne, 287, 292
Arnolfini, Giovanni, and his Bride, 44
Art Institute of Chicago, 33
Arthritis and Rheumatism (publication), 186
arthritis, 145, 180, 186, 187
Artwear, 190
asthma, 187
Astro-Trimmer, 162
At Last, Inc., 297
atherosclerosis, 224, 238
Atlas of Men, 109
Atomic Balm, 166
ATP, 67, 68
Ayds, 139

B

Babylonians, 15
baldness, 145
Banner, Lois, 49
Banyankole, 15
Barnard, Dr. Neal, 84
Barney's New York, 190
barnstorming, 52
Barnum, Phineas T. Museum, 132
basal metabolic rate (BMR) 215, 216
Battle of Hastings, 3, 4
Beatty, Warren, 146
Beauty and the Beast, 30

Beauty Myth: How Images of Beauty are Used Against Women, 30
Being Fat—Is It Such a Crime?, 273
benzedrine, 137
benzocaine, 139
Beowulf, 3
Berger, Dr. Stuart, 184, 207
Beth Israel Medical Center, 157
Betrayers of the Truth: Fraud and Deceit in the Halls of Science, 83
Better Business Bureau, 123
Better Sweaters, 164
Bible, 22, 164
Big Beautiful Woman (BBW), 295
Biotherm's Serum Contour, 157
birth control pills, 85, 144
Bod for '90, 288
Body Love, 272
body wrapping, 168
bodybuilding, 55, 56, 57
Bosch, Hieronymous, 32, 33
Boule de Suef, 28
boxing, 55
brain disorders, 94
Brain, Dr. Robert, 36
Branden, Dr. Nathaniel, 269, 271
breast cancer, 85, 224
breast enhancement surgery, 43
Breasts are Here to Stay, 290
Brillat-Savarin, Jean-Anthelme, 28
brown adipose tissue, 71, 223
Bruegel, Pieter, the elder, 34, 35, 47
Bruges, 31
Brut, 41
Bryant, Lane, 295
Budweiser, 18
bulimia nervosa, 193, 195, 196, 197, 198, 199, 201, 202, 203, 282, 286
Burke, Delta, 292
bustle, 46
Butler, George, 55
Butterball, 230
Byres, Sean M., 190

C

cacogenics, 17
Caesar, Julius, 119
caffeine, 211
calcium, 214
Callaway, Dr. C. Wayne, 217
Campbell, Stephen, 86, 88
Canterbury Tales, 22, 104
Cardiovascular Center, New York University-Cornell, 233
cardiovascular disease, 137, 141, 176, 181, 212, 223, 276
Carter, Dixie, 292
Catherine's Stout Shop, 295
cellulite, 156, 157, 158
Center for Disease Control, 261
Center of Science in the Public Interest, 228
Certo, Sir Dominic, 58
Charles I, 48
Charles II, 48
Chaucer, 22, 28, 104, 118
Chemical Corner: Let's Stop Kidding *Ourselves*, 58
Cher, 199, 252
chlorofluorocarbons (CFCs), 279
cholesterol, 77, 78, 176, 182, 210, 223, 226, 229, 230, 231
Chorus Line, 50
Christo, 278
chylomicrons, 70
circulatory system, 69
Circulation, 183
Clark's Reducing Salts, 158
Coca-Cola, 51, 52
collagen, 57, 241
colon cancer, 162, 210, 224
Columbia University, 102, 223
Come Out, Come Out, Wherever You Are, 295
Comptrex, 138
congestive heart failure, 143, 185
constipation, 253
Consumer Product Safety Commission, 124
Consumer Reports, 207, 213
Consumers Union, 207
Contac, 138
convulsions, 138, 167
Cooper Clinic, Dallas, 245
Cooper, Fran, 190
Cosmopolitan, 222, 288, 290, 293
Craig, Roger, 260
Crazy People, 125
Cro-Magnon men, 12
Cromwell, Oliver, 48

Cupid, 109
curvature of the spine, 199
Curves are Back!, 288

D

Dalrymple, 52
David, 142
de Beauvoir, Simone, 282
de La Bruyere, Jean, 297
De Maupassant, Guy, 28
Decorated Body, The, 36
Department of Health and Human Services, 179
depression, 192, 241, 242, 262, 268, 276
Designing Women, 292
Detroit Institute of Arts, 26
Dexatrim, 138
diabetes, 138, 143, 162, 180, 185, 186, 187, 212, 233, 239
Diabetes and Obesity, 184
Diabetes, Obesity, and Vascular Diseases, 184
diarrhea, 167
Diet Fast, 218
Diet, 120 Year, 207
Diet, 35 Plus, 207
Diet, Dr. Adkins, Revolution, 207
Diet, Beverly Hills, 207
Diet, Beyond Pritikin, 207
Diet, Calories Don't Count, 208
Diet, Complete Scarsdale Medical, 207
Diet, Diet-type Weight-Loss, 207
Diet, Dr. Berger's Immune Power, 207
Diet, Eat Healthy, 207
Diet, Eat to Succeed, 207
Diet, Elizabeth Takes Off, 207
Diet, Fat to Muscle, 207
Diet, Fit for Life, 207
Diet, Hilton Head Metabolic, 207
Diet, I Love New York, 207
diet, liquid protein, 217
diet, liquid formula, 217
Diet, Macrobiotic, 207
Diet, Medical Makeover, 207
Diet, Pray Your Weight Away, 207
Diet, Rice Report, 207
Diet, Two-Day, 207
dietary fiber, 229
digestive system, 69
digitalis, 137
Dimetapp, 138
Disraeli, Benjamin, 87
diuretics, 137, 140, 211
Diurex, 140
diverticulitis, 162, 210
Doberman, 262
Don't Diet, 181
Donahue, Phil, 3, 63, 291, 292
Doublespeak, 149
Drabinsky, Elizabeth, 190
Drenowski, Dr. Adam, 220
Dublin, Louis I., 117, 171, 174
Duchess of Windsor, 59
Durer, Albrecht, 25, 27, 109
Dynamic Life Essence, 151
dysmenorrhea, 140

E

Eating disorders, 191, 197, 198
Eating Disorders in Focus, 200
Eating Disorder Service, Newington (CT) Children's Hospital, 200
Eating Right Pyramid, 212, 213
Egan, Dr. Brent, 233
Einstein, Albert, 92
electrolysis, 112
electric muscle stimulators (EMS), 259
Eleveine, 139
embolism, 160
endocrine system, 141, 144
endorphins, 261
Environmental Protection Agency, 278
epileptic seizures, 197
Equal Rights, 53
Ernsberger, Dr. Paul, 159, 185
Eros, 110
Eskimos, 22
Essence, 222
estrogen, 142
eugenics, 17
Eve, 27, 158

F

Fair Oaks Hospital, Summit, N.J. 220
farthingale, 45
Federal Trade Commission, 122, 151, 219
Felitti, Vincent, 217
Ferrell, Conchata, 274
Fiber Trim, 161

Fiber-Rich, 161
50-Plus, 222
fish oil, 226
Flaws and Fallacies in Statistical Thinking, 86, 88
fluoride, 95
Food and Drug Administration, 61, 62, 124, 146, 150, 162, 228
food labeling, 229
Founders Society, Detroit Institute of Arts, 26, 35
Framingham (MA) project, 180
Francis, Bev, 56, 57
Frankenstein, 143, 190
Franklin, Benjamin, 83
Frederick's of Hollywood, 296
Freedman, Rita, 272, 293
Freud, 110
Fugler, Howard, 190
Fussell, Samuel, 56

G

Gaines, Charles, 55
Galateas, 190
gall bladder, 77, 221
Garden of Earthly Delights, The, 32, 34
gastric balloon implant, 159
genetics, 17
Georgetown University, 218
Gerontology Research Center, 175
giantism, 98
Gibson, Charles Dana, 49
Gibson girl, 49
Gillette, Dr. Robert D., 145
ginseng, 145
Glamour, 200, 289
glucose, 68, 69, 72, 83, 185, 216
glycerol, 70, 71, 72, 76, 216
glycerine, 70
glycogen, 68, 69, 70, 208, 216
Godey's Ladies Book, 50
Goebbels, Joseph, 124
Gold's Gym, 251
Gold, Tracey, 199
gonorrhea, 186
Good Housekeeping, 222
Goodman, John, 292
Goodrum, 52
gout, 144, 224, 233
Grapefruit-Plus, 138
Great Depression, 115
greater omentum, 75
Greek Goddess, 24
Greeley, Father Andrew M., 127
Grenada, 150
Grover's Tasteless Chill Tonic, 50
Growing Pains, 199
Guisewite, Cathy, 294
Gurin, Joel, 186
gynecomastia, 142

H

Hai Karate, 41
Hamlet, 178
Happy to Be Me Doll, 297
hardening of the arteries, 10, 238
Harper's Bazaar, 222
Harvard, 133
HCG, 141
headaches, 141, 167
Health, 172, 173
Healy, Bernadine P., 84
heart attack, 81, 183, 234
heart disease, 138, 180, 181, 183, 187, 231
Heart Failure, 231
heatstroke, 81
Height-Weight-Mortality Ratio Table, 171
Heimel, Cynthia, 18
Herbalite International, 150
herpes, 224
hiatal hernia, 197
high blood pressure, 96, 138, 140, 180, 183, 185, 186, 187, 239
High Self-Esteem Toys, Inc., 297
high-density lipoproteins, 238
Hippocrates, 101
Hippocratic oath, 128, 130
Hitler, Adolf, 67, 124
HIV, see also AIDS, 276
Holmes, Oliver Wendell, 85
Hooke, Robert, 95
hormonal disorders, 94
Hottentot, 73
House of Representatives, 218
How to Raise Your Self-Esteem, 269
How to Tell the Liars from the Statisticians, 95
human chorionic gonadotropin, 141

human growth hormone (HGH), 98, 131, 142, 143, 144
Hunger-Plus, 138
hypercholesterolemia, 232
huypertension, 96, 180, 184
hypochondriasis, 192
hypothalamus, 234
hysteria, 192

I
Idealistic Male and Female, 27
iliopsoas muscles, 256
immune deficiency, 159
implants, 112
infertility, 194
Ingres, Jean Auguste Dominique, 31
Inside Edition, 207
insomnia, 137
Institute for Aerobic Research, 245
Institute of Human Nutrition, Columbia University, 223
insulin, 176, 185
International Federation of Bodybuilders, 58
International Journal of Obesity, 180
International Sportsmedicine Institute, Los Angeles, 211
intestinal blockage, 159
intestine stapling, 159
Irish Minnie, 28
iron, 41, 214
Irving, Washington, 29
Is Shakespeare Dead? ,126

J
Jagger, Mick, 30
jaw-wiring, 159
Jefferson, Thomas, 248
Johnson, Ben, 142
joint disorders, 81
Journal of American Academy of *Actuaries*, 277
Journal of American Medical Association, 145, 156
Journal of American National Strength and Conditioning, 252
Just My Size, 296
juvenile delinquency, 106

K
Kaiser Permanente, 217
Kaplan, Jay, 182
Keen and colleagues, 184
Kessler, David, 146
ketones, 216
Keys and colleagues, 192
Kidney, 75, 141, 167, 214
  diseases of, 76, 138, 141, 144, 211
  stones, 211, 224
kinesthetic sensations, 263, 264
King, Jr., Martin Luther, 270
Kirland, 44

L
L'Eggs, 296
L.A. Law, 274
labels, 229
lab-scam, 83
Ladies' Home Journal, 50
LaLanne, Jack, 255
Lancet, 84, 183
Landers, Ann, 120, 290
Lane Bryant, 297
Laragh, Dr. John, 233
Learning to Love Your Body, 293
Learning to Love Your Body At Last, 288
LeBrun Vegee-LeBrun, Louis Elisabeth, 26
lecithin, 77
Legend of Sleepy Hollow, 29
Leno, Jay, 139
Leonard, "Sugar" Ray, 92
Life magazine, 49
Lilien, Copie, 297
linolenic acid, 226
lipophobia, 189, 202
lipoproteins, 70, 71, 238
lipoprotein lipase, 71, 72, 73, 217
liposuction, 43, 59, 157, 160, 161
liquid protein diet, 129, 217
liver, 77, 176, 197
Lives, 119
Louvre Museum, 26
low-density lipoproteins, 238
low-impact aerobics, 248
Luganis, Greg, 92
lungs 197
  cancer of, 76
Lutz, William, 149, 150

lymphatic system, 70
lysine, 224

M

Mackie, Bob, Sportswear, 190
Mademoiselle, 222
Maine, Margo, Ph.D., 200
male hormones, 57
male pattern baldness, 57
malnutrition, 159
Mammrae900 ™, 61
Mandrell, Barbara, 287
mannitol, 227
Mark Eden Bust Developer, 61
Marlowe, Christopher, 27
Married...With Children, 199
Martial, 37
mastectomy, 283
Mature Legance, 296
McMurray, Robert G., 242
Medical College of Wisconsin, Milwaukee, 233
Medifast, 217, 219
Meehan, Vivian, 199
Memling, Hans, 31
  Museum, 31
menopause, 240
menstruation, 199
Merrill, Charles E. Company, 172
metabolic abnormalities, 98
metabolic diseases, 94
metabolism, 68, 226, 237
Metropolitan Life Insurance Company, 117, 171, 172, 178
Metropolitan Life Insurance Mortality Tables, 176, 177, 203, 289
Metropolitan Museum of Art, 25
Michelangelo, 35, 36, 142
Mirage, 292
Miss America, 46, 201, 293
Miss Big and Beautiful, 293
Mississippi State Chemical Laboratory, 162
mitochondria, 71
Mitsushima, Kazuko, 190
Monroe, Marilyn, 54, 92
Moore, Thomas, 231
Morgan, Dr. Brian, 223
morphine, 262
Mothers Against Drunk Drivers (MADD), 281
Mr. Universe, 263
Ms America, 58
Ms Olympia, 56
Muldoon, Matthew, 182
Muscle and Fitness, 58
Muscle: Confessions of an Unlikely *Bodybuilder*, 56, 63
Museum Bogmans-van Beuningen, 31
Museum of Modern Art, 33
My Sin, 41
myelin sheaths, 77

N

NAAFA Newsletter, 126
Nader, Ralph, 124
National Anti-vivisection Society, 84
National Association to Advance Fat Acceptance (NAAFA), 125
National Association of Anorexia Nervosa and Associated Disorders, 199
National Association for Hospital Development, 129
National Cancer Institute, 95, 224
National Cattlemen's Association, 213
National Coalition on Television Violence, 278
National Collegiate Athletic Association, 142
National Council Against Health Fraud—Task Force on Victim Redress, 124
National Football League, 143
National Gallery, 44
National Geographic Magazine, 28
National Institute of Health, 83, 84
National Institute on Aging, 175
National Institute on Alcohol Abuse and Alcoholism, 276
National Library of Medicine, 94
National Milk Production Federation, 214
National Opinion Research Center, 127
National Research Council, 210
Natural History Museum, Vienna, 16
Nature's Rival Company, 59
Nautilus, 252
Nazi, 67
NBC, 139
NEA, Inc. 6

Neanderthals, 12
Nero, 24
New England Journal of Medicine, 183, 231
Night Court, 37
NoDoz, 139
norepinephrine, 185
normal curve, 90
Normal Distribution of Scores, 90
North American Syndicate, 244
Northeastern University, Boston, 259
Nutri-System, 221
Nuwer, Hank, 295
Ny Carlsberg Glyptotch, Copenhagen, 24

O

O'keeffe, John, 29
Office of Research on Women's Health, 84
Office of Scientific Integrity, 83
Oh! Such Style, 296
omega-3s, 226
omentum, 75
Onassis, Christina, 120
Optifast, 217, 219
Organic Gardening, 222
Orwell, George, 127
osteoarthritis, 186
osteoporosis, 199, 224, 239, 240
Ovid, 27

P

pannier, 45, 46
Papp, 44
Parade Magazine, 264
paranoid schizophrenia, 137
Parents, 222
parotid glands, 196
Parton, Dolly, 252
Passion, 41
Passions of the Mind, 92
Pavarotti, Luciano, 92
Pavlov, 13
peascod belly, 47
Penney, J.C., 295
Pentagon, 150
People, 199
Pep-Back, 139
Perlman, Itzak, 92
Permathene-12, 138
pernicious anemia, 159
Peruna, 59
petroleum jelly, 75
phenylpropanolomine, 138
pheromones, 40, 41
Philosopher in the Kitchen, The, 28
Phoenix Natural Fiber Cookie, 161
phospholipids, 76, 77
Physician's Committee for Responsible Medicine, 84
Physician's Desk Reference (PDR), 58
phytoplankton, 279
Picasso, Pablo, 33
  Seated Nude by, 182
Pinnochio, 47
pituitary gland, 143, 144, 234
Plakinger, Tina, 58
Playboy, 18, 36, 37, 149, 201, 288
Plutarch, 119
Pollock, Dr. Michael, 251
Popeye, 274
potassium, 167, 197
Prado Museum, 32
pregnancy, 10, 72
premenstrual syndrome (PMS), 240
Prentice-Hall, Inc., 88
President's Council on Physical Fitness and Sports, 264
Prevention, 222
Prolamine, 138
prostate cancer, 224
Proverbs, 22
Psychology Today, 242
Pudd'n Wilson, 269
Pumping Iron: The Art and Sport of *Bodybuilding*, , 263
Pumping Iron II: The Unprecedented Woman, 55
Purdue University, 288
Pygmalion, 190

Q

Queen's Lace, 296

R

Radiance, 159, 295
Raphael, Sally Jessy, 37, 200, 281, 293
Reader's Digest, 222
Reader's Guide to Periodic Literature, 50, 116
Redbook, 222

Reebok, 261
Reiset, Madame, and her Daughter, 31
Renoir, Auguste, 26
Return of the Female Form, 288
rheumatic fever, 186
rhinoplasty, 43
Rich, Louis, 230
Rivera, Geraldo, 3
Roarin' Twenties, 285
Robertson, Dr. Donald, 211
Roller machines, 165
Roman Catholic Church, 34
Roosevelt, Franklin, 67
Roseanne, 292
Roundheads, 48
Royal College of Physicians, 95
Royal Statistical Society, 95
royal jelly, 145
Rubens, Peter Paul, 25
Runyon, Kim, 297
Russell, Lillian, 49
Russell, Sharon, 273
Rutkowski, Diane, 55

S

saline implants, 61
salivary glands, 196
Sallmeyer, Hans, 140
San Francisco Giants, 260
saturated fat, 77, 229
Sauna Belt, 162
Scavullo, Francesco, 190
Schwartzeneggar, Arnold, 252
Sears, Roebuck, 59, 60, 260
Seated Nude, 33
Seated Bather, 26
sebaceous oil, 74
Second Sex, The, 282
Seduction, 41
Seneca, 53
serotonin, 182
set-point for fat, 234, 235, 237
Seven Countries Study, 181
Shakespeare, 119, 283
Shakespeare Alive!, 44
Shaw, Carole, 295
Shedd, Reverend Charles W., 207
Sheldon, William, 102, 105, 106, 109, 110, 111
Sherman, Dr. John E., 157
shin splints, 81
Shirburn Ballads, 22
shock, 160
Sickle cell anemia, 97
silicone gel implants, 62
Simmons, Richard, 282
Simpson, Wallis, 59
Sinaikin, Dr. Philip, 220
SintJans Hospitaal, 31
Sistine Chapel, 35, 36
skin cancer, 279
Slim-Mint Gum, 139
Slim-Skins, 163, 164
Slim With Fiber, 161
Society of Actuaries, 175
somatotypes, 105, 109, 111, 112, 113, 132
Somnours' Tales, 118
sorbitol, 227
Southwest Bariatric Nutrition Center, 211
Soviet Union, 270
Spiegel, 296
Sports Illustrated, 255
spot reducing, 258
St. Elizabeth Family Health Center, 145
St. Ursula, 31
Stanford University, 239
Stare, Frederick, 133
Start Exercising—and Stick With It, 264
Statistical Bulletin, 172, 177
Stay Trim Gum, 139
Stein, Gertrude, 85
Step 'n Fetchit, 270
steroids, 57, 58, 76, 77, 78, 140
Steroids: The Rambo Drug, 58
Stevens, Ray, 262
Stimucin, 139
stomach cancer, 159
stomach stapling, 159
Stowe, Harriet Beecher, 49
Streep, Meryl, 92
stress fractures, 81, 199
stress hormone, 185
stroke, 137, 138, 181, 239
suicide, 276
Super Odrinix, 138
Sweet Sixteen, 295
Sweet Sweat, 166

syphilis, 186
Syracuse Cancer Research Institute, 275

T

Taller, Herman, M.D., 208
Taylor, Elizabeth, 120
testosterone, 10, 142, 240
They Shoot Fat Women, Don't They?, 292
Thinz: Back to Nature Pills, 139
Third World, 206
Thompson, Roger, 190
Thoughts on Thighs, 290
Thyroid, 137, 138, 141, 143, 234
thyroxine, 141]
Tonight Show, 139
toxic shock syndrome, 61
triglycerides, 70, 71, 76, 226
Trim-Jeans, 163
tryptophan, 146
tuberculosis, 186
Tufts University, 251
  Diet and Nutrition Letter, 230
Turkey products, comparison, 230
Turkish Goddess, 24
Twain, Mark, 126, 269
20/20 TV Show, 273
Twiggy, 191
Twilight Zone, 39

U

U.S. Department of Agriculture (USDA), 213, 228
U.S. Olympic Committee, 142, 143
ulcer, 137, 159, 187
Ultrafast, 219
United States Marine Corps, 1
United Science of America, Inc. (USA, Inc.), 133
Universal Press Syndicate, 294
University of California, Berkeley, 93
University of Chicago, 127
University of Cincinnati Medical College, 64
University of Florida, 251
University of Michigan, 220
University of Minnesota, 192
University of North Carolina, Chapel Hill, 242
University of Pennsylvania, 206
University of Pittsburgh, 182
University of Sydney (Australia), 180
uterine cancer, 224

V

V-Fashions, 296
valium, 147
Van Eyck, Jan, 43, 44
Van Tassel, Katarina, 29
vasopressin, 141
Vegee-LeBrun, Madame and her *Daughter*, 26
Venus, 15, 16, 22, 27
Venus and Adonis, 25
Venus of Willendorf, 15, 16, 23, 107
Viet Nam, 277
Vikings, 3
Virkkunen, M., 182
Vitamins, 212, 214
Vogue, 50, 116
von Bulow, Claus and Sunny, 147
Voy, Robert, M.D.

W

Wadden, Dr. Thomas, 206
Walgreen's Cold Capsules, 138
water intoxicatino, 167
Wedding Dance, 34, 35
Weider, Joe, 151
Weight Watchers, 231
What a Young Woman Ought to Know, 64
Whelan, Dr. Elizabeth, 231
Whitman, Walt, 22
William the Conquerer, 3
Wimpy, 274
Winfrey, Oprah, 3, 234, 272, 287
Wolf, Noami, 30
Woman, 288
Woman's Home Companion, 59
Wood, Dr. Peter, 239
Wood, Grant, 33
Wood-Allen, Mary, 64
Wooley, Dr. Susan C., 64
World Health Organization, 197
World War II, 54, 217
Wright, Thomas, 22
Wyden, Rep. Ron, 218

XYZ

Xylitol, 227
zinc, 214, 221

☐ **The Physician Within** by Catherine Feste. Here internationally renowned health motivation specialist, Cathy Feste, focuses on motivating those with a health challenge, and anyone else, to stay on their regimen and follow healthy behavior.
004019, ISBN 0-937721-19-0, $8.95

☐ **Whole Parent/Whole Child: A Parent's Guide to Raising a Child with a Chronic Illness** by Patricia Moynihan, R.N., P.N.P., M.P.H., and Broatch Haig, R.D., C.D.E. Everything parents of children with chronic health conditions need to know is here. With authority, insight, and compassion, this book shows you how to be the kind of parent you want to be and how to help your child lead the fullest life possible.
004051, ISBN 0-937721-53-0, $9.95

☐ **I Can Cope: Staying Healthy with Cancer** by Judi Johnson, R.N., Ph.D., and Linda Klein. This book is a clear, comprehensive resource for anyone whose life has been touched by cancer. And it's by Judi Johnson, co-founder of the American Cancer Society's internationally acclaimed "I Can Cope" program, which helps over 40,000 people a year.
004026, ISBN 0-937721-28-X, $8.95

☐ **Making the Most of Medicare: A Personal Guide Through the Medicare Maze** by Arthur R. Pell, Ph.D. Finally, a book that actually helps overcome the government red tape associated with Medicare. It shows what can and cannot be expected from Medicare and provides easily understood explanations of Medicare policies—plus tips on how to use them for optimum advantage.
004071, ISBN 0-937721-66-2, $11.95

☐ **Retirement: New Beginnings, New Challenges, New Successes** by Leo Hauser and Vincent Miller. From two internationally renowned motivational speakers, trainers, and retirees comes a book that will help you achieve new goals in retirement. It's a plan of action that charts a course to successful, rewarding, and active retirement.
004059, ISBN 0-937721-59-X, $5.95

☐ **Fast Food Facts** by Marion Franz, RD. This revised and up-to-date best-seller shows how to make smart nutritional choices at fast food restaurants—and tells what to avoid. Includes complete nutrition information on more than 1,000 menu offerings from the 32 largest fast food chains.
Standard-size edition 004068, ISBN 0-937721-67-0, $6.95
Pocket edition 004073, ISBN 0-937721-69-7, $4.95

☐ **Convenience Food Facts** by Arlene Monk, RD. Includes complete nutrition information, tips, and exchange values on over 1,500 popular name-brand processed foods commonly found in grocery store freezers and shelves. It helps you plan easy-to-prepare, nutritious meals.
004081, ISBN 0-937721-77-8, $10.95